THE ULTIMATE GUIDE TO RED LIGHT THERAPY,
REVISED EDITION

THE ULTIMATE GUIDE TO

Red Light Therapy,

REVISED EDITION

THE BREAKTHROUGH SOLUTION FOR ANTI-AGING, WEIGHT LOSS, MUSCLE GAIN, INFLAMMATION REDUCTION, AND PEAK PERFORMANCE

Ari Whitten, M.S.

CONTRIBUTIONS BY DR. MICHAEL HAMBLIN

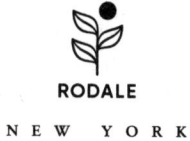

RODALE

NEW YORK

Rodale Books
An imprint of Random House
A division of Penguin Random House LLC
1745 Broadway, New York, NY 10019
rodalebooks.com | randomhousebooks.com
penguinrandomhouse.com

An earlier edition of this work was self-published by the author in 2018.

Library of Congress Cataloging-in-Publication Data
Names: Whitten, Ari author
Title: The ultimate guide to red light therapy / by Ari Whitten, M.S.
Other titles: Ultimate guide to redlight therapy
Description: First edition. | New York, NY: Rodale, [2025] |
Includes bibliographical references and index. |
Identifiers: LCCN 2025026375 (print) | LCCN 2025026376 (ebook) |
ISBN 9780593736555 hardcover | ISBN 9780593736562 ebook
Subjects: LCSH: Phototherapy | Color—Therapeutic use | Red—Health aspects
Classification: LCC RM840 .W45 2025 (print) | LCC RM840 (ebook)
LC record available at https://lccn.loc.gov/2025026375
LC ebook record available at https://lccn.loc.gov/2025026376

Printed in the United States of America on acid-free paper

1st Printing

2026 Rodale Books Edition

BOOK TEAM: Managing editor: Allison Fox • Production manager: Richard Elman •
Copy editors: Stuart Calderwood and Lori Newhouse •
Proofreaders: Megha Jain and Caryl Weintraub

The authorized representative in the EU for product safety and compliance is
Penguin Random House Ireland, Morrison Chambers, 32 Nassau Street,
Dublin D02 YH68, Ireland. https://eu-contact.penguin.ie

How to Use This Book

This book is packed with scientific research, technical details, and practical guidance on red and near-infrared light therapy. But here's the important thing: You don't need to read it all. Frankly, unless you're passionate about understanding the science very deeply, I don't recommend it—the scientific and technical detail may be overwhelming for many readers.

I suggest reading the introduction and chapter 1 to get an overview of what red and near-infrared light therapy are, and perhaps at least skimming chapter 2 on physiological mechanisms to understand how it works. In chapter 3, which covers dozens of types of health benefits from using red and near-infrared (NIR) light therapy, read the specific sections on the types of benefits that you're trying to achieve and don't worry about the ones not of interest to you. From there, feel free to skip around to the sections of the book that interest you—you may wish to learn about the technical details that determine the efficacy of red and NIR light treatments, or you may wish to skip directly to the practical how-to guidance for using it to achieve anti-aging effects in your skin, or amplify the benefits you get from exercise, or any number of other specific benefits you may be looking to achieve. You do not need to read this book from cover to cover—for most readers, especially those seeking practical guidance rather than scientific detail, a selective approach will serve you much better. There is no "right way" to read this book. Treat it as a reference manual, not a novel. It's perfectly fine to skip around to the sections that you want to learn about.

Think of this book as your personal guidebook to red and NIR light therapy—one that adapts to your needs and interests. Whether you're a science enthusiast or health professional who wants to understand every mechanism and pathway, or someone who just wants to know which device to buy and how to use it for a specific health-related goal, this book is designed for you.

For the science-minded reader: If you want to truly understand the nitty-gritty details—the cellular mechanisms, the physics of light penetration, the nuances of dosing protocols—then by all means, read every chapter. You'll find comprehensive explanations of how and why red and NIR light therapy works at every level of biology, as well as extensive research and technical guidance on effective dosing and device selection.

For the practical reader: If you're primarily interested in achieving specific benefits of red and NIR light therapy and don't care about details of biochemical mechanisms, or biphasic dose responses, or all the technical nuances of different ways of doing red and NIR light therapy, that's perfectly fine. Skip directly to the how-to sections on device selection and treatment protocols for your specific goals. You'll find simple, clear, actionable guidance without needing to wade through the science.

For everyone in between: Most readers will fall somewhere in the middle. You might want to understand the basics of how red and NIR light therapy works, then jump to specific applications that matter to you. The book is structured to support this approach—each section stands on its own.

Don't let the density of information overwhelm you. The detailed science is there if you want it, but if you just want practical guidance on what device to get and how to use it, you can skip straight to that.

Your experience with this book can be as deep or as light as you choose. It's intentionally designed to serve as both a comprehensive scientific resource and a practical quick-reference guide.

Use it however serves you best.

Disclaimer

IMPORTANT: THIS BOOK IS FOR EDUCATIONAL PURPOSES ONLY

The materials and content in this book are for general information and education only and are not intended to be a substitute for professional medical advice, diagnosis, or treatment. While I've worked hard to provide helpful information for many different health concerns, none of the information in this book should ever be interpreted as a claim of treatment or cure of any particular medical condition.

ABOUT THE RESEARCH

This book discusses research about red and NIR light therapy, also called photobiomodulation (PBM), an emerging and rapidly evolving science. As you read this book, it's important to understand that I share my best understanding of the current research, but that new discoveries are being made all the time.

Many topics within the field of PBM do not have a scientific consensus. They are contentious and hotly debated, because the current evidence isn't strong enough to allow us to draw solid conclusions, and different experts often have varying views on how to interpret the research. I have tried to accurately and fairly represent the spectrum of opinions and perspectives while discussing any such topic. Even in cases where I may not fully agree with a particular view, I have tried to charitably present that perspective.

What we know today may change significantly as new studies are published, and many aspects of this therapy are still being actively studied and debated by scientists. While I've done my best to provide a comprehensive analysis of the available research, my interpretation may not be the only valid one, and other experts in the field may have different views on various aspects of this therapy. The science in this field continues to evolve, and future research will undoubtedly refine or even overturn some of the information presented here.

PRODUCT INFORMATION AND RECOMMENDATIONS

In the device selection guide section of this book, I discuss various devices and products based on my experience and honest assessment. Full transparency: I have affiliate relationships with virtually all of the major PBM device companies. This is a standard relationship in which I receive a commission if you purchase a device through my links or use my discount codes. This is at no extra expense to you—in fact, it typically provides you with a discount.

These relationships don't influence my recommendations in this book. I am not currently a part owner of or consultant to any brand mentioned in this book, and I have no financial incentive to recommend one brand over another since I maintain affiliate relationships with virtually all the major device manufacturers and receive similar commissions from them.

Also, please note that while I discuss many PBM device types and brands, there are no personal affiliate links or discount codes in this book, and I recommend devices from a wide array of brands—many of which I have no affiliate relationship with at all. There's no need to use my affiliate links or discount codes for any purchase, but if you'd like to support my work, you can find my unique affiliate links and discount codes on my website.

All of this is to say that no financial conflicts of interest have influenced any of the information in this book, including device recommendations. These are based solely on my honest assessment of the devices I believe are currently best for particular types of goals. As I explain in the device selection guide, there are new and better devices coming to the market almost every month, and since I cannot easily update this book after publishing, I will keep an updated list of my current device recommendations on my website.

One more important note on device selection: Results can vary significantly among individuals, and what works well for one person may not work the same way for another. My recommendation for a particular type of device for a particular benefit should not be interpreted as a guarantee that the device will help with specific conditions or symptoms that you may have. As with starting a new diet, exercise regimen, meditation practice, or pharmaceutical, individual results will vary.

RESPONSIBILITY AND UNDERSTANDING

All of the information in this book is published in good faith and for general information purposes only. I make no warranties about the completeness, reliability, or accuracy of this information. Nothing in this book should be considered a guarantee of benefit or medical claim. As with any other intervention (e.g., a drug, a diet, an exercise program, or medical device), there are potential risks of harm. (Generally speaking, the risks from red and NIR light therapy are exceedingly small, but potential harm is still possible.) Any action you take upon the information in this book is strictly at your own risk. If you have any particular medical condition, always consult a healthcare professional for guidance about your specific situation.

SPECIAL THANKS

I want to give special acknowledgment to Dr. Michael Hamblin, Ph.D., who has made large contributions to this book. Dr. Hamblin's credentials in the field of PBM are unparalleled:

- Former professor at Harvard Medical School (now retired)
- Former principal investigator at the Wellman Center for Photomedicine at Massachusetts General Hospital
- Author of more than 1,000 peer-reviewed publications in PBM
- Author and editor of major clinical textbooks on PBM therapy
- Recognized globally as one of the world's leading authorities, and the most prolific researcher in the entire field of PBM

I consulted with Dr. Hamblin extensively as I was developing this Version 2.0 of the book, and while doing a series of consultations and interviews over many months, we developed a very fruitful relationship that ultimately led to him becoming an editor and co-author of this book. Dr. Hamblin has overseen and edited many hundreds of pages of my writing for this project (including a great deal of content that didn't make the cut into this book), and has also contributed much of his own writing in numerous sections of this book.

Given that PBM is still an emerging field with many unanswered questions, an enormous amount of complexity, and many differences of opinion among PBM experts and clinicians on everything from mechanisms to dosing parameters to the best devices to use, I knew it was essential to collaborate with leading PBM researchers to ensure accuracy and minimize errors in my interpretation of the evidence. While some of my own ideas and interpretations of the evidence may differ in some cases from others (which is guaranteed because there is no consensus view on many aspects of PBM, and there are significant differences of opinion about various PBM topics even among the top experts in this field), I wanted him to make sure that what I wrote in this book was as accurate as possible. My main goal of collaborating with Dr. Hamblin was to ensure that I created a book that was comprehensive, scientifically accurate, and accessible to the average reader with no background in this topic.

Dr. Hamblin has been wonderful to work with as a co-author, and I'm deeply grateful to him for generously contributing his time and incredible expertise to help me make this book vastly better than the original edition.

(A quick note on language: Though Dr. Hamblin is a co-author, I've chosen to use "I" rather than "we" throughout most of the book since I describe many personal opinions, device experiences, and my personal conversations with experts that would make constantly switching between pronouns unnecessarily clunky.)

I also want to give heartfelt thanks to Dr. Mark Cronshaw for his invaluable insights. He's one of the most brilliant minds in the world when it comes to understanding the complex science of PBM dosimetry—a researcher, professor, and clinician on the leading edge of PBM applications. His commitment to bridging the gap between scientific research and clinical practice aligns perfectly with the goals of this book.

In writing this book, I spent close to 20 hours in conversation with Dr. Cronshaw (many published on my podcast), where he guided me through the nuances and complexities of key areas in PBM science. Dr. Cronshaw's deep understanding of how light interacts with biological tissues, combined with his clinical experience applying these principles to patient care, has added tremendous depth to this work. His insights on the biophysics of light penetration, tissue optics, dosimetry, and the practical realities of delivering effective doses to target tissues have been particularly valuable in helping me understand several critically important and contentious topics in PBM science.

I am deeply grateful to Dr. Cronshaw for his generous contribution of time, expertise, and careful attention to detail that has made this book more comprehensive, accurate, and scientifically robust. I particularly appreciate how even in areas where we initially disagreed, he would playfully challenge my thinking and guide me toward a deeper understanding of the science. Beyond his brilliant insights, he's also an absolute joy to work with—

extraordinarily kind and blessed with a wonderful sense of humor.

I cannot thank both of these brilliant PBM experts enough for helping me make this book far better than I could have achieved alone.

Contents

The Essential Role of Light in Human Health

Imagine a drug that could speed healing, enhance brain function, reduce inflammation throughout the body, boost cellular energy production, improve athletic performance, help you lose fat and build muscle, improve your metabolic health and immune function, and even slow the aging process. All without significant side effects. A compound so remarkable that if it existed in pill form, pharmaceutical companies would race to patent it, doctors worldwide would prescribe it to millions, it would generate billions in revenue, and it would be widely regarded as a "miracle drug." Here's the extraordinary truth: This "drug" already exists—but not as a pill. It's red and near-infrared (NIR) light.

Over the past several decades, researchers have published more than 6,000 studies documenting the remarkable health benefits of red and NIR light therapy (photobiomodulation, or PBM for short). Yet despite it being one of the most signifi-cant health discoveries of the last 50 years, most people have never heard of it.

For most people, the very concept that specific types of light interact with human cells or play a significant role in human health seems somewhat bizarre. This skepticism reveals a crucial gap in our understanding of human biology.

Our species has evolved over countless millennia under a giant ball of fire in the sky, some 93 million miles away, and this glowing orb has shaped our biology in profound ways. All humans, from our earliest ancestors until recent generations, have lived most of their lives under open skies, their bodies moving through daily cycles of bright sunlight and firelight's glow. This ancient relationship with light shaped far more than just surface-level changes like tanning or pupil dilation; it built essential mechanisms into our cellular machinery that control everything from energy production to immune function, cellular regeneration, hormonal health, DNA repair, and metabolic health.

When most people think about light, they think of it in terms of the simple binary of light versus darkness: Light lets us see; darkness obscures. Many people are familiar with the basic concept that sunlight leads to vitamin D synthesis in our bodies, through ultraviolet light interacting with compounds in our skin. And there is also growing awareness of the role of light, particularly the blue wavelengths of light, entering the eyes and influencing our circadian rhythms. But the relationship between light and human health runs far deeper than this. Every cell in your body is, directly or indirectly, influenced by light in your environment, either through immediate interactions or slower biological effects that manifest over minutes, hours, and days.

The idea that light penetrates our skin and influences our cells—playing a vital role in human health—isn't some fringe theory or crazy New Age idea. Science is revealing that humans are far more dependent on light for optimal biological function than has been previously understood. This isn't speculation—it's grounded in hard science, now documented in thousands of peer-reviewed studies. Just as a plant withers without sunlight, humans also rely on light to be healthy, though in less obvious ways. Our cells require regular exposure to specific wavelengths of light to function optimally, and though it's less outwardly obvious than in a plant

when we are deprived of that light, it takes a profound toll on our health nonetheless.

Let's consider food as an analogous situation. We all know that we need to consume food in order to be healthy—we require certain types of nutrients in certain amounts, and if we get poor proportions of nutrients in our diet or consume too much junk food (which is a combination of being too poor in beneficial nutrients and too rich in harmful compounds that our body doesn't need), we become unhealthy. You may be familiar with the concept of "essential nutrients." An essential nutrient is a substance that the body absolutely requires to function properly but cannot synthesize on its own (or cannot make in sufficient quantities), meaning it must be obtained from external sources like food or the environment. When we lack an essential nutrient, we develop specific deficiency symptoms that can only be resolved by obtaining that particular nutrient—for instance, without vitamin C we develop scurvy, without essential amino acids we can't build proteins properly, and without iron we can't produce healthy red blood cells. What makes a nutrient "essential" isn't just that it's beneficial, but that it's absolutely required for life, causes clear deficiency symptoms when lacking, and serves a unique biological role that cannot be filled by other substances.

Most of us are unaware that just as our body depends on certain nutrients from food—proteins, vitamins, minerals, fatty acids—it also requires specific wavelengths of light to be healthy. We might call these "light nutrients," and like essential nutrients, our bodies need them in certain amounts to function properly. These wavelengths trigger unique biological effects that cannot be replicated by any other stimuli—making them as essential to our cellular health as vitamin C or omega-3s are to our overall wellness.

Our ancestors didn't have to think about this, because their outdoor lives provided ample exposure to sunlight during the day. But in just a few generations, we've dramatically altered this relationship, and the magnitude of this light deficiency in modern environments is staggering. Step outside on a sunny day, and your body is bathed in 10,000 to 100,000 lux of full-spectrum light. Step into your office, home, or school, and that drops to a mere 100 to 500 lux—a reduction of up to a thousandfold. Today, we spend over 90 percent of our lives in artificial environments, resulting in an enormous reduction in light exposure compared to what our ancestors had. And that's just considering overall light intensity—it says nothing of the differences in exposure to specific wavelengths of light, like red and NIR, blue, far-infrared (FIR), and ultraviolet (UV) light, between outdoor and indoor light.

Modern artificial lighting provides a severely impoverished spectrum of light, lacking many of the wavelengths our bodies have evolved to use for specific biological functions. Fluorescent lights and light-emitting diodes (LEDs), while energy-efficient, emit an unnatural spectrum that bears little resemblance to the sunlight our bodies expect and need.

Even more problematically, we've completely inverted our natural light exposure patterns. Our ancestors spent their days under bright, full-spectrum sunlight and their evenings in the warm, red-wavelength glow of fires. In contrast, we spend our days in dimly lit buildings under artificial lighting that lacks vital wavelengths, then expose ourselves to bright, blue-rich light from screens and LED lighting well into the night. This inversion of our natural light-dark cycles disrupts our circadian rhythms at a fundamental level, throwing off the intricate timing mechanisms that coordinate countless biological processes.

The vast majority of people living in the modern world are suffering from chronic mal-illumination and aren't even aware of it. This has widespread effects on our brain and organ function, immune system, energy levels, mood, neurotransmitter balance, hormone levels, metabolic health, and virtually every major system of our bodies. Like a diet of processed junk food that leaves us overfed yet undernourished, our modern lighting environment bombards us with artificial light while depriving us of the specific wavelengths our bodies need to function properly. We get too much of the wrong kinds of light, too little of the right kinds, and receive it at all the wrong times. This mal-illumination affects every aspect of our biology, from brain function and neurotransmitter production to hormonal signaling, immune system function, and cellular energy production.

Research has revealed the devastating scope of this problem. Sunlight deficiency has been linked with numerous diseases, such as:

- Neurodegenerative diseases like Alzheimer's, dementia, multiple sclerosis, and Parkinson's[1–4]
- Dozens of types of cancers[5–8]
- Obesity[9, 10]
- Diabetes[9]
- Metabolic syndrome[10]
- Heart disease[9]

There is even research that suggests that low levels of sun exposure are a risk factor for human health equivalent to that of being a cigarette smoker![11] A Swedish study looked at nearly 30,000 women for 20 years (note: studies with this many people that are this long-term are exceedingly rare) and found that **women with the lowest sun exposure had a twofold-higher rate of death compared to the women with the most sun exposure, a similar magnitude of increased mortality risk as smokers have compared to non-smokers!**[12]

Adding insult to injury, our evening exposure to artificial light actively compounds these problems. The blue-rich light from our phones, tablets, computers, TVs, and LED lighting doesn't just keep us awake—it triggers a cascade of biological disruptions. Artificial light exposure at night (from electronic devices like phones, TVs, computers, indoor lighting, etc.) have been linked with numerous diseases, like:

- Several types of cancers[13, 14]
- Depression and many mood disorders[15]
- Fat gain, obesity, diabetes, and metabolic syndrome[16–18]
- Insomnia and poor sleep[19]

This crisis of mal-illumination represents one of the most significant yet underappreciated public health challenges of our time. The artificial lighting environments we've created in our homes, workplaces, and schools are fundamentally incompatible with our biological needs, creating a form of environmental mismatch that rivals poor nutrition in its impact on human health. Put simply, most peoples' light-exposure habits in the modern world are the equivalent of eating an all-McDonald's diet—chronically deprived of essential elements needed for optimal health.

While most people are familiar with vitamin D deficiency from lack of sun exposure, and many have heard about blue light's effects on sleep, these well-known issues are merely the visible tip of a much larger iceberg of biological disruption.

The field of photobiology—the study of light's effects on living systems—has transformed our understanding of how light interacts with human biology. Over the past several decades, we've discovered that just as nutritional science revealed the crucial role of various food nutrients in human health, photobiology is unveiling the essential nature of specific light wavelengths for human health and healing.

Photobiomodulation (PBM) (modifying biology with light), a branch of photobiology focusing on the therapeutic effects of light, has emerged as one of the most significant health discoveries of the last 50 years. This field has documented how specific wavelengths of light can trigger beneficial biological effects, from enhanced cellular energy production to accelerated healing. When most people hear this, they react with understandable skepticism. After all, the idea that light could penetrate our skin and influence our cellular machinery seems almost like science fiction. But again, this isn't just theory—we now have a mountain of scientific evidence elucidating the intricate mechanisms by which these effects occur.

But to talk of "light" having effects on human biology is somewhat nebulous—just as it would be to talk of the effects of "food" on the human body. What kind of food are we talking about? Broccoli or doughnuts, fish or French fries, blueberries or Twinkies? These things act in different ways. Similarly, light of the wrong type, in the wrong place, wrong dose, or wrong timing, can have damaging effects (from DNA damage in the skin, to macular degeneration in the eyes, to artificial light at night causing metabolic and hormonal havoc). Specific wavelengths can also have profoundly beneficial effects on our cellular function and overall health.

Think of your cells as sophisticated solar panels, each containing different types of specialized light-sensitive components. These cellular structures have evolved over millions of years to capture and utilize specific wavelengths of light in distinct ways. All forms of electromagnetic radiation—from radio waves to visible light to gamma rays—interact with matter in specific ways. Our bodies are no exception. We've evolved sophisticated mechanisms to detect, respond to, protect ourselves from, and benefit from various parts of the electromagnetic spectrum.

Over the last few decades, scientists have slowly revealed that these wavelengths interact with our cells in remarkably specific ways. Most important, we're beginning to understand that when we have deficiencies or excesses of certain wavelengths (or when light exposure is mistimed), it can trigger cascades of biological effects that influence everything from cellular-energy production to systemic inflammation, to overall metabolic health, to hormone levels, and much more.

Many people don't realize that inadequate exposure to red and NIR light is perhaps one of the most problematic of these light-nutrient imbalances. These wavelengths of light play crucial roles in cellular-energy production, tissue repair, and systemic inflammation—processes that affect every aspect of our health.

I think that one reason why red and NIR light deficiencies have been so easily overlooked is that the effects are extremely subtle, despite being widespread throughout every cell in the body. When you get inadequate ultraviolet exposure, you develop measurable vitamin D deficiency, with established and well-understood harmful effects. When you get too much blue-light exposure at night and insufficient amounts during the day, you are noticeably more tired, irritable, foggy-headed, hungry, and negatively affected in a host of other systemic ways by circadian dysregulation.

Yet, when you get inadequate red and NIR light exposure, the effects are more subtle, generalized, and insidious, gradually affecting cellular and systemic health without being immediately noticeable. Red and NIR light play a crucial role in mitochondrial function, supporting energy production, reducing oxidative stress, and promoting cellular repair. Without adequate exposure, the body's ability to maintain optimal cellular health declines over time. You may not experience obvious symptoms right away (certainly none that you've been taught to attribute directly to a deficiency of red and NIR light exposure), and there is no specific biomarker associated with red and NIR light exposure (as is the case with vitamin D and sunlight), but the cumulative impact could manifest as slower recovery, chronic fatigue, reduced resilience to stress, impaired immune function, or even accelerated aging.

Because these effects impact the body at a cellular level rather than through a single, easily identifiable deficiency or system, they are harder to directly associate with a lack of red and NIR light. This makes it easier for both individuals and healthcare systems to overlook their significance, even though they quietly underlie many aspects of systemic health. Basically, the absence of adequate red and NIR light doesn't create dramatic immediate dysfunction but subtly chips away at the body's capacity to thrive.

To truly understand how red and NIR light exert such profound effects on human biology, let's first explore the broader context of the full electromagnetic spectrum.

This spectrum spans an enormous range—from the infinitesimal wavelengths of gamma rays (0.0001 nanometer [nm]) to the long waves of radio signals stretching over meters.

Light, the part of the spectrum we can see, occupies just a tiny slice of this range—from roughly 400 to 700 nm. Pass sunlight through a prism and you'll see it split into the familiar colors of the rainbow—red, orange, yellow, green, blue, indigo, and violet (ROY G. BIV, for easy memorization). These visible wavelengths span from 400 to 700 nm.

The Electromagnetic Spectrum

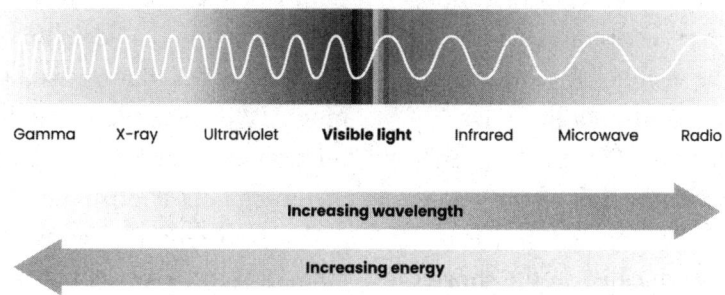

Gamma   X-ray   Ultraviolet   **Visible light**   Infrared   Microwave   Radio

Increasing wavelength

Increasing energy

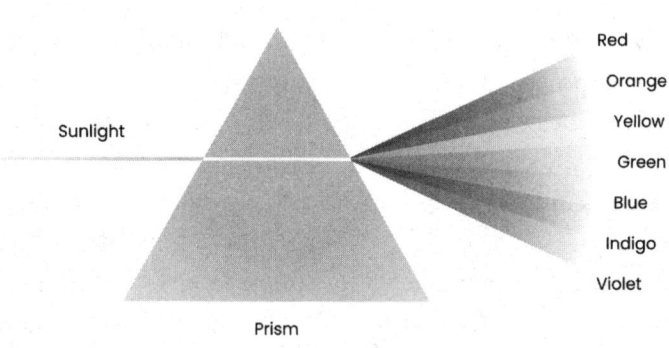

Sunlight

Prism

Red
Orange
Yellow
Green
Blue
Indigo
Violet

Visible Spectrum

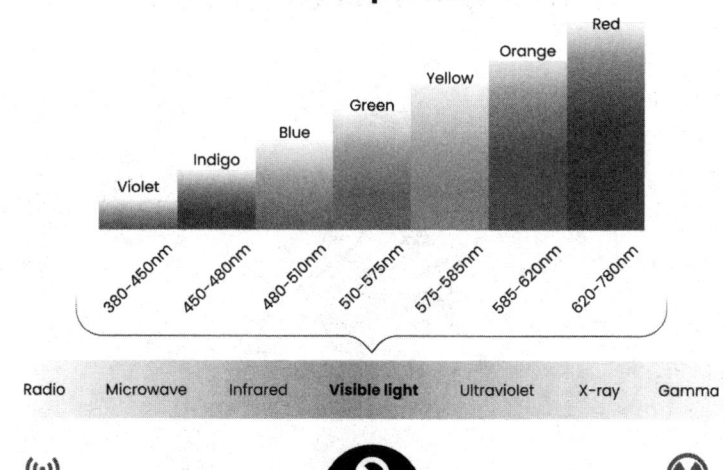

Violet
Indigo
Blue
Green
Yellow
Orange
Red

380–450nm   450–480nm   480–510nm   510–575nm   575–585nm   585–620nm   620–780nm

Radio   Microwave   Infrared   **Visible light**   Ultraviolet   X-ray   Gamma

At the lowest end of the visible light spectrum are the deep violets (around 400 nm), with ultraviolet (UV) radiation existing below that (<400 nm). At the highest end of the visible light spectrum is red light, which goes from a little over 600 to approximately 700 nm. Above the visible light spectrum is NIR, from about 700 to 1,400 nm (but for therapeutic PBM, the focus is typically on the shorter end, from 700 to 1,000 nm). Beyond that comes mid-infrared and then far-infrared (FIR) energy.

Hidden within this vast spectrum lies a remarkable discovery: Specific ranges of electromagnetic radiation can powerfully influence human biology. Each of these "bioactive" wavelengths interacts with our cells in distinct ways.

UV light, particularly in the range of 290 to 400 nm, has biological effects that extend far beyond its well-known role in vitamin D synthesis. When UV light strikes the skin, it triggers a complex series of photochemical reactions that begin with the conversion of 7-dehydrocholesterol to previtamin D3. But this is just the beginning. UV exposure also modulates the production of numerous other compounds, including beta-endorphins, nitric oxide, and various immunomodulatory molecules. Recent research has revealed that UV exposure influences the composition and function of the skin microbiome, affects the production of antimicrobial peptides, and modulates systemic immune responses.

Moving into the visible spectrum, blue light, ranging from 380 to 500 nm, serves as the primary regulator of our circadian rhythm, but its effects extend far beyond simple sleep-wake cycles. When blue light strikes specialized melanopsin-containing retinal ganglion cells, it triggers a cascade

The 5 Types of Bioactive Light

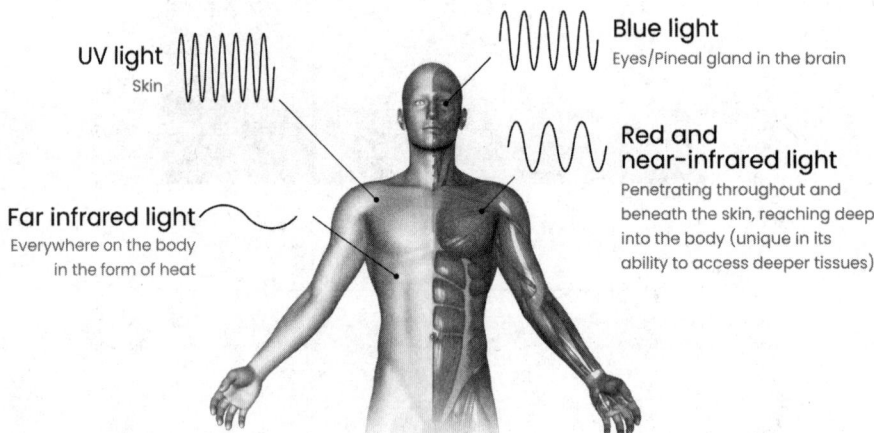

UV light
Skin

Blue light
Eyes/Pineal gland in the brain

Red and near-infrared light
Penetrating throughout and beneath the skin, reaching deep into the body (unique in its ability to access deeper tissues)

Far infrared light
Everywhere on the body in the form of heat

of biological events that influence the entire endocrine system. These cells connect directly to the suprachiasmatic nucleus—our master biological clock—which then orchestrates the timing of countless physiological processes. The implications are profound: Blue light exposure patterns influence everything from hormone production and neurotransmitter balance to metabolic rate and immune function. Modern research has shown that proper timing of blue light exposure can enhance cognitive performance, improve mood, and even influence weight regulation through its effects on metabolic hormones. (Blue light also has other effects, such as sterilization of surfaces by killing bacteria, and is widely used in helping to control the bacteria that contribute to acne as well as other applications.)

At much longer wavelengths, FIR light (3,000 to 15,000 nm) adds another dimension to "light nutrition" through its thermal and non-thermal biological effects. This wavelength range influences tissue function primarily through its interaction with water molecules, affecting cellular water structure and molecular bonds. These effects extend beyond simple heating, influencing blood-flow patterns, cellular metabolism, and the expression of heat shock proteins that play crucial roles in cellular protection and repair. Research has shown that FIR exposure can improve cardiovascular function, enhance detoxification processes (sweating is a key pathway of detoxification), and influence mitochondrial function through mechanisms distinct from those of red and NIR light.

Among all bioactive wavelengths, red and NIR light hold a unique distinction: They can penetrate far deeper into human tissue than any other wavelength. This remarkable ability exists because of what scientists call the "optical window" or "therapeutic window" in human tissue—a specific range of wavelengths, roughly from 600 to 1,000 nm. This window exists because of the unique interaction between different wavelengths of light and the major molecules in our tissues. At shorter wavelengths, light is strongly absorbed or scattered by hemoglobin in our blood and melanin in our skin. At longer wavelengths, water becomes the dominant absorber. But in between—precisely where red and NIR light fall—there's a "window" where light can pass through these barriers much more easily, traveling several centimeters into the body to reach deep tissues.

Once in those deeper tissues, red and NIR light trigger unique and powerful biological effects—interacting with the mitochondria of the cells, altering gene expression, and other mechanisms that enhance cellular-repair mechanisms, reduce inflammation, improve collagen synthesis, and accelerate wound healing, among other health benefits we'll explore in the coming sections.

These unique effects of red and NIR light aren't just a coincidence of physics;

Penetration of Different Wavelengths

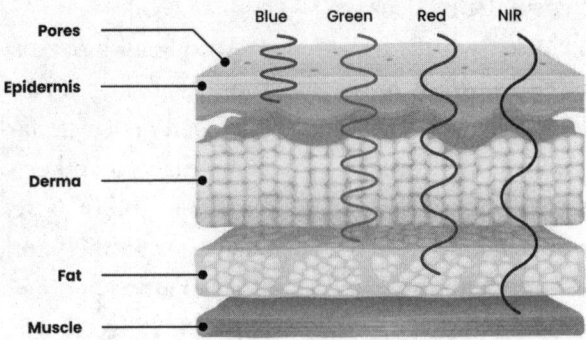

it's the result of millions of years of evolution. The fact that our bodies maintain this "window" of transparency to red and NIR light, combined with the presence of cellular mechanisms that respond specifically to these wavelengths, suggests that these kinds of light played a crucial role in our biological development. Just as our eyes evolved to see visible light because that was most useful for survival, our deeper tissues evolved this transparency to red and NIR light because these wavelengths provided important biological benefits. The therapeutic applications of these effects are remarkably broad, from enhancing muscle recovery and athletic performance to improving brain function and metabolic health to enhancing wound healing, all working through natural biological mechanisms that our bodies have evolved to utilize over millions of years.

Before delving into the science and practical uses of red and NIR PBM ther-apy, let's zoom out to the broader picture again. The field of photobiology has revealed that human biology requires specific wavelengths of light to function properly. Yet our modern lifestyle has created a state of mal-illumination, where we're not only deprived of essential light wavelengths but also exposed to excessive amounts of the wrong types at the wrong times.

Within this landscape of "light nutrients" that our physiology is designed to benefit from, red and NIR light are widely regarded as the primary focus of PBM. Over the last several decades, a large body of scientific research (thousands of studies) has emerged showing that red and NIR light have remarkable therapeutic effects on human biology. While the sun has been our ancestral source of these wavelengths, modern science has allowed us to harness them more precisely through specific devices for PBM.

The remarkable effects of this therapy

aren't arbitrary—they stem from millions of years of evolution, during which every cell in our bodies developed sophisticated mechanisms to capture and utilize these specific wavelengths of light. These aren't just beneficial wavelengths—they are essential "light nutrients" that our cellular machinery depends on, just as it depends on oxygen and glucose.

Think of it this way: Just as we would never expect a plant to thrive in darkness, or our bones to stay strong without vitamin D, our cells cannot function optimally without adequate exposure to these specific wavelengths of light. When we apply red and NIR light therapeutically, we're essentially correcting a deficiency—one that affects nearly every person living in the modern indoor world.

The recognition of light as an essential nutrient represents a fundamental shift in our understanding of human health. It forces us to reconsider our modern indoor lifestyle, where we've inadvertently created a state of chronic "light malnutrition." By understanding these wavelengths as crucial nutrients that our cells need for optimal function, we can better appreciate why their therapeutic application can have such profound effects on human health and healing.

Through precise application of these wavelengths in therapeutic doses, we can now go beyond simply correcting deficiencies. Modern PBM technology allows us to leverage these ancient cellular mecha-

nisms to achieve an astounding range of benefits, thoroughly documented by scientific research:

CELLULAR HEALTH AND REGENERATION

- Enhance mitochondrial function and cellular energy production
- Accelerate healing and tissue repair
- Stimulate stem cell proliferation
- Reduce systemic inflammation

PHYSICAL PERFORMANCE AND RECOVERY

- Enhance strength, muscle mass, and athletic performance
- Speed muscle recovery and reduce exercise-related soreness
- Accelerate healing from injuries and wounds

ANTI-AGING AND AESTHETICS

- Reduce wrinkles and improve skin tone through increased collagen production
- Promote hair growth
- Improve body composition

BRAIN AND METABOLIC HEALTH

- Enhance cognitive function and mood
- Support brain health and sleep quality
- Improve metabolic and cardiovascular health
- Strengthen immune-system response

The focus of this book is to serve as a practical guide to understand the foundational principles of PBM using red and NIR light and the science underlying its physiological mechanisms. By providing an overview of the scientific literature on its many health benefits, readers can gain an understanding of the principles that determine the efficacy of treatment, while also offering a selection of PBM devices and how to use them effectively for a wide variety of specific purposes.

THE ULTIMATE GUIDE TO RED LIGHT THERAPY, REVISED EDITION

CHAPTER ONE

A History of Red and Near-Infrared Light Therapy

Throughout human civilization, light has been revered not just as a source of illumination, but as a profound healer. Ancient civilizations across the globe recognized the sun as sacred—a life-giving force worthy of worship and reverence. From the solar deities of Egypt to the sun-honoring rituals of indigenous cultures in the Americas, our ancestors intuitively grasped the sun's vital role in health and healing. Though they lacked our modern scientific understanding of the precise physiological and biochemical mechanisms, they recognized a fundamental truth about light's relationship to living things—an insight that led to healing traditions that modern science is now validating and explaining at the molecular level.

The therapeutic use of light—what we now call "photomedicine" or "photobiomodulation" (PBM)—has documented roots stretching back over three millennia.

In India, the ancient Hindu text Atharva Veda, written around 1400 BCE, contains some of the earliest written references to healing practices involving sunlight. These weren't just spiritual rituals but systematic approaches to treating various ailments through controlled light exposure.

As remarkable as these ancient practices are, some researchers propose that our relationship with healing light may extend millions of years farther into our evolutionary past. Iain Mathewson proposed this intriguing hypothesis in his paper "Did human hairlessness allow natural photobiomodulation 2 million years ago and enable photobiomodulation therapy today? This can explain the rapid expansion of our genus's brain."[1]

While scientists had previously attributed human hairlessness to better temperature regulation through sweat glands or increased vitamin D production from UV exposure, Mathewson offered a revolutionary perspective. He argued that "the penetration of red/NIR light into mitochondria-rich muscles could release systemic mediators that stimulated human brain growth over millions of years." This could potentially explain why the timeline of human hairlessness coincides with our species' dramatic brain development.

Moving from evolutionary theory to recorded history, humans have been consciously harnessing light's healing properties for thousands of years.

As civilizations developed across the ancient world, three grand traditions of medicine emerged, each incorporating light therapy in different ways: traditional Chinese medicine, Indian Ayurveda, and ancient Egyptian medicine.[2]

In ancient Egypt, Ra, the sun god, was revered as a source of primal life-giving energy. Ra was depicted as a ram-headed sun god wearing a sun disc and sailing across the heavens in daylight from east to west in a celestial boat. The Pharaoh Amhotep IV of the eighteenth dynasty (1801–1792 BCE) even established a monotheistic religion centered on sun worship. In Heliopolis, a city on the Nile delta, devotees invoked their sun god with fervent and solemn incantations in order to cure illnesses and prevent disease.

The healing power of sunlight was acknowledged even in biblical texts. The Talmud recognized that the sun "carries healing in its wings" (Malachi 3:20). A story tells of Jacob limping due to an accident, and when "the Sun rose upon him," Rabbi Berachaya interpreted this to mean, "The sun shone upon him in order to heal him."

In Ayurvedic medicine, sunbathing—called "Atapaseva"—was prescribed for various conditions. As traditional texts explain: "Atapaseva is very useful for lightening the body, increasing the agni and treating bhrajaka pitta. Many conditions can be improved by sitting in the sun; certain types of eczema, psoriasis, arthritis, depression and water retention to name a few. Lying in the sun and meditating upon the solar plexus, is a wonderful shaman for kapha and vata."[3]

The Greeks and Romans also recognized sunlight's therapeutic value. Hippocrates taught that "water and sunshine were blended together in the human body to produce the best health." Romans enjoyed sunbaths in their solaria (called Heliosis), typically followed by cold sponging. The Roman physician Caelius Aurelianus, writing in the fifth century, prescribed sunbaths for a wide range of diseases.

In medieval times, the fascinating "red treatment" became a standard approach to smallpox. The method involved wrapping patients in red cloth, surrounding them with red decor and curtains, and providing only red foods and drinks. John of Gaddesden, a royal physician to Edward I of England who died in 1361, wrote:[4]

. . . Let a scarlet or red cloth be taken and the variolous [pox-ridden] patient be wrapped in it completely—as I did with the son of the most noble king of England when he suffered those diseases . . . I made everything about his bed red . . . it is a good cure and I cured him in the end without the marks of smallpox.

This practice persisted for centuries. Even Queen Elizabeth I was wrapped in a red blanket when she contracted smallpox in 1562, and early modern smallpox wards featured red walls, red curtains, and red lamps—an early example of using specific light wavelengths for therapeutic purposes.

EARLY MODERN DEVELOPMENTS

The therapeutic use of sunlight continued into more recent centuries, with reports of light therapy appearing more frequently in medical literature. In 1735, Fiennius described a case in which he cured a cancerous growth on the lip using a sunbath. As long ago as 1774, Faure and other French surgeons reported the cure of leg ulcers through sun exposure. In 1776, LePeyre and LeConte found that "sunlight concentrated through a lens accelerated wound healing and destroyed tumors."

There were also reports that sunlight had beneficial effects on internal conditions. In 1782, Harris used "sunlight-exposed mollusk shells to improve a case of rickets." Gauvain in 1815 and Bonnet in 1840 recommended sunlight treatment for chronic joint inflammation.[5] Indeed, in 1845, Bonnet first reported that sunlight could be used to treat tuberculous arthritis (a bacterial infection of the joints).

The scientific understanding of light's biological effects began to emerge in the early nineteenth century. Two pioneering scientists, Theodor von Grotthuss (1785–1822) and John William Draper (1811–1882), independently discovered what became known as the Grotthuss-Draper first law of photochemistry: "that light must be absorbed by a specific chemical substance in order for a photochemical reaction to take place." This fundamental principle laid important groundwork for our modern understanding of how light interacts with biological tissues.

THE VITAMIN D CONNECTION

Theobald Adrian Palm (1848–1928), a physician from Edinburgh, Scotland, who traveled to Japan, made a crucial observation that would eventually lead to our understanding of vitamin D. While in Niigata, he noticed that rickets—a disease then thought to be caused by poverty, poor diet, overcrowded housing, or even poor soil—was remarkably rare among Japanese children, especially those living in sunny climates.

Palm boldly challenged the prevailing theory, noting: "Rickets is a disease of civilization, and is so frequently found in the large cities of America and Europe that it is doubtful whether the children of the poorer classes ever wholly escape it."[6] He recommended treating children with rickets using sunbaths and relocating them to sunnier regions. His observations eventually contributed to the discovery of vitamin D in 1920, the "sunlight vitamin" that could be synthesized in the skin through UVB exposure.[7]

Leonard Findlay (1878–1947), a pediatrician at Glasgow University, made similar observations and ultimately suggested that rickets was caused by a lack of sunlight, exercise, and fresh air. In his review of rickets etiology, Findlay concluded that:[8]

> Rickets is a disease of the temperate zone, being very rare, and, in fact, practically unknown, in tropical and subtropical countries. The staple diet in these climates is anything but nourishing, the people living mainly on rice, or some other cereal, exactly the kind of food which is supposed in this country to generate the disease.

This discovery represented one of the first scientific validations of light's biological impact on human health. Modern research has vastly expanded our understanding of vitamin D's role beyond bone health. We now know that vitamin D functions more like a hormone than a traditional vitamin, influencing hundreds of genes and virtually every tissue in the body. Vitamin D receptors are found throughout the cardiovascular system, immune cells, muscles, brain, and endocrine system.

Recent studies have linked optimal vitamin D levels to improved immune function, reduced inflammation, better mood regulation, and even longevity. The capacity to produce vitamin D through UVB exposure—a mechanism that requires precisely the hairless skin that Mathewson highlighted in his evolutionary theory—remains a perfect example of how light directly influences our biochemistry. This relationship between sunlight and vitamin D production demonstrates the profound molecular dialogue between light and human biology that continues to be explored in modern PBM research.

Arnold Rikli (1823–1906), a Swiss entrepreneur who became ill working with chemicals in his father's leather factory, developed his own "helio-hydroscopic treatment centers" in Bled, Slovenia.[9] These centers involved exposing the body to water, air, and sun—a philosophy captured in his famous quote: "Water is good, air is better, but light is best of all." By 1906, Rikli's approach had helped make Bled one of the best tourist destinations in the Austro-Hungarian Empire.

Nils Ryberg Finsen (1860–1904), born in the Faroe Islands, revolutionized light therapy and became the third recipient of the Nobel Prize in Physiology or Medicine in 1903. Finsen developed the "Finsen Lamp," a large electric carbon arc lamp with a system of filters and lenses that produced concentrated beams of light. He initially used red light to treat smallpox patients by reducing inflammation and preventing scarring.

A breakthrough came when one of Finsen's engineers, Niels Mogensen, who suffered from tuberculosis of the skin (lupus vulgaris) with severe facial lesions, showed dramatic improvement after just 4 days of treatment with Finsen's ultraviolet light.[10] This led to the establishment of the Medical Light Institute in Copenhagen in 1896, where, between 1886 and 1901, an impressive 83 percent of the 804 tuberculosis patients treated were cured, with only 6 percent showing no improvement.

Interestingly, researchers in 2005 discovered that Finsen's device likely delivered UVA and blue light rather than UVB as originally thought, suggesting that the tuberculosis bacteria contained enough free porphyrins to be killed by these wavelengths through photodynamic action.

In his Nobel Lecture in 1903, Finsen reflected on his personal connection to light therapy:

> My disease has played a very great role for my whole development. The disease was responsible for my starting investigations on light. I suffered from anemia and tiredness, and since I lived in a house facing the north, I began to believe that I might be helped if I received more sun. I therefore spent as much time as possible in its rays. As an enthusiastic medical man I was of course interested to know what benefit the sun really gave.

After Thomas Edison invented the electric light bulb in 1879, John Harvey Kellogg (1852–1943)—businessman, inventor, and physician—began applying electric light for therapeutic purposes at the Battle Creek Sanitarium in Michigan. To overcome Michigan's frequently cloudy skies, Kellogg constructed his first "incandescent electric light bath" in 1891 and exhibited it at the World's Columbian Exposition in Chicago in 1893.

Kellogg's 1910 book, "Light Therapeutics: a practical manual of phototherapy for the student and the practitioner, with special reference to the incandescent electric-light bath," described applications of electric light to various body parts including the spine, chest, abdominal region, and joints.[11] Under his guidance, the Battle Creek Sanitarium expanded dramatically, treating just 106 patients in 1866 but 7,006 by 1906.[12]

Oskar Bernhard (1861–1939), a Swiss surgeon, made a serendipitous discovery about sunlight's healing properties in 1902. When treating a patient with severe knife wounds whose surgical incision had burst open and was healing poorly, Bernhard tried an unusual approach:[13]

As I entered the hospital one beautiful morning, and the sun shone warmly through the open window, while a refreshing and stimulating atmosphere filled the whole ward, the thought suddenly occurred to me of exposing this large wound to the sun and air; for the mountain peasant of the Grisons also exposes fresh pieces of flesh to the sun and dry air to preserve them, and in this way makes a nourishing and tasty food, the well-known "Bindenfleisch." So I resolved to try this antiseptic and drying effect of the sunlight and air on the living tissues. Then, to the great astonishment of the staff, I had the bed put to the open window and laid the large wound open. By the end of the first hour and a half's exposure there was a marked improvement noticeable, and the wound presented quite a different appearance.

This success led Bernhard to establish his own private clinic for sunlight therapy at St. Moritz in 1905, featuring south-facing balconies to maximize sun exposure.[14]

Similarly, Auguste Rollier (1874–1954) opened a clinic in Leysin, Switzerland, specializing in treating non-pulmonary tuberculosis with carefully controlled sun exposure.[15] Rollier recommended gradually building up to "a daily total of two to three hours in the summer months, and three to four hours in the winter," and also successfully treated soldiers with intractable war wounds from World War I.

By May 1928, light therapy had reached such popularity that *The Times of London* published a forty-page supplement entitled "Sunlight and Health," filled with photographs, illustrations, and advertisements. As Tania Anne Woloshyn noted in her book *Soaking Up The Rays*, the supplement was intended to "enable, not merely reflect, the widespread acceptance and legitimization of therapeutic light and to cement the so-called innate connection between sunlight and health within the minds of its readership."[16]

However, not everyone was convinced

that heliotherapy could work in Britain. Physicians Eleanor and William Russell wrote in 1925:[17]

> It is very difficult and almost impossible to practice heliotherapy in this country, owing to its low altitudes and its climatic conditions. The moisture-laden atmosphere and the smoky air filter out practically all the therapeutic rays of the sun, particularly in our large cities, and especially in winter, so that the sunlight we get is almost free from these rays.

A transformative advancement came in 1917 when Albert Einstein proposed the concept of "population inversion and stimulated emission"—a state where more atoms or molecules are in an excited, light-emitting state than in a light-absorbing state.[18] This theoretical groundwork eventually led to the development of lasers.

The first working laser was produced in 1960 by Theodore Maiman at Hughes Research Laboratories in California, using a synthetic ruby crystal that emitted pulsed coherent light at 694 nm.[19] At a press conference at the Hotel Delmonico in New York on July 7, 1960, Maiman announced:

> Thank you, and good morning, ladies and gentlemen. We are here today to announce to you that man has succeeded in achieving a goal that scientists have sought for many years. For the first time in history a source of "coherent" light has been attained. This is another way of saying that the long-sought "laser" is no longer an elusive dream, but is indeed, an established fact.

THE BIRTH OF PHOTOBIOMODULATION

The medical applications of lasers were soon explored, with Paul E. McGuff at Tufts New England Medical Center investigating their use in treating tumors. However, it was Endre Mester (1903–1984), a Hungarian professor at Semmelweis Medical University in Budapest, who serendipitously discovered the healing effects of low-power laser light in 1965.

In the 1960s, Mester was using red-light lasers to kill tumor cells implanted into laboratory animals.[20] He was trying to repeat McGuff's successful research in Boston. Interestingly, Mester's laser only had a small fraction of the power output of McGuff's device and thus was insufficient to kill the tumor cells.

But Mester observed a fascinating phenomenon: "He noticed that the skin wounds made during the implantation of the tumors healed dramatically faster in the animals being treated with the red light compared to the animals not being treated with light. The light actually caused damaged cells to heal faster!"

He also observed that "hair growth was also stimulated" in the treated animals. This accidental finding led Mester to explore the effects of low-power laser beams on wound healing in humans with diabetes, venous insufficiency, and rheumatoid arthritis.[21] His pioneering work in revealing the anti-inflammatory and pain-relieving effects of laser therapy earned him recognition as the "Father of Photobiomodulation."

Indeed, this discovery of the power of red light to speed up healing and regeneration of human cells has now been confirmed by hundreds of studies.

Russian scientist Tiina I. Karu (born 1945) further advanced the field by investigating the photobiological mechanisms of low-power laser beams. She was the first to highlight the role of mitochondria and cytochrome C oxidase as photoreceptors in living cells and identified some of the signaling pathways that could be triggered by exposure to red and NIR light.[22]

In 1962, Nick Holonyack at General Electric's Advanced Semiconductor Laboratory invented the first visible light-emitting diode (LED), earning him the title "Father of the light-emitting diode."[23] Though initially overshadowed by laser technology, LEDs eventually became crucial in light therapy when Harry Whelan at the Medical College of Wisconsin used NASA-promoted LEDs to treat oral mucositis lesions in pediatric leukemia patients.[24]

The advantages of LEDs—ease of home use, cost-effectiveness, safety, and wide availability—have since led them to largely replace lasers in therapeutic applications. Most comparative studies between lasers and LEDs using the same optical parameters have concluded "there is little difference between them" in terms of therapeutic effectiveness.[25]

In the 1990s, NASA began exploring this technology as well. They were initially using red-light LED technology for growing plants during shuttle missions. But once it was discovered that these lights also affected human cells, NASA started testing and refining the technology with the idea to use it to help astronauts maintain muscle and bone mass, as well as to treat chronic wounds.

Since these early days, PBM and low-level laser/light therapy (LLLT) have grown into robust fields of research. The body of scientific evidence has expanded exponentially, with thousands of studies now documenting the effects of red and NIR light on biological systems. This remarkable accumulation of research spans disciplines from cellular biology and neuroscience to sports medicine and dermatology.

The breadth of documented benefits is equally impressive, and ranges from cellular effects—increased collagen, stem cell activation, and enhanced mitochondrial function—to clinical outcomes like accelerated wound healing, pain reduction, and improved cognitive and athletic performance, to the treatment of arthritis, depression, Parkinson's disease, sports injuries, chemotherapy-induced oral mucositis, hair loss, acne, and dozens of other conditions.

By 2015, the terminology for this field had evolved from "low-level laser therapy (LLLT)" to "photobiomodulation therapy (PBMT)".[26] This shift reflected several important developments in the field. A major driving factor was indeed the growing prominence of LED devices, which had proven to be as effective as lasers in most applications while being more affordable, safer, and easier to use in home settings. As research repeatedly confirmed that coherent laser light was not necessary for therapeutic effects, and that the key factors were wavelength, dosage, and treatment parameters rather than the light source itself, the term "laser therapy" became increasingly inaccurate for describing the broader field.

Additional factors in this terminology evolution included the recognition that "low-level" was an imprecise descriptor (what constitutes "low" was never clearly defined), and the growing understanding that light therapy sometimes works by inhibiting certain biological processes rather than stimulating them.[27] The consensus term "photobiomodulation therapy" better encompassed the field's diverse applications, light sources, and biological mechanisms. (Note that **while photobiomodulation is technically broader, when most people say "photobiomodulation" they're typically referring to red and NIR light therapy.** The other wavelengths are typically more specialized applications rather than the core of what PBM represents therapeutically.)

Red and NIR light therapy devices have been FDA-approved for several purposes, including anti-aging, hair-loss reversal, acne treatment, pain relief, slow-to-heal wound treatment, and fat loss. This FDA approval demonstrates the abundance of research showing benefits, because the therapy has to be proven both safe and effective in numerous trials to gain such approval.

The field of PBM continues to evolve with ongoing investigations into optimal dosing parameters, treatment protocols, and novel applications. As technology advances, more affordable and effective devices are becoming available to clinicians and consumers alike, democratizing access to this powerful therapeutic approach.

From ancient sunlight rituals to modern LED devices, the therapeutic application of red and NIR light represents one of humanity's oldest and most enduring healing traditions—one that continues to evolve with our advancing scientific understanding. What began as intuitive practices based on observation has now been validated through rigorous scientific inquiry, revealing that our ancestors' reverence for light's healing power was indeed founded on a profound biological reality.

How Photobiomodulation Works: The Mechanisms and Pathways of Red and NIR Light Therapy

How do waves of light transform into powerful signals that can heal and restore the body? The journey of a photon from a light wave traveling through space to a catalyst of cellular healing is a complex and fascinating process.

Since researchers first began investigating low-level laser therapy in the 1960s and 1970s, the precise mechanisms of how photobiomodulation (PBM) "works" have been somewhat mysterious and hotly debated in the scientific community. Researchers knew red and near-infrared (NIR) light produced remarkable health benefits, but understanding exactly how light interacts with cells proved challenging. Over the past two decades, significant breakthroughs have dramatically clarified these mechanisms, revealing a nuanced and intricate biological communication system. Even since the first version of this book was published in 2018, our collective understanding of PBM mechanisms has advanced significantly—enough to re-

quire a near-complete rewrite of this section. And it's also likely that our current scientific understanding is still in its adolescence, and much more will be uncovered in the coming decades.

Before diving into the mechanisms of PBM, it's crucial to shift how we typically understand medical interventions. Most of us have been taught to think about how things work in the body through a pharmaceutical lens—where a treatment acts on a discrete mechanism, targeting one specific receptor, enzyme, or biochemical pathway. A precise, linear intervention: one molecule blocking or activating a specific target.

But this just isn't how PBM works. As research continues to expand on PBM, scientists are uncovering an impressively diverse array of cellular and systemic mechanisms through which red and NIR light exert their beneficial effects. Rather than acting through a single pathway or mechanism, red and NIR light influence multiple biological systems simultaneously, triggering cascades of effects throughout the body.

This complexity has unfortunately led to some skepticism and a relatively slow acceptance of PBM in conventional medicine. Medical researchers often question how exactly it works, expecting a simple, linear answer that light photons interact with one particular kind of receptor and trigger a specific mechanism or two. But then they're often frustrated by responses describing complex cascades of effects at many different layers of our physiology—because their opinion may be something along the lines of "if you can't tell me the exact mechanism of how it works, then it's not really scientific." Some PBM researchers are trying to fit things into a conventional mold, reducing PBM down to two or three very discrete "mechanisms" (e.g., cytochrome c oxidase [CCO], etc.). While this kind of reductionistic thinking can, on one hand, lead to valuable specific knowledge, it can also sometimes obscure the bigger picture in another sense—in the same way that reducing the effects of sunlight down to just "vitamin D" or reducing the effects of exercise down to "muscle growth" or reducing meditation down to "lowering stress levels" misses their profound systemic impacts.

This multitude of mechanisms and pathways may lead to skepticism among the mainstream medical thinkers trying to pin down a particular "mechanism" of "how PBM works." But ironically, as you'll soon see, the fact that PBM affects so many pathways and mechanisms throughout our biology is what makes it so powerful. Like other fundamental biological inputs, such as exercise or eating a nutritious and diverse diet, PBM can influence health more deeply and broadly than any single-pathway intervention ever could.

Rather than affecting a specific mechanism unique to a particular medical condition in a highly targeted way, PBM is more like a complex biological orchestrator. Just as a workout or a nutritious meal triggers countless mechanisms and affects many layers of our biology, PBM works in a similarly multifaceted way. While a drug might block a specific receptor or inhibit a particular enzyme, light triggers a network of responses. These responses ripple through our physiology, affecting cells both locally and systemically. From local tissue growth factors to collagen production, to changes in inflammatory cytokines and immune function, to blood chemistry, metabolic function, and even stem cell activation, PBM creates a comprehensive, multi-layered biological response in our bodies.

These mechanisms span from the subcellular to the systemic level, including profound effects on mitochondrial function and cellular energy production, modulation of the immune system's inflammatory responses, optimization of metabolic processes, activation of stem cells, enhancement of cellular growth and regeneration, improvements in vascular function and blood flow, regulation of hormone production, and even modulation of gene expression. The complexity of these overlapping and interconnected pathways helps explain why red and NIR light can benefit such a wide range of conditions and tissues.

The full picture of how these various mechanisms interact continues to be elucidated, with new discoveries happening all the time that expand our understanding of light's biological effects. But what's crucial to grasp is that light isn't just a medical intervention like a drug designed to target specific disease mechanisms. Rather, it works through a web of complex interconnected pathways forged by our ancient evolutionary partnership with light—a relationship that has shaped how our bodies function over millions of years, long before *Homo sapiens* even existed. Using a reductionist lens, we can break things down into parts and mechanisms (like the way we talk about drugs) and talk about how PBM works in a particular medical condition via a particular mechanism. But remember that in the big picture, the way red and NIR light interact with human biology is typically far more complex and multifaceted than our simplistic mechanism-based models typically imply.

When red and NIR light penetrate your tissues, they trigger a cascade of biological effects that flows from the molecular level outward—first affecting individual cells, then spreading through tissues, entire organs, and ultimately orchestrating beneficial changes throughout the entire body. What begins at the smallest scale ripples through every layer of your physiology.

Now let's explore the key changes induced by PBM, tracing the process from the initial nano-level interactions between photons of light and biological molecules to whole-body systemic transformations.

MOLECULAR CHANGES: THE FOUNDATION OF LIGHT THERAPY

Research has identified dozens of specific molecular pathways that respond to, or are indirectly influenced by red and NIR light, including various signaling cascades, transcription factors, and genetic regulators. This extensive network of molecular responses helps explain the diverse therapeutic effects observed with light therapy.

We'll explore many of these pathways in detail shortly, but here is an overview:

- **CCO:** This molecule in your mitochondria absorbs light directly, acting as a primary photoreceptor.
- Adenosine triphosphate (**ATP**): An energy-carrying molecule, often

referred to as "the energy currency of life," providing more power for cellular functions.

- **NITRIC OXIDE (NO):** Released after light exposure, it improves blood flow and cellular signaling.
- **CALCIUM:** Light changes how this important messenger moves in cells, triggering various healing responses.
- **REACTIVE OXYGEN SPECIES (ROS):** In small amounts, these act as signaling molecules that activate protective pathways.
- **MELATONIN:** PBM has profound and surprising effects on melatonin levels in our cells.
- **WATER:** Cellular water structure and hydrogen bonding may be influenced by PBM exposure, affecting how cells function.
- **GROWTH FACTORS:** Light stimulates production of compounds like vascular endothelial growth factor (VEGF), brain-derived neurotrophic factor (BDNF), and transforming growth factor beta-1 (TGF-beta 1) that promote healing.

CELLULAR CHANGES: HOW YOUR CELLS RESPOND

These molecular changes lead to important shifts in how your cells function.

- **INFLAMMATION CONTROL:** Immune cells shift from promoting inflammation to supporting healing.
- **CELL PROTECTION:** Cells become more resistant to damage from toxins and stress.
- **ENHANCED REPAIR:** Cells grow, divide, and move more effectively to heal damaged tissues.
- **PROTEIN SYNTHESIS:** Production of essential proteins like collagen increases.
- **STEM CELL ACTIVATION:** Your body's master repair cells become more active and effective.
- **GENE EXPRESSION:** Light exposure changes which genes get turned on or off.

TISSUE AND ORGAN SYSTEM EFFECTS

As cellular changes accumulate, entire tissues and organ systems begin to respond:

SKIN AND CONNECTIVE TISSUE
- Increased collagen and elastin production

- Better wound healing with less scarring
- Improved skin tone and reduced wrinkles

MUSCLES
- Enhanced energy production for better performance
- Faster recovery after exercise
- Improved glucose metabolism

BRAIN AND NERVOUS SYSTEM
- Reduced inflammation in neural tissue
- Better blood flow to the brain
- Support for neuron growth and new connections
- Relief from pain and improved mood

HAIR FOLLICLES
- Extended hair-growth phase
- Activated hair-growth cells

- Enhanced blood circulation to hair roots

BONES AND JOINTS
- Stimulation of bone-forming cells
- Enhanced mineral deposition
- Reduced joint inflammation

IMMUNE SYSTEM
- Balance between pro- and anti-inflammatory responses
- Improved function of immune cells
- Better clearance of damaged cells and pathogens

ADIPOSE TISSUE
- Enhanced fat breakdown
- Changes in fat-related hormone production
- Improved metabolic activity in fat cells

SYSTEMIC (WHOLE-BODY) EFFECTS

Ultimately, these changes combine to create whole-body benefits:

- Skin rejuvenation
- Faster wound and injury healing
- Reduced systemic inflammation
- Optimized mitochondrial function
- Enhanced stem cell activity
- Improved athletic performance
- Better circulation
- Hormonal balance

- Accelerated recovery
- Strengthened immune health
- Increased energy and reduced fatigue
- Better stress adaptation
- Anti-aging effects
- Increased cellular resilience
- Pain reduction
- Improved body composition
- Autoimmune modulation
- Improved microbiome diversity
- Optimized metabolic health

- Improved sleep quality
- Enhanced brain function

This progression from molecular interactions to whole-body effects explains why PBM can benefit so many different conditions. By enhancing fundamental cellular processes, light therapy helps your body function better at every level.

It's also important to recognize that light doesn't simply activate specific mechanisms in an unregulated way where it "pushes" all cells into a uniform response. Instead, it generally works as a *regulator* of various functions, helping dysfunctional or damaged cells restore balance while maintaining normal function in healthy cells. Here's how Dr. Hamblin described this important point:[1]

The biomodulation achieved by PBM allows it to be applied in situations that can be apparently paradoxical because it can sometimes be used to stimulate cells and tissues, and in other situations it can inhibit the same biological effect. For this reason, PBM is referred to by many researchers as a regulator or modulator because it restores the organism to homeostasis.

This complexity highlights how red and NIR light can impact the body at multiple levels, setting off cascades of changes that modify cellular function both at the initial site of exposure and in distant tissues via systemic mechanisms, affecting both cellular health in the tissues directly exposed to the light, and overall systemic health.

THE TWO LAYERS OF PBM EFFECTS: INITIAL INTERACTIONS AND DOWNSTREAM BIOLOGICAL CASCADES

Now that we've got an overview of the many effects of PBM across the different levels of our physiology, let's dive in to the specifics of how it all works. We'll do this in two parts, breaking down the fundamental mechanisms first and then looking at the broader physiological changes that follow.

The first layer is the true "mechanisms" of PBM in the purest sense. These are essentially the "molecular switches" that the photons of light directly interact with to initiate a response in our cells—it's the

meeting of photon and biology.

Research has identified several key molecular targets where this happens, with the four most widely recognized being:

1. **CCO:** A crucial enzyme in the mitochondrial electron transport chain that absorbs red and NIR light to enhance ATP production and cellular metabolism.
2. **TRANSIENT RECEPTOR POTENTIAL VANILLOID 1 (TRPV1) ION CHANNELS:** Light-sensitive calcium channels that

regulate pain perception, inflammation, and cellular signaling.

3. **TGF-BETA 1:** A signaling molecule activated by light that promotes tissue repair, immune modulation, and collagen production.

4. **WATER (NANOSTRUCTURED WATER CLUSTERS):** Light absorption may alter water viscosity within cells, affecting mitochondrial efficiency and cell function.

The second layer to this story is everything that happens after these molecular switches are activated—the cascade of changes at the cellular level and throughout the body that actually result in various kinds of health benefits.

In the following sections, we'll explore each of these fundamental mechanisms and pathways in detail, outlining how light initiates these processes and leads to widespread health benefits.

THE FOUR FUNDAMENTAL MECHANISMS OF PHOTOBIOMODULATION: WHERE LIGHT MEETS BIOLOGY

The 4 Mechanisms of Photobiomodulation

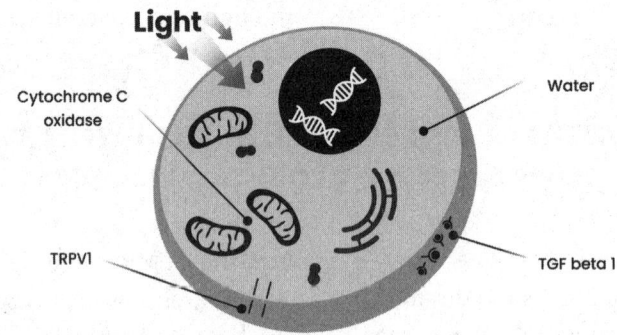

Light

Cytochrome C oxidase

Water

TRPV1

TGF beta 1

Mechanism #1: The Electron Transport Chain and Cytochrome C Oxidase

Think of your cells as tiny power plants. At the heart of each cell are mitochondria—small structures that generate the energy your body needs to function. Inside these mitochondria is something like an assembly line for energy production called the electron transport chain. Workers on this assembly line (electron transport chain complexes) pass electrons from one to another, creating energy at each step.

One of the most well-documented mechanisms of PBM involves the interaction of red and NIR light with one particular "worker" on this assembly line: cytochrome c oxidase (CCO)—a key enzyme in the mitochondrial electron transport chain (ETC). This enzyme has specific absorption peaks in the red and NIR regions of the spectrum, triggering a series of biochemical reactions that enhance cellular metabolism and energy production.[2]

The process begins at the molecular level when photons are absorbed by CCO's copper and heme centers, leading to a change in the enzyme's electronic structure. This photoexcitation increases the rate of electron transfer in the ETC, directly enhancing the proton gradient across the inner mitochondrial membrane. The result is a significant boost in ATP production—your cell's primary energy currency.

There's also a critical role of nitric oxide (NO) in this process of how red and NIR light bolsters CCO activity. Mitochondria need CCO to bind with oxygen to produce ATP, but NO competes with oxygen for binding, slowing ATP production. This isn't to say that NO is harmful (quite the opposite; it has numerous beneficial effects throughout the body). Rather, excessive NO competing with oxygen within mitochondria can cause dysfunction.

PBM may release NO from CCO, freeing up oxygen to restore efficient energy production.[3, 4] In other words, light could knock the NO out and let the oxygen in, which would allow CCO to resume the use of its oxygen molecules and thus promote efficient mitochondrial function. This process is like removing a roadblock so traffic can flow freely again, allowing your cellular energy production to proceed more efficiently.

While this remains under investigation, studies suggest that light-induced NO dissociation enhances cellular respiration.[5]

In short, red and NIR light hits a critical enzyme in your cellular power plants, changes its structure, and helps it work better by removing a molecular traffic jam. This leads to improved cellular energy production.

While researchers are still investigating some of the nuances of the mechanisms, there's clear agreement that red and NIR light ultimately enhances mitochondrial energy production.

Beyond just producing more ATP, light therapy creates small, controlled increases in reactive oxygen species (ROS)—such as superoxide and hydrogen peroxide. Think of these as cellular messenger molecules that activate repair mechanisms and beneficial gene expression. While too much ROS can be harmful (like excessive oxidative stress), these mild increases actually support your body's antioxidant defenses and make cells more resilient.

So why does this central effect on mitochondria matter? Quite simply, because mitochondria fuel nearly every biological function within cells and serve as a type of biological "hub" or "headquarters" for regulating cellular health.[6] No matter what cell type, whether muscle cells, heart cells, thyroid gland cells, skin cells, or brain cells, they depend on mitochondrial energy production to do their job well. So as a generalization, anything which improves mitochondrial function in those cells will tend to make that organ system function better. And it seems that human biology is very much designed in such a way that light is one of the fundamental inputs that enhances mitochondrial function.

This also helps explain what might seem too good to be true: how one therapy can help so many different conditions. Since every cell contains mitochondria, and virtually all cellular functions depend on energy, improving the "power supply" of cells throughout your body can enhance many different physiological processes simultaneously. It's not that light is a magical cure-all; rather, it's enhancing a basic biological function–cellular energy production—that affects everything else.

Mechanism #2: TRPV1 Ion Channels
Another key mechanism of PBM involves the Transient Receptor Potential Vanilloid 1 (TRPV1) ion channel, a protein that acts as a bridge between red and NIR light exposure and the body's healing processes. Initially identified as the receptor responsible for sensing heat and the spiciness of chili peppers,[7] TRPV1 is far more than a simple heat sensor—it also responds to mechanical forces and specific wavelengths of light, making it a potentially critical player in PBM.

When red and NIR light (600 to 1,000 nm) enters the body, TRPV1 channels can be activated in two main ways:

- **DIRECT PHOTORECEPTION:** Light-sensitive proteins on TRPV1 interact with photons, triggering the channel to open.[8]
- **HEAT-INDUCED ACTIVATION:** The mild warming effect of PBM (raising tissue temperature to ~43°C, or ~109°F) can also activate TRPV1.[9]

When TRPV1 channels open, calcium ions flood into the cell, setting off a chain reaction of biological effects. Calcium serves as a messenger molecule, influencing:

- **GENE EXPRESSION:** Calcium triggers transcription factors that regulate DNA activity, instructing cells to repair and regenerate.
- **MITOCHONDRIAL FUNCTION:** Calcium enhances ATP production, providing energy for cell growth and tissue repair.[10]
- **CELLULAR STRESS RESPONSE:** TRPV1 helps cells regulate inflammation and oxidative stress, protecting against damage.

On a broader scale, TRPV1 activation by PBM triggers numerous tissue-level effects. According to one group of researchers,[11]

> The PBM process works with chromophore CCOs and [TRP] ion channels to raise secondary messengers like calcium ions, cAMP, and ROS. These secondary messengers play a vital role in initiating the activation of transcription factors and signaling molecules, which subsequently trigger downstream signaling cascades leading to profound photobiological effects within the cell.

TRPV1 plays a role in circulation, modulation of pain signals, and neuroplasticity.[12–14] However, the relationship between TRPV1 and PBM appears complex and context-dependent. Research suggests that depending on specific conditions, wavelengths, and tissues involved, PBM may either activate or inhibit TRPV1 channels. Some studies indicate that certain wavelengths in the red to mid-infrared range might modulate TRPV1 activity in ways that could contribute to pain relief. Also, when tissues are warmed to approximately 43°C or 109°F (which can occur with some PBM applications), TRPV1 activation may influence mitochondrial function while potentially affecting inflammatory responses through mechanisms that might involve mast cells and histamine release. These varied effects could partially explain the diverse outcomes observed with PBM therapy, including both anti-inflammatory and tissue-regenerative effects. However, it's important to note that the specific mechanisms connecting TRP-V1, mitochondrial function, and clinical outcomes of PBM are still being investigated, and much more research is needed to fully elucidate the role of TRPV1 in mediating the effects of PBM.

Mechanism #3: TGF-Beta 1 and Cellular Regeneration

Another of the key pathways activated by red and NIR light is Transforming Growth Factor Beta 1 (TGF-beta 1), a powerful signaling molecule that drives tissue healing and regeneration.[15] Normally, TGF-beta 1 exists in an inactive state, but when exposed to red and NIR light, it becomes activated and ready to stimulate repair processes.[16]

Once activated, TGF-beta 1 signals cells to repair damaged tissue, build new cells, and regulate inflammation.[17] It also ensures that different cells in the body communicate properly, coordinating the healing process. This makes it a vital part of how PBM helps the body recover from injury and stress.

Dr. Praveen Arany has been a pioneer in this field, and I've had the pleasure of interviewing him on my podcast. Here's what he had to say about his group's discovery of TGF-beta 1 and its interaction with red and NIR light:[18]

My research actually started there. I asked "How can you use light and improve wound healing?" The wound is a very dynamic environment with lots of cells and changes that actually are very attractive for many reasons. I found that to be my playground, if you will, for beginning to understand how light works. In that process, we actually discovered one of the other mechanisms, which turns out to be a growth factor called TGF-beta 1. This growth factor is extremely important for many different processes, but specifically for wound healing.

Now, this growth factor turns out to be present normally in the body, in all of our tissues, in an inactive, latent form. That is where I think we saw the opportunity. Now, this growth factor is present but is not activated. That's where we found, after lots of very careful investigation, that a single amino acid, a single methionine on that growth factor is actually responsible for sensing light. We make that analogy of rhodopsin in your eye. We don't have electronic sensors in our eyes; how come we are able to see? . . . That's where, if you look very carefully, you will see that there is actually a molecule called rhodopsin in your eye that is capable of sensing light.

If you can have one molecule that is capable of enabling vision, we thought, why would it not be possible to look for other molecules? That's where we found this growth factor TGF-beta 1. After very careful investigations in the lab, in vitro, which is in cell culture and cells, to animal mod-els, which we very carefully investigated, we found that there is a single amino acid in this growth factor that is responsible for the light sensitivity.

The signaling cascade of TGF-beta 1 is not limited to individual cells—it propagates effects throughout tissues by altering cellular behavior, modifying the extracellular environment, and coordinating the activities of various cell types. Here are some examples of how it works across different tissues and organ systems:

- **CONNECTIVE TISSUE:** In tendons, ligaments, and cartilage, TGF-beta 1 boosts collagen production, particularly types I and III, which are essential for structural integrity.[19, 20] It also promotes the reorganization of collagen fibers, strengthening these tissues and making them more resilient.
- **MUSCLE TISSUE:** TGF-beta 1 activates satellite cells, the muscles' stem cells, enabling them to repair damaged muscle fibers.[21] It also supports the growth of new blood vessels, improving oxygen and nutrient delivery to healing tissues.
- **SKIN:** In skin tissue, TGF-beta 1 accelerates wound healing by increasing dermal thickness, promoting collagen synthesis, and guiding the remodeling of the extracellular matrix for better quality repair.[22]

- **BONE:** TGF-beta 1 stimulates osteoblasts, the cells responsible for building bone, aiding in the formation and mineralization of new bone matrices.[23] This is particularly important for fracture healing and bone regeneration.
- **IMMUNE FUNCTION:** TGF-beta 1 helps regulate inflammation by triggering anti-inflammatory pathways while suppressing excessive immune activity that can lead to tissue damage.[24] It also supports the recruitment and activation of immune cells like macrophages, which aid in clearing debris and coordinating the repair process. By modulating immune activity, TGF-beta 1 ensures that healing occurs in a controlled, effective manner without unnecessary tissue damage.
- **STEM CELL ACTIVATION:** TGF-beta 1 is a key regulator of stem cell activity. It "wakes up" dormant stem cells, directing them to sites of tissue damage and guiding their differentiation into specific cell types needed for repair.[25, 26] This ensures that new cells integrate effectively into the tissue environment, supporting regeneration and restoring function.

The TGF-beta 1 pathway may be the key pathway in how red and NIR light therapy can harness the body's natural repair mechanisms. By stimulating repair, reducing inflammation, and sending stem cells where they're needed, it plays a major role in how PBM helps improve recovery, immune function, skin health, wound and injury healing, and any other scenarios where cellular regeneration is critical.

Mechanism #4: Water as a Photoacceptor ("Nanostructured Water")

Water isn't just a passive substance in our cells; it may play an active role in how red and NIR light influences biology. Research suggests that water inside cells absorbs red and NIR light, changing its properties in ways that could improve cellular function.

We typically think of water simply as a medium for chemical reactions, but emerging research suggests it may directly influence biological processes. When exposed to red and NIR light, the viscosity (thickness) of water changes, making it more fluid. Imagine trying to swim through Jell-O versus regular water: Movement is much easier in a thinner liquid. Similarly, if the water in and around cellular structures becomes less resistant, biological processes can run more smoothly.

This type of structured water was originally described as a "fourth phase of water" by Gerald Pollack,[27] where water near cell membranes absorbs light and changes how proteins and enzymes within those cell membranes function. This nanoscopic layer of water is called the "exclusion zone water" or "EZ water," which differs from ordinary "bulk water" that exists away from cellular surfaces.[28]

This effect is most pronounced within mitochondria. Several studies have suggested that light-activated water layers inside mitochondria make ATP production more efficient by allowing key enzymes to move more freely and by reducing friction in tiny molecular motors that produce ATP.[29–31]

While this theory is still being explored, it suggests another way PBM may benefit the body: not just by stimulating mitochondria directly, but also by altering the water that surrounds them. If further research validates this mechanism, it could reshape our understanding of how light therapy enhances cellular function and overall health.

THE HORMETIC RESPONSE, CELLULAR STRESS-RESISTANCE, AND GENE EXPRESSION CHANGES

PBM also works in part because it slightly "stresses" your cells. While this might sound like a bad thing, it's actually a powerful way to boost cellular health. Hormesis is when mild stress makes living systems stronger by activating their natural protective mechanisms. Just like how exercise stresses muscles (and bones, and the heart, and blood vessels) to make them stronger and improve their function, or how intermittent fasting challenges cells to become more efficient and resilient, PBM applies controlled cellular stress that prompts your body to repair, strengthen, and improve its overall resilience.

When red or NIR light reaches cells, it stimulates mitochondria to temporarily produce more ROS—molecules that act as messengers for cellular adaptation. While high levels of ROS can be damaging, this mild, controlled increase activates protective responses that help cells function better over time.

The body responds to this stress in several ways:

- **INFLAMMATION CONTROL:** PBM turns on pathways that reduce excessive inflammation and support healing. In damaged or inflamed tissues, PBM suppresses NF-κB, a kind of master switch for inflammation, and thereby helps shift the body toward a more anti-inflammatory state.[32]

- **ANTIOXIDANT PRODUCTION:** The body increases natural antioxidants like superoxide dismutase and glutathione to protect cells from damage. This is primarily a result of PBM increasing nuclear factor erythroid 2-related factor 2 (Nrf2), a key sensor of ROS that up-regulates internal antioxidant defenses in response.[33]

- **HEAT SHOCK PROTEINS:** These specialized proteins help repair damaged cells and maintain protein health in response to stress, such as the adaptive stress created by PBM.[34]
- **GROWTH-FACTOR SIGNALING:** PBM also activates a variety of growth-factor pathways that act like cellular construction crews in response to ROS. These pathways help repair damaged tissue, create new blood vessels through mediators like VEGF, and support nerve health through factors like BDNF.
- **MITOCHONDRIAL EFFICIENCY:** The temporary increase in ROS signals mitochondria to grow stronger, produce more energy, and enhance function.

PBM reveals a fascinating mechanism of cellular communication in which mitochondria play a much more active role in gene expression than was previously understood. When exposed to red and NIR light, mitochondria trigger specific genetic changes that enhance cellular resilience and repair.

Research has shown that PBM specifically upregulates genes involved in:[35–37]

- Antioxidant defense (such as genes coding for superoxide dismutase and glutathione)
- Mitochondrial biogenesis and function
- Anti-inflammatory processes
- Cellular repair mechanisms
- Protein folding

The Hormetic Response to Photobiomodulation

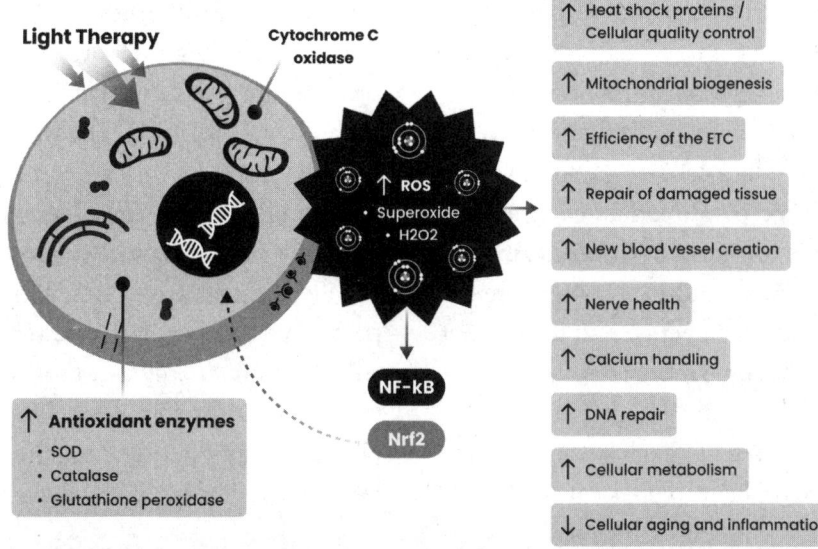

This happens through a process called retrograde signaling, in which mitochondria send signals back to the cell's nucleus that influence gene expression. Whereas DNA has been thought of as the sole commander of cellular function, mitochondria can now be seen as active communicators that respond to environmental signals like light. This challenges our traditional understanding of genetic control, showing how external factors can directly influence which genes are turned on or off. This is "epigenetics"—how signals from the environment and one's behaviors influence gene expression.

What makes PBM particularly powerful is that it doesn't just temporarily alleviate symptoms like an anti-inflammatory or painkiller drug would. Instead, it stimulates lasting adaptations at the cellular level that lead to greater resilience against stressors and an enhanced capacity to produce energy. For example, PBM has been found to activate the Nrf2 pathway, a critical genetic regulator that turns on genes responsible for protecting cells against oxidative stress. This leads to increased production of protective enzymes that help neutralize harmful free radicals and reduce cellular damage. Cells develop enhanced antioxidant capacity, becoming more resistant to various forms of stress; their mitochondria become more efficient at producing energy; and their repair mechanisms become more robust. This creates a kind of cellular "toughening" effect, similar to how regular exercise makes our bodies more resilient to physical challenges.

However, proper dosing is key, due to what's commonly called the "Goldilocks zone" of PBM. Too little light exposure fails to trigger sufficient ROS production to initiate the beneficial stress response. On the other hand, too much light can overwhelm the cell's adaptive capabilities and potentially cause damage.

This explains why larger doses and more powerful devices aren't always better in PBM therapy, and why finding the optimal dose is crucial for therapeutic success. Just like in exercise, where too little effort yields no results and too much can cause damage to the body, PBM requires balance.

The discovery of these hormetic mechanisms has highly significant implications for how we use PBM therapy. It explains why regular, appropriately dosed treatments can lead to cumulative improvements in cellular function: Each session triggers adaptive responses that gradually build upon one another.

Understanding the hormetic response provides insight into why PBM can have such diverse beneficial effects, from reducing inflammation to accelerating healing. The initial ROS-mediated stress response triggers not just protective mechanisms but also regenerative ones, activating pathways involved in tissue repair, cell survival, and energy metabolism. This creates a comprehensive cellular response that can improve tissue function and resilience across multiple systems in the body.

NITRIC OXIDE

When exposed to red and NIR light, biological systems release nitric oxide (NO), a crucial signaling molecule that acts as a vasodilator, helping to increase local blood flow, which enhances oxygen and nutrient delivery to tissues.

PBM triggers NO release through multiple pathways, including direct stimulation of endothelial NO synthase (which is crucial for vascular health and for facilitating blood flow), photodissociation from heme proteins, and conversion of nitrite to active NO under hypoxic conditions.[40–44]

In wound healing, nitric oxide contributes to several processes, including stimulating collagen production, promoting blood vessel formation, reducing inflammation, and supporting tissue regeneration. Notably, PBM has been consistently shown to increase NO production in human skin and improve endothelial function through NO-mediated mechanisms.[38–40]

At the cellular level, NO plays a role in various protective mechanisms. It influences mitochondrial respiration, helps manage oxidative stress, and supports cellular energy metabolism. These interactions occur within a careful balance—beneficial in controlled amounts, but potentially harmful if excessive.

NO plays an important role in maintaining blood vessel health, helping blood vessels relax and preventing excessive clotting, and inadequate levels of endothelial NO synthase have been linked to the development of cardiovascular disease.[40]

More research is needed, but these effects on blood circulation and vascular function may be a critical mechanism by which PBM exerts its therapeutic benefits.

EXTRA-PINEAL MELATONIN: A KEY CELLULAR DEFENSE MECHANISM

Most people know melatonin as a sleep hormone produced by the pineal gland. But this is only part of the story. There are two additional layers to the melatonin story that few people are aware of and are only beginning to be understood by science. The first is that melatonin has many more functions in the body than simply promoting sleep. The second is that melatonin isn't only produced by the pineal gland—the story is far deeper.

Melatonin isn't just a "sleep hormone." It turns out that it's also an incredibly potent antioxidant with critical roles in protecting mitochondria from oxidative stress (and likely other functions as well). Melatonin is believed to be one of the first antioxidant molecules to develop in response to rising atmospheric oxygen levels. This is thought to have occurred more than two billion years ago, long before it played a role in regulating circadian rhythms or sleep.[45, 46] The microorganisms that developed this powerful defense against oxidative stress were the ancestors of our very own mitochondria. To this day, our mitochondria produce most of the melatonin in our bodies, and they preferentially accumulate it when it is taken up from outside the cell, as would occur with the nightly flood of melatonin from the pineal gland, or with consumption of melatonin supplements. [47, 48] While blue light delivered into the brain through our eyes is the primary governor of pineal melatonin levels, melatonin is still secreted in the absence of blue light.

Evolution of Melatonin Over the Millennia

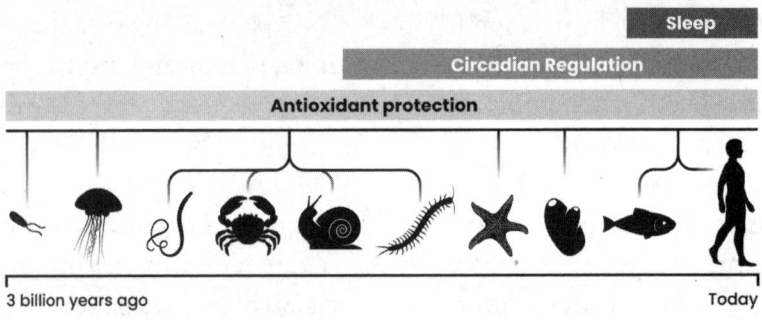

Manchester et al. *J Pineal Res.* 2015; 59(4): 403-19.

But the story of melatonin actually goes much deeper than this. It turns out that melatonin isn't just a hormone produced in the pineal gland and circulated in the bloodstream. Groundbreaking research by scientists like Russell Reiter and Dun-Xian Tan has revealed that melatonin is not limited to the pineal gland but is also produced directly *within mitochondria* across *virtually all cells* of the body, where it serves to protect the cell from damage. Even more remarkably, it turns out that red and NIR light stimulate cells to produce this intracellular melatonin.[49]

While more research is needed to elucidate the role of localized melatonin production in the effects of PBM, it's reasonable to logically speculate that by stimulating mitochondrial melatonin production, PBM helps cells recover, maintain energy, and defend themselves against damage. This makes melatonin more than just a sleep hormone—it's a vital defense molecule that can be enhanced through light therapy, helping cells heal, thrive, and perform at their best. It's likely that this will turn out to be a key pathway of how red and NIR light works to enhance cellular healing and regeneration.

As of now, the way we understand it is that when red and NIR light penetrates tissues, it generates mild, transient oxidative stress—a hormetic signal that prompts mitochondria to ramp up antioxidant defenses, including the production of melatonin. While harmful in large amounts, the NIR-induced low level of oxidative stress serves as a signal leading to the upregulation of antioxidant molecules that protect mitochondria, such as melatonin. Melatonin is affected by exercise, something that very few people seem to be aware of. Under normal dim-light conditions, melatonin increases by just 0.15 pg/mL per minute. This is our healthy circadian rhythm in action. Yet, after the onset of intense exercise, melatonin levels increase 33 times faster, by 5 pg/mL per minute, plateauing when serum melatonin concentrations are two to three times higher than the nightly peak (~200 pg/mL).[50]

Plasma Melatonin Transit Response
(Exercise vs Circadian)

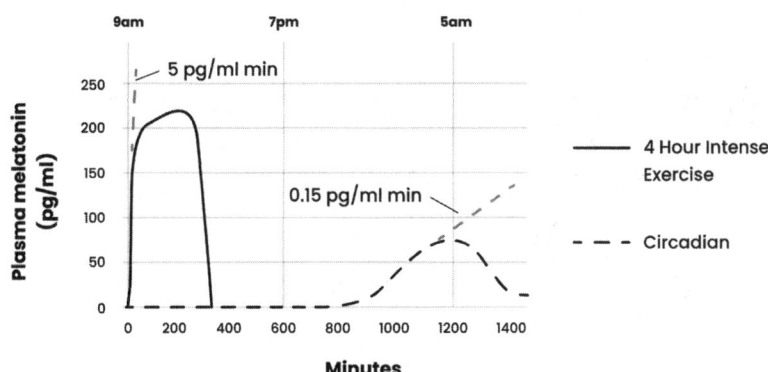

It's likely that the increase in melatonin originated from the mitochondria within muscle tissue as a means of helping the mitochondria cope with the high energy demands of exercise (and consequential increased oxidative stress). NIR light does the same thing! Moreover, this type of melatonin production would occur rapidly and thus could provide immediate protection to minimize cellular injury.

This "extra-pineal" melatonin acts locally within mitochondria, where it is most needed, scavenging free radicals and preventing oxidative damage to mitochondrial DNA, proteins, and membranes. Unlike traditional antioxidants, melatonin is uniquely positioned for this task, as it is both water- and fat-soluble, allowing it to move freely within and across cell structures.

This localized production is rapid and adaptive, likely offering immediate protection to cells during periods of increased energy demand. For example, studies have shown that intense exercise also dramatically increases melatonin levels in muscle mitochondria to help mitigate oxidative stress from heightened energy production.[50]

Ample research has already shown that melatonin provides powerful protection against oxidative stress:

- **ANTIOXIDANT POWER:** Melatonin is twice as effective as vitamin E and four times more potent than glutathione or vitamin C in neutralizing free radicals.[51] Its structure allows it to neutralize multiple types of free radicals and then transform into additional antioxidant molecules, essentially making it a "multi-action" antioxidant.[52]

- **MITOCHONDRIAL BIOENERGETICS:** Melatonin helps maintain and regulate the electron transport chain, reduces electron leakage, and supports consistent ATP production, creating a positive feedback loop of improved mitochondrial efficiency and reduced oxidative stress.[53, 54]

- **NEUROPROTECTION:** Melatonin has been shown to shield mitochondria in brain cells, protecting against the oxidative and nitrosative stress-induced mitochondrial dysfunction seen in neurodegenerative diseases like Alzheimer's, Parkinson's, and Huntington's.[55]

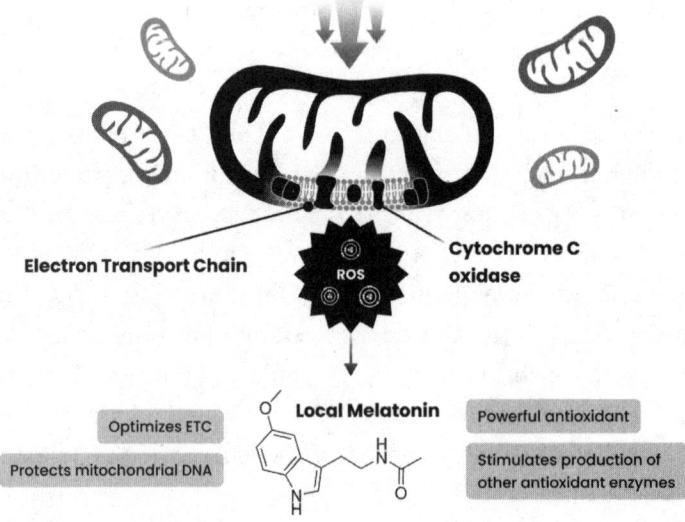

Red & Near-Infrared Light Leads to Extra-Pineal Melatonin Production

Electron Transport Chain

ROS

Cytochrome C oxidase

Local Melatonin

Optimizes ETC

Protects mitochondrial DNA

Powerful antioxidant

Stimulates production of other antioxidant enzymes

- **ANTI-AGING POTENTIAL:** By reducing oxidative stress, protecting mitochondrial DNA, and maintaining cellular energy production, melatonin may play a role in slowing the aging process and mitigating age-related diseases.[56]

Importantly, melatonin can directly prevent free-radical damage *within* the actual mitochondria—a function unique to melatonin, since virtually no other "antioxidant" can do this.[57] Melatonin's structure allows it to be soluble in both water and lipids, making it capable of easily passing through and protecting cell membranes and the cellular machinery within. Its antioxidant protection is potent, being twice as powerful as vitamin E and four times more powerful than glutathione or vitamin C.[58]

Within the mitochondria themselves, melatonin provides protection against oxidative stress that's as good as or better than the antioxidant molecules (MitoE and MitoQ) that have been synthetically designed to accumulate within mitochondria at concentrations 500 times what would occur naturally.[59]

Another fascinating quirk about melatonin is that not only can it neutralize a wide array of free radicals, but it can also catalyze the formation of several other powerful internal antioxidant molecules thereafter, essentially making it a sort of hydra antioxidant that can defend against excessive free radicals in many different ways.[52] Melatonin increases the production and activity of other antioxidant enzymes like glutathione peroxidase, superoxide dismutase, and catalase.[60] You can think of it as basically "recharging" your internal antioxidant defense system.

Melatonin: a 4-in-1 Antioxidant

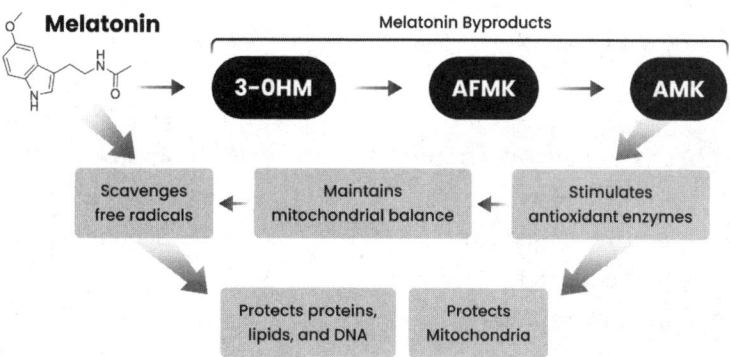

Melatonin's ability to protect mitochondria and the cells that house them from oxidative stress is so powerful that its structure has remained unchanged throughout billions of years of evolution. It is one of nature's best ideas, perfectly suited to the job at hand.

And remember, not only is mitochondrial health critical to our energy levels, but poor mitochondrial health is implicated in numerous diseases and even aging itself.[61] So the fact that red and NIR light supports melatonin production both at the level of the pineal gland, and likely much more importantly, at the cellular level throughout the body, may have far-reaching benefits to us for increasing energy levels (and preventing fatigue), slowing aging, and preventing disease.

GROWTH FACTORS

In addition to TGF-beta 1, which acts as one of the primary molecular "switches" activated by PBM, light therapy triggers the release of numerous other growth factors that contribute to healing and regeneration. These growth factors are essential proteins that guide cellular repair, tissue regeneration, and the restoration of normal function. And it's likely that they play key roles in the regenerative and healing effects of PBM. Here is an overview of just a few of the tissue-specific growth factors known to be stimulated by PBM:

- **BASIC FIBROBLAST GROWTH FACTOR (bFGF):** Supports cell growth, tissue repair, and blood vessel formation to deliver oxygen and nutrients[62]
- **VASCULAR ENDOTHELIAL GROWTH FACTOR (VEGF):** Promotes new blood vessel growth, essential for healing and regenerating oxygen-deprived tissues[63]

- **BRAIN-DERIVED NEUROTROPHIC FACTOR (BDNF):** Enhances brain cell growth, repair, and neuroplasticity, supporting cognitive function[64]
- **INSULIN-LIKE GROWTH FACTOR-1 (IGF-1):** Stimulates muscle and bone repair, improving strength and resilience[65]
- **PLATELET-DERIVED GROWTH FACTOR (PDGF):** Aids wound healing and collagen production, strengthening tissues[66]
- **NERVE GROWTH FACTOR (NGF):** Supports nerve regeneration and helps repair the nervous system[67]
- **BONE MORPHOGENETIC PROTEINS (BMPs):** Stimulate bone growth and fracture healing, reinforcing bone structure[68]

Importantly, these growth factors don't work in isolation. Instead, they create a synergistic network, amplifying and sustaining one another's effects through feedback loops. For example, VEGF not only promotes blood vessel growth but also supports the delivery of other growth factors to the injury site. Similarly, bFGF can stimulate the production of VEGF, enhancing angiogenesis and tissue repair. This interconnected system ensures that PBM's effects are more potent and long-lasting than the action of any single growth factor alone.

PBM orchestrates growth factor release in a carefully timed sequence. The process begins within minutes to hours of light exposure, as early-response genes are activated and ROS initiate signaling pathways. Over the next hours to days, secondary waves of growth factors are released, amplifying the initial response. Finally, long-term effects such as tissue remodeling and structural reinforcement unfold over days to weeks. This precise timing ensures that each phase of tissue repair is supported optimally.

PBM Triggers Important Growth Factors

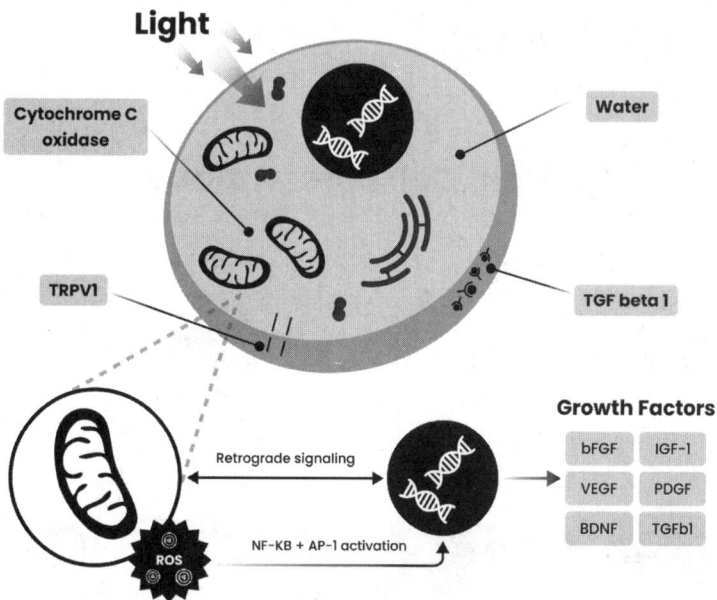

PBM's ability to stimulate multiple growth factors—including tissue-specific growth factors in many different types of tissues in the body—helps explain why it is effective for so many conditions—from wound healing and nerve regeneration to muscle recovery and brain function. Rather than targeting a single mechanism, PBM enhances the body's natural ability to repair itself through many layers of mechanisms involved in mediating cellular protection and regeneration.

One of the most fascinating aspects of PBM therapy is its ability to mobilize and activate the body's own repair system through stimulating stem cells. These remarkable cells, often called the body's "master cells," can transform into the specific types of cells needed to repair damaged tissues—whether that's new skin cells for wound healing, muscle cells for injury recovery, or blood cells to support immune function. They likely serve as a critical (and often overlooked) pathway of how red and NIR light deliver lasting therapeutic benefits.

Stem cells reside in protected microenvironments, or "niches," within tissues such as bone marrow, fat, skin, muscles, and even the brain. These niches are typically low-oxygen (hypoxic) environments to protect stem cells from oxidative stress and DNA damage, ensuring their long-term regenerative potential. This hypoxic state keeps the cells relatively quiescent, relying on glycolysis—a less efficient form of energy production that doesn't require oxygen—to meet their minimal energy needs. PBM disrupts this equilibrium in a controlled and beneficial way, driving stem cells out of their niches and into action.[69–73]

Stem Cell Differentiation

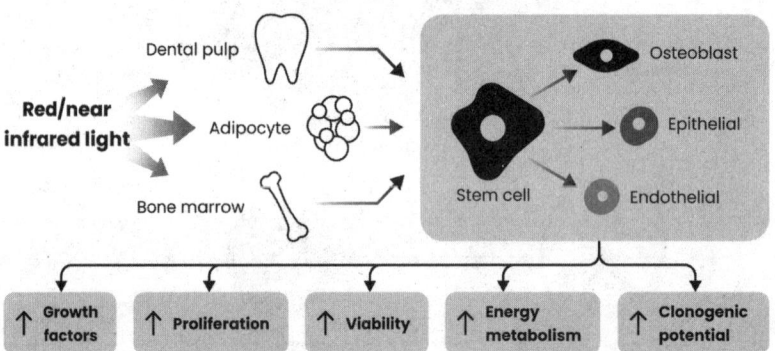

PBM doesn't just mobilize stem cells; it also enhances their regenerative potential by influencing gene expression. Research shows that light exposure can upregulate genes involved in cell survival and proliferation while promoting differentiation-specific programs depending on the cellular context. Studies have demonstrated increased expression of stem cell markers, proliferation-related genes, and lineage-specific differentiation factors following PBM treatment, suggesting that the therapy primes stem cells for more effective tissue repair.[74]

PBM also influences the stem cell microenvironment or "niche" in important ways. The therapy stimulates the production of various growth factors and signaling molecules that help guide stem cell behavior. For example, light exposure can increase the production of factors like bFGF and VEGF, which help create an environment conducive to tissue repair. These factors act like molecular beacons, helping direct stem cells to where they're needed and supporting their survival and function once they arrive.

Activated stem cells contribute to healing and regeneration through two primary mechanisms:

- **DIRECT REPAIR:** Stem cells differentiate into the specific cell types required for tissue repair, replacing damaged or lost cells. For example, they might become keratinocytes in skin, neurons in the brain, or myocytes in muscle.
- **SECRETOME PRODUCTION:** Perhaps even more importantly, stem cells release a "secretome"—a cocktail of bioactive molecules that includes growth factors, anti-inflammatory mediators, and extracellular matrix proteins. This secretome creates a regenerative environment, reducing inflammation, promoting tissue remodeling, and enhancing healing.

By activating stem cells, PBM stimulates genuine tissue regeneration, as opposed to simply masking symptoms or providing short-term relief of pain like a painkiller drug. If you do PBM on your injured knee joint, for example, you're not just reducing inflammation and getting pain relief—you're stimulating growth factors and stem cells in the area to help repair the damage. This regenerative process helps restore tissue structure and function, delivering durable improvements for conditions involving degeneration, chronic inflammation, or injury. It's not just symptomatic relief—it promotes actual cellular healing.

SYSTEMIC VS. LOCAL EFFECTS: HOW LIGHT INFLUENCES CELLS IT NEVER TOUCHES

The traditional understanding of PBM was straightforward: You would shine light on a particular area of the body and the light would directly interact with those cells to stimulate healing or the desired effect. For example, shining light on a wound or injured tendon so that those specific cells receiving the light were stimulated to repair. This direct, localized effect made intuitive sense and certainly produces measurable benefits.

However, clinicians began observing

something unexpected. Patients were reporting improvements in areas of their bodies that were nowhere near the treatment site. For example, when treating lower-back pain, patients might report that their chronic shoulder pain went away. When treating an arthritic joint on one side of the body, the corresponding joint on the opposite side sometimes showed improvement as well.

These observations have led scientists to recognize that PBM operates through two distinct mechanisms:

- **LOCAL EFFECTS:** Direct healing at the treatment site where light photons are actually absorbed by cellular components (particularly mitochondria), triggering immediate biochemical changes in those specific cells.

- **SYSTEMIC EFFECTS:** Healing benefits that appear in distant tissues through secondary signaling mechanisms, with no direct light exposure. These effects occur when illuminated cells release signaling molecules that travel through the bloodstream or neural pathways to influence distant tissues and organs.

While the emphasis has historically been on the direct effects of light on the cells it interacts with, it may turn out that the systemic effects are (at least in some cases) even more important. This systemic signaling represents a paradigm shift in our understanding of how PBM works.

THE EVIDENCE FOR SYSTEMIC EFFECTS OF PBM

Sometimes this idea arouses skepticism. It's one thing to grasp the idea that light can affect cells, but the idea that light could affect cells it never even interacts with often arouses skepticism. In fact, it's not as strange an idea as it might seem. You're already familiar with many other examples of how light delivered on one area of the body can affect the entire system. Vitamin D from ultraviolet light is of course a simple, well-accepted example of this, as is nitric oxide from ultraviolet light, and as is even blue-light photons triggering systemic effects via the circadian pathways of the brain. So it is far from novel that light can affect the entire system of the body. It's happening inside of us every day without us realizing it.

As far as red and NIR light, researchers have conducted experiments with animals that clearly demonstrate these whole-body effects:

- An Australian research group studying Parkinson's disease applied light to the lower back and hind legs of mice while covering their heads with aluminum foil.[75] Remarkably, they found that the beneficial effects were comparable to when light was directed at the head. They extended this research to nonhuman primates, demonstrating that light applied to the abdomen or legs of monkeys with Parkinson's disease provided neuroprotective benefits.[76]

- Researchers at UNINOVE in São Paulo, Brazil, pioneered what they call "transcutaneous tail vein photobiomodulation" in rodents.[77] They have shown that this approach is beneficial in animal models of muscle injury,[78] spinal cord injury,[79] and peripheral nerve injury.[80]

- Scientists investigating the "photobiomodulation of the gut microbiome" have applied light to the abdomens of mice and rats, altering their gut-microflora composition.[81] This intervention affects the gut-brain axis, improving cognitive function and showing promise for treating Alzheimer's disease.[82]

These systemic effects extend beyond laboratory animals, with several key human studies providing convincing evidence:

- One of the earliest reports described a triple-blind clinical trial examining PBM for healing superficial wounds in volunteers.[83] Two wounds were created (one on each arm), with one wound receiving either a single treatment with an 820-nm laser or a sham laser, while the other wound remained untreated. Not only did the PBM-treated wounds heal faster than the sham-treated wounds, but remarkably, the untreated wounds opposite the real laser-treated wounds also healed faster than the control wounds.

- Phil Gabel, a physical therapist in Australia, conducted a study on patients with chronic lower-back pain and concurrent depression.[84] Patients received either therapeutic exercise alone or exercise plus PBM directed at the lower back using a combined 660-/850-nm laser. While both groups saw significant improvements in back pain, only those receiving PBM showed improvement in depression symptoms, suggesting benefits beyond simple pain relief.

- The same Australian group studying Parkinson's disease extended their research to human patients.[85] Seven Parkinson's disease patients received PBM treatments to the abdomen and neck three times weekly for 12 weeks in a clinical setting, followed by 33 weeks of at-home treatment. Participants demonstrated measurable improvements in balance, cognition, fine motor skills, and olfactory function.

Now let's examine some of the mechanisms (at least those currently known) that help explain how red and NIR light can induce systemic effects.

Mechanisms of Light-Mediated Systemic Effects

For PBM to produce systemic effects, light absorption must generate substances or signals that travel from the area of the body the light interacted with to other areas of the body, and that stick around long enough (before being broken down) to travel from the treatment site to distant tissues.

- Dr. Hamblin described this in his 2018 textbook by saying:
- [T]here is considerable evidence of the systemic effects of PBM, which means that application to one site of the body can produce an improvement of a condition in another distant body part that did not receive light. Systemic effects can be explained by local effects of light that can be transferred to other sites through the circulating blood, via the lymphatic system, or via the nervous system.

Several possible mechanisms explain how this occurs:

Stem Cells as Mediators of Systemic Effects

We previously discussed stem cells in the context of local effects, where light activates and mobilizes stem cells in the treated tissue (e.g., using PBM on your knee joint to stimulate local stem cells). But the effects of PBM on stem cells actually go beyond the treatment site. There are two distinct effects of PBM on stem cells:

1. **LOCAL ACTIVATION:** When light penetrates tissues at the treatment site, it stimulates resident stem cells to proliferate and differentiate, accelerating local repair.

2. **SYSTEMIC MOBILIZATION:** Simultaneously, PBM triggers the release of stem cells from reservoirs like bone marrow into the bloodstream. These mobilized stem cells travel throughout the body, homing in on areas of injury or inflammation—even in tissues that never received direct light exposure.

The critical distinction here is that not only does light stimulate and mobilize stem cells in the areas of tissue that the light interacts with (e.g., stimulating stem cells in the muscle or joint or organ you're directing light on), but it also causes the release of stem cells into *circulation*.

For example, research by Uri Oron's team has demonstrated that shining light on skin overlying the tibia bone effectively mobilizes stem cells into circulation.[86] Once PBM mobilizes stem cells into circulation, they then travel through the bloodstream, detecting distress signals from damaged or degraded tissues anywhere in the body. They migrate to where they're needed most, whether that's damaged heart tissue, inflamed joints, or compromised neural tissue. Once they arrive, they adapt to the local environment and begin the work of repairing and regenerating the affected area. For example, a study by Oron et al. shined 10 mW/cm² of red light onto the exposed tibia bone (to reach the stem cell–rich marrow) of rats for 100 seconds at 20 minutes and 4 hours following a heart attack. He and his team found that the marrow released many stem cells into circulation, which responded to biological signals from the damaged heart and immediately started using their regenerative properties to reduce scarring and stimulate the growth of new arteries.[87] In other words, PBM stimulated stem cells in the *leg* to help repair the injured *heart*! Oron's research has confirmed the therapeutic power of this mechanism in multiple conditions: heart attack recovery,[88] Alzheimer's disease,[89] and kidney injury.[90]

This systemic effect allows PBM to enhance healing in untreated areas, making it much more than a localized treatment. It creates a body-wide increase in circulating stem cells, ready to support repair wherever they're needed. Importantly, this helps explain why so many people who start doing PBM on their body often notice "strange" and "coincidental" healing of other areas in their body that didn't even receive any light. This is crucial to understand: PBM's effects aren't limited to cells that directly interact with the light. Through stem cells circulating in the bloodstream, PBM can stimulate healing throughout the entire body.

I believe that we'll eventually come to understand stem cells in circulation as a key factor in mediating the benefits of PBM. For this reason, even when you have goals for a particular body part (e.g., facial skin anti-aging or treating an injured joint), I strongly encourage you to also leverage these powerful systemic effects. In the final section of the book on device selection, I'll talk about the specifics of how to maximize these systemic benefits of stem cells—how to boost the level of stem cells in your body to help repair damaged cells wherever they may be in your body.

Immune System Modulation

One of the most significant systemic effects of PBM is its ability to shift the inflammatory response by altering immune-cell function. Research by Dr. Hamblin has shown that PBM influences macrophage polarization, shifting the macrophages from an inflammatory (M1) state to a healing (M2) state.

This shift occurs through fascinating changes in cellular metabolism. Proinflammatory M1 macrophages primarily rely on glycolysis (a less efficient form of energy production) and have a dysfunctional Krebs cycle, which is replaced by an alternative metabolic pathway. These metabolic patterns support their inflammatory activities, including the production of reactive oxygen species and nitric oxide. In contrast, anti-inflammatory M2 macrophages show increased mitochondrial respiration through oxidative phosphorylation, maintain an intact Krebs cycle, and have lower levels of glycolysis.

PBM appears to directly influence this metabolic balance by increasing oxidative phosphorylation in the mitochondria of M1 macrophages, essentially switching them toward the M2 phenotype. This metabolic shift triggers their transformation from pro-inflammatory to anti-inflammatory and pro-healing activity. Similar polarization states exist in neutrophils (N1 pro-inflammatory and N2 anti-inflammatory), though these have not been as extensively studied in relation to PBM.

This immune modulation represents a powerful mechanism by which localized light therapy can create systemic anti-inflammatory effects throughout the body, helping to explain how PBM in one area can reduce inflammation in distant tissues and organs.

Metabolic Effects

PBM appears to influence metabolic functions beyond the local treatment area, potentially contributing to some of its observed systemic benefits. Research suggests several ways PBM may affect metabolic processes throughout the body:

PBM may contribute to blood sugar regulation. Some research suggests it can improve glucose uptake in cells and reduce inflammatory factors associated with insulin resistance, which could help with metabolic efficiency in certain conditions.

There's evidence that light therapy may influence hormonal activity. Studies have observed effects on stress-hormone patterns, on circadian rhythm factors, and potentially on growth-hormone activity—which plays a role in tissue-repair processes.

PBM appears to affect oxidative balance within cells. It seems to stimulate the body's natural antioxidant responses, potentially helping cells better manage oxidative stress and maintain healthier function.

Light therapy may also modify inflammatory responses. Research indicates that PBM can influence the balance between pro-inflammatory and anti-inflammatory signaling, potentially supporting more efficient resolution of inflammatory processes.

These metabolic influences, while still being investigated, may help explain how PBM applied to one area might contribute to benefits observed in other parts of the body. More research is needed to fully understand these systemic metabolic effects, but the existing research will be discussed in depth in the next chapter.

Blood-Mediated Systemic Effects

One approach to triggering PBM's systemic effects involves exposing blood to therapeutic light. This can occur through various approaches, both direct and indirect. Some researchers have explored delivering light directly into the bloodstream using fiber-optic catheters inserted into veins, an approach known as intravascular laser irradiation of blood, which has been studied extensively in Russian medical literature.[91]

Because inserting needles into veins is considered invasive by many practitioners, gentler, non-invasive methods have been developed. These include shining light through intact skin onto superficial veins in the wrist, inside the nostrils, or under the tongue—areas where blood vessels run close to the surface.[92] Since red and NIR light penetrate through the skin effectively, this allows for easy blood exposure without needing invasive procedures. (In contrast to certain wavelengths of light like UV that don't penetrate the skin, where invasive medical methods may be needed to irradiate the blood.)

In recent years, whole-body LED light beds have become increasingly popular for general health-and-wellness treatments. These devices expose large portions of circulating blood to therapeutic light wavelengths as blood flows through vessels near the skin surface and likely maximize systemic benefits that are mediated via the skin and blood.

Several components in the blood may help carry light's healing effects throughout the body:

1. **MITOCHONDRIA:** As discussed, PBM powerfully modulates mitochondria. This includes mitochondria in cells in the bloodstream. While red blood cells lack mitochondria, each platelet contains five to eight mitochondria, and white blood cells contain even more.[93] Researchers recently discovered that human blood also contains cell-free circulating mitochondria not contained within cells.[94] These free mitochondria may be particularly important for systemic effects of light therapy, as they can absorb light directly in the bloodstream and potentially influence distant tissues.

2. **RED BLOOD CELLS AND IMMUNE CELLS:** When PBM is applied to any area of the body with significant blood flow, the blood itself is effectively treated. Blood is constantly circulating through the treated area, where it is being exposed to red and NIR wavelengths of light. As blood passes through the treated area, several key changes occur. First, red blood cells and platelets become more flexible and less likely to clump together, improving their ability to navigate through small capillaries and deliver oxygen to tissues, especially in people with circulation problems.[1] Though lacking mitochondria, red blood cells contain hemoglobin, which absorbs light readily. PBM can improve how red blood cells flow and function,

especially in people with circulation problems.[95] PBM also affects white blood cells, particularly their inflammatory signaling patterns. One of the most significant changes is in how it shifts immune function from a pro-inflammatory phenotype toward an anti-inflammatory phenotype.[2-3] As treated blood circulates throughout the body, it carries these modified immune cells and their signaling molecules to every tissue.

3. **GROWTH FACTORS:** TGF-β is a protein that promotes cell growth and healing. Light therapy can activate the dormant form of TGF-β by producing mild oxidative signals.[96] Once activated, this protein can travel through the bloodstream to help healing throughout the body.[97, 98]

4. **STEM CELLS:** As described previously.

5. **MELATONIN:** As discussed previously, red and NIR light stimulates melatonin secretion (in addition to stimulating it at the intracellular level). This molecule evolved as a protective antioxidant billions of years ago, long before its role in sleep cycles. Light-induced melatonin has widespread effects, reducing inflammation, activating protective genes, and even influencing gut bacteria composition, creating another potential pathway for whole-body benefits.

6. **NO:** NO is important for many healing responses triggered by light therapy.

However, its brief lifespan in the bloodstream raises questions about whether it can travel far enough from the treatment site to create widespread effects.

The Nervous System Pathway

The circulatory system may not be the only route through which PBM's beneficial effects spread throughout the body. The nervous system likely plays a significant role in some circumstances, particularly through effects on autonomic nervous system regulation.

Research suggests that PBM can influence heart rate variability, a key biomarker of autonomic function. Several clinical studies have shown that transcranial PBM applications can increase heart rate variability and enhance parasympathetic activity, promoting a relaxation response and improved stress resilience. This autonomic modulation is further supported by a 2022 study examining full-body PBM therapy in NCAA "Power 5" conference female soccer players.[99] Using OURA rings to monitor players throughout a competitive season, researchers found significant autonomic nervous system effects following PBM sessions: Average heart rate was lower the night after treatment, while heart rate variability showed trending increases. Remarkably, these improvements occurred despite athletes averaging 40 minutes less sleep following PBM sessions. This suggests that full-body PBM therapy may enhance recovery through autonomic modulation, potentially reducing the body's need for sleep-based restoration.

Some people believe that light can be used similarly to traditional acupuncture, which has long been recognized for its systemic effects through nervous system modulation. Indeed, focused laser beams have been used to perform "laser acupuncture" by targeting established acupuncture points. Similarly, when treating painful conditions in the limbs, many experienced practitioners apply light not only to the painful area but also to the spine (particularly the dorsal root ganglia), neck, and head. This approach recognizes the interconnected nature of the nervous system and leverages neural pathways to enhance therapeutic outcomes. Studies from China have provided additional evidence for PBM's effects on the autonomic nervous system through acupoint stimulation. Research has demonstrated that laser therapy applied to specific acupuncture points can significantly modulate autonomic function. For example, laser treatment on the Neiguan (PC6) acupoint, located on the inner forearm, has been shown to decrease sympathetic nervous system tone, helping shift the body toward a more parasympathetic-dominant state.[99] These findings align with traditional Chinese medicine principles while providing a modern neurophysiological explanation for how targeted light therapy can create systemic effects through neural pathways.

Another study, of whole-body PBM and anaerobic cycling, found that while PBM didn't improve immediate performance, athletes were able to sustain significantly higher heart rates during exercise and showed improved heart rate variability the following morning compared to placebo conditions.[100] This combination of higher exercise intensity followed by enhanced recovery markers suggests that PBM positively influences autonomic nervous system function during both exertion and recovery phases.

A study on sacral PBM for colonic dysmotility found that pure sacral laser treatment significantly increased parasympathetic nervous system activity while reducing sympathetic stress, as measured by heart rate variability.[99] In a case study, a patient with chronic constipation who couldn't have spontaneous bowel movements for 5 years regained this ability after eight treatment sessions, with measurable improvements in autonomic nervous system function. Another 2022 study found a similarly powerful effect of sacral PBM on the autonomic nervous system of people with problems defecating, and that it strongly increased parasympathetic tone (and reduced sympathetic tone) as shown by heart rate variability.

Numerous studies have shown improvements in athletic performance and recovery after exercise with pre-exercise PBM.[101] It's very possible that at least some of this effect is mediated via changes in the nervous system.

Some studies have also demonstrated

that PBM can influence the stress response by helping normalize hypothalamic-pituitary-adrenal axis function and affecting levels of stress hormones like cortisol.[102, 103] This neuroendocrine modulation provides another pathway through which localized light therapy could create systemic effects.

Skin-Mediated Effects

Beyond its role as a simple barrier, the skin functions as a sophisticated neuroendocrine organ—what some researchers have called "a brain on the outside."[104] The complex physiology and biochemistry of skin plays a crucial role in PBM's systemic effects.

The skin contains its own autonomous self-regulating neuroendocrine system composed of hormonal and neuropeptide networks with corresponding receptors.[104] These are produced and expressed by various skin cells including keratinocytes, melanocytes, Langerhans cells, and Merkel cells. This complex network allows the skin to detect, integrate, and respond to diverse environmental signals, including light.

When PBM is applied to the skin, it can trigger these neuroendocrine pathways, creating responses that extend far beyond the treatment area. Light exposure can stimulate the production of various neurotransmitters, neuropeptides, and hormones that travel through the bloodstream or neural pathways to affect distant tissues. The skin is also tightly networked to central stress axes, contributing to the maintenance of whole-body homeostasis.

In conversation, PBM researcher Dr. Cronshaw put particular emphasis on the importance of the complex physiology and biochemistry of skin in mediating the benefits of PBM:

Far from skin being just a protective outer covering, it is now considered to be like the outer part of the brain. There is a complex two-way traffic between our skin and the sensors of the peripheral nerves to the spine and the brain. There are light-sensitive receptors in skin, and aside from being the site for the manufacture of vitamin D on exposure to UV light, other wavelengths in the blue-to-NIR stimulate the production of a wide range of important neurotransmitters, steroids, and hormones. These include serotonin (the so-called "happiness" neurochemical) as well as noradrenaline (the "Get up and go, go" drug) and dopamine (the "reward/compulsion" drug). These light-generated agents are powerful mediators of our mood as well as having systemic effects on our physiology. Although the skin does not have "eyes," it has lots of light-receptive sensors the full effects of which are still undergoing research investigation.

It's likely we'll see much more research elucidating the skin's role in mediating the effects of PBM in the coming years.

As you can gather, PBM can alter many pathways that mediate whole-body effects, which act on cells that the light photons never directly reach. So now we extend our understanding of how light interacts with our biology from the microlevel of the initial molecular mechanisms, up to the cascades of events triggered inside those cells, to then ultimately altering the whole body.

THE CASCADING EFFECTS OF PHOTOBIOMODULATION: A MULTI-LEVEL PERSPECTIVE

The beauty of PBM lies in how a simple interaction between light and cells creates layers of beneficial effects that build upon one another. At the cellular level, we've seen how light therapy triggers the mitochondria to produce more energy, activates signaling pathways, and creates that beneficial mild oxidative stress we discussed earlier. These effects combine to enhance all aspects of cellular function—from energy production to DNA repair to protein synthesis. As we have explored, this "cellular workout" strengthens the cell's natural protection systems while shifting activity away from inflammatory patterns toward healing.

At the tissue level, these cellular improvements create the effects we've discussed throughout—better blood flow through NO release, immune system shifting from M1 to M2 states, and the mobilization of stem cells from their bone marrow niches. We've seen how these mechanisms improve healing across many tissue types: Skin becomes healthier as collagen production increases (explaining the anti-aging effects); wounds close with less scarring; and damaged muscles, nerves, and other tissues recover more efficiently. These mechanisms create a web of interconnected effects that support and amplify one another.

At the whole-body level, these local changes combine to create systemic benefits. Chronic inflammation—the silent driver behind heart disease, diabetes, neurodegenerative conditions, and accelerated aging—decreases throughout the body. The endocrine system recalibrates, optimizing hormone production that governs everything from sleep quality and stress resilience to sexual function and energy levels. Metabolic health improves as cells become more efficient at processing nutrients and maintaining healthy blood sugar levels. Our cells develop enhanced resistance to oxidative damage and environmental stressors. And crucially, the sustained mobilization of stem cells into circulation creates an ongoing regenerative presence throughout the body. These cellular repair specialists continuously

The Cascading Effects of Photobiomodulation

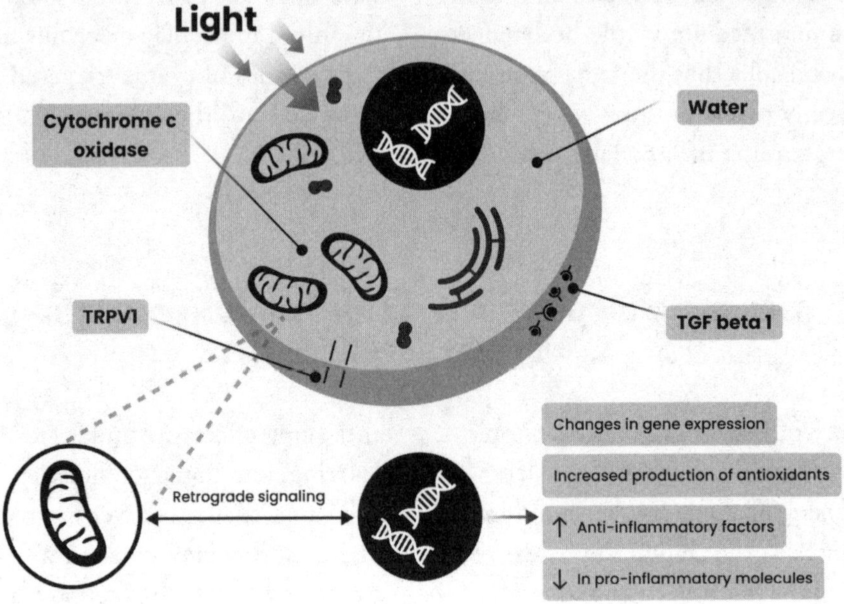

Light

Cytochrome c oxidase

Water

TRPV1

TGF beta 1

Retrograde signaling

Changes in gene expression

Increased production of antioxidants

↑ Anti-inflammatory factors

↓ In pro-inflammatory molecules

Tissue Response

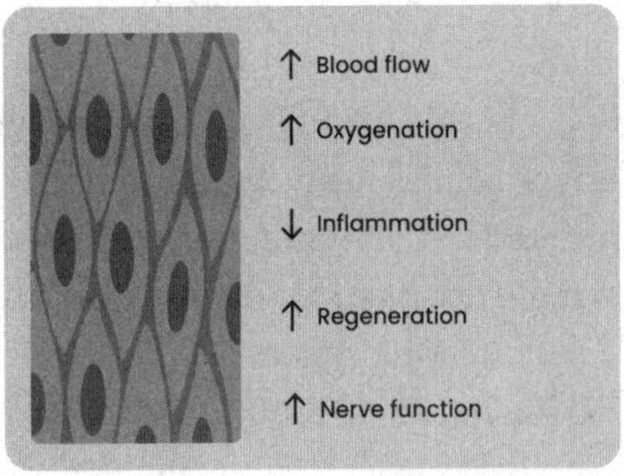

↑ Blood flow

↑ Oxygenation

↓ Inflammation

↑ Regeneration

↑ Nerve function

Systemic Response

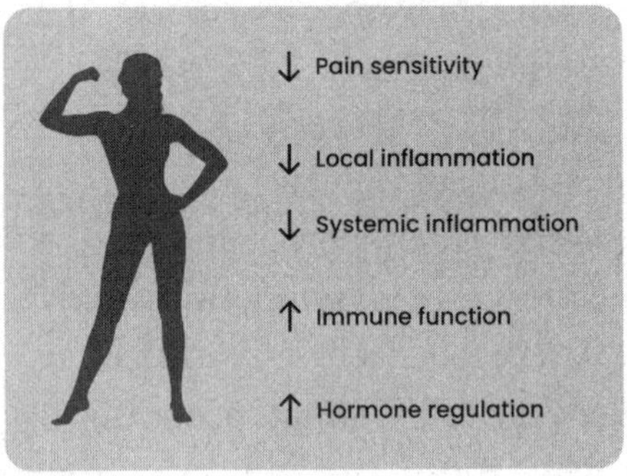

↓ Pain sensitivity

↓ Local inflammation

↓ Systemic inflammation

↑ Immune function

↑ Hormone regulation

Overview

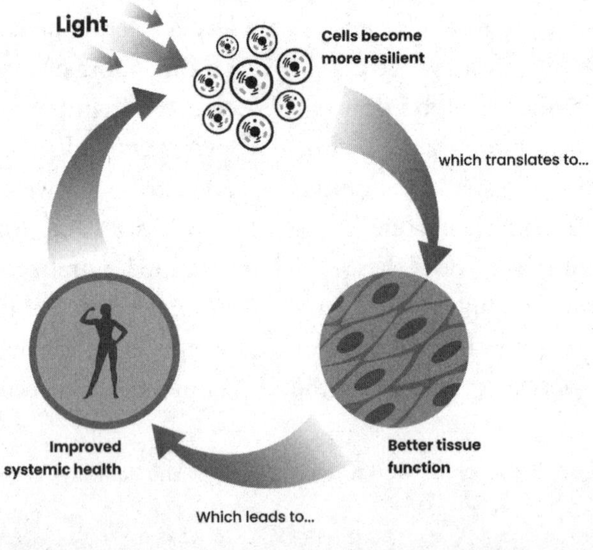

Light

Cells become more resilient

which translates to...

Improved systemic health

Better tissue function

Which leads to...

patrol for damaged tissues, worn-out cells, and areas needing renewal, providing a natural anti-aging and healing mechanism that operates 24/7.

Perhaps most remarkably, all of this complexity emerges from something beautifully simple: specific wavelengths of light interacting with our cells in ways that evolution has refined over millions of years. In an age where medical interventions often involve complex pharmaceuticals with lengthy lists of side effects, PBM offers a different path; one that provides the very wavelengths of light our bodies evolved to harness for healing and regeneration. By understanding and harnessing these natural photobiological processes, we gain access to a powerful tool for enhancing health, accelerating healing, and potentially slowing the aging process itself.

CHAPTER THREE

The Benefits of Red and Near-Infrared Light Therapy

An ever-growing body of research over the last decade has looked into how red and NIR light therapy (PBM) can improve health. Amazingly, this research has reported benefits in virtually every organ system in the body. It can help you to reduce signs of aging on your face, build muscle, lose fat, improve brain health, regrow hair, amplify the results you get from your workouts, reduce cellulite, hasten recovery after injury, improve joint health, reduce pain, increase energy levels, improve fertility, help heal traumatic brain injuries, improve sleep, improve the function of your immune system, reduce your blood sugar levels, speed wound healing, improve your overall metabolic health, and lower inflammation—and much more.

The scope of these benefits might seem extraordinary, but they're all grounded in solid scientific evidence. Let's dive into more than thirty documented ways red and NIR light can transform your health.

COMBAT SKIN AGING AND GET MORE YOUTHFUL SKIN

Because PBM stimulates both collagen and elastin production, combats fine lines and wrinkles, as well as the appearance of scars, surface varicose veins, acne, and cellulite, PBM is fast becoming recognized as a safe and welcome alternative to injections and surgery.

As we age, we produce less collagen, which results in the appearance of fine lines and wrinkles due to thin, dry skin. Red and NIR light penetrates deep into the dermis layer, stimulating cells that produce collagen; this new collagen moves to the surface of the skin, reducing the fine lines and wrinkles.

Collagen is important—not just for giving us youthful skin and helping us avoid that saggy look around the neck and jowls—but also to keep the *entire* body youthful, resilient, strong, and vital. In fact, collagen is the most abundant protein in the entire body. Even more important than the skin's appearance, collagen is also what gives our muscles, skin, blood vessels, bones, and digestive system the healthy tissue that they need to function properly.

In some medical schools in Europe, physicians put a lot of emphasis on keeping the extracellular matrix (the fibrous protein that surrounds and supports our cells) healthy, and dysfunction in the extracellular matrix is seen as a major contributor to disease. Why is this important? Because collagen is an integral part of the extracellular matrix, and red and NIR light are integral in supporting the collagen networks of our body.[1]

Repairing damage caused by UV radiation requires that skin be able to repair cellular and DNA damage, much as it does when healing from wounds. Red light does this extremely well through stimulating collagen synthesis and fibroblast formation, anti-inflammatory action, stimulation of energy production in mitochondria, and even stimulating DNA repair.[2]

According to a review of red and NIR light for skin rejuvenation, every primary cell type of the skin barrier (including immune-cell residents) responds to light in beneficial ways.[3]

A wealth of human studies has proven that red and NIR light can reverse the signs of aging, repair damage from UV rays, and reduce the appearance of fine lines, wrinkles, and even hard-to-remove scars.

A 2013 issue of *Seminars in Cutaneous Medicine and Surgery* featured a review of the research that highlighted dozens of studies proving that red and NIR light can reduce the signs of aging.[4]

Red Light and Collagen Production

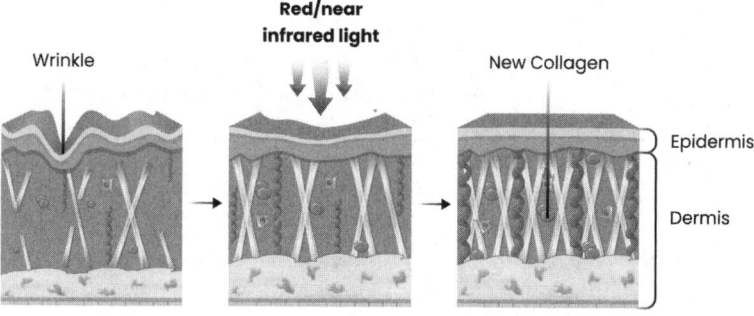

Another review of the research by Harvard professor Dr. Hamblin, reported that red and NIR light can:

- Reduce the signs of skin damage, DNA damage, and aging caused by UV rays[5]

- Reduce wrinkles[6]
- Reduce colored patches, hyperpigmentation, and skin discoloration[4]
- Enhance collagen synthesis and collagen density (Research has shown it can enhance production of collagen by 31 percent.)[7, 8]
- Accelerate repair in the epithelial layer of the skin[9]
- Combat other skin conditions like acne, keloids, vitiligo, burns, herpes virus sores, and psoriasis[5]
- Speed wound healing by enhancing skin-tissue repair and growth of skin cells[10]

A clinical review of phototherapy for psoriasis highlighted one study that used exclusively red and NIR light for the treatment of plaque psoriasis[11] and showed that two 20-minute sessions for 4 to 5 weeks resulted in 60- to 100-percent clearance rates without any significant side effects.[12]

In one study using an at-home facial mask delivering 445- and 630-nm wavelengths, young adults with mild-to-moderate acne saw significant improvements in their acne severity after daily 15-minute sessions for 8 weeks—24-percent reduction in inflammatory lesions, 20-percent reduction in noninflammatory lesions, and 19-percent improvement in overall acne scoring.[13] (Note: Blue light is effective for treating acne but may be overall pro-aging at the level of the skin. So if the goal is skin

CELL TYPE	EFFECTIVE WAVELENGTH(S)	EFFECT OF LIGHT EXPOSURE
Keratinocytes	590 nm 633 nm 830 nm	Strengthens adhesion, renews keratinocytes, and improves epidermis quality
Melanocytes	633 nm 830 nm	Normalizes pigment synthesis, reduces over-darkening, and potentially helps with repigmentation of depigmented areas
Fibroblasts	590 nm 633 nm 830 nm	Stimulates fibroblasts to produce high-quality collagen and elastin, and improves dermal extracellular matrix homeostasis and structure
Mast cells	830 nm 633 nm (lesser extent)	Accelerated wound-healing transitions, earlier and more efficient remodeling, and better alignment of new fibers
Macrophages	830 nm 633 nm (lesser extent)	Photoactivates macrophages, enhancing target identification, chemotaxis, debris clearance, and efficiency. Increases FGF release significantly, creating a more favorable extracellular matrix for fibroblast activity during the proliferative stage
Neutrophils	830 nm	Recruits neutrophils to normal skin, even without pathogens present. These neutrophils release trophic factors that support wound healing and enhance extracellular matrix function.

anti-aging, I'd advise use of a pure red or red and NIR device.)

In a clinical trial of a home-use LED device for facial rejuvenation in middle-aged adults with signs of photo-aging, a facial mask providing 637- and 854-nm wavelengths with total irradiance of 25 mW/cm² (a measure of the light intensity we'll discuss in detail in later sections of the book) for 9 minutes (13.5 J/cm²), was used twice per week for 8 weeks. The red and NIR light improved skin elasticity, hydration, and texture (roughness to smoothness).[14]

In another clinical trial, women with mild-to-severe neck wrinkles used an at-home LED collar to deliver 630- and 850-nm wavelengths at 25 mW/cm² for 9 minutes (13.5 J/cm²) per day, daily for 16 weeks. The red and NIR light improved neck wrinkling, skin hydration, and skin elasticity without affecting thyroid function.[15]

When applied directly to the under-eye region, use of an LED device emitting 633- and 830-nm wavelengths daily for 6 weeks improved under-eye wrinkles, texture, dark circles, bags, pigmentation, and erythema.[16] All the participants reported a high degree of comfort, ease of use, and satisfaction with the eye device.

In women with treatment-resistant melasma, microdermabrasion followed by 940-nm pulsed LED treatment with 90 mW/cm² for 5 minutes (13.5 J/cm²) reduced pigmentation and melasma severity by 46 percent compared to microdermabrasion alone.[17]

While virtually all of this research is conducted in women, men benefit, too. Use of an LED face mask emitting 633-, 830-, and 1,072-nm wavelengths for 6 weeks has been shown to improve fine lines and wrinkles, skin texture, and youthful appearance specifically in men.[18]

Reverse Skin Aging and Get Youthful Skin

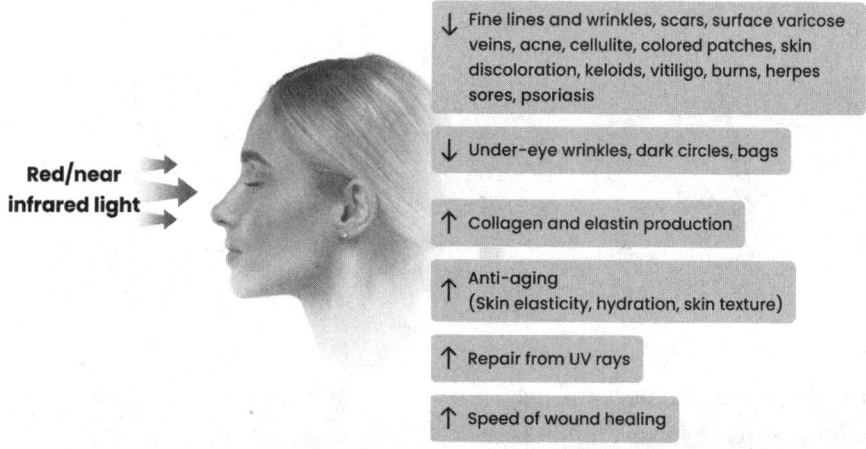

Red/near infrared light

↓ Fine lines and wrinkles, scars, surface varicose veins, acne, cellulite, colored patches, skin discoloration, keloids, vitiligo, burns, herpes sores, psoriasis

↓ Under-eye wrinkles, dark circles, bags

↑ Collagen and elastin production

↑ Anti-aging (Skin elasticity, hydration, skin texture)

↑ Repair from UV rays

↑ Speed of wound healing

In summary, red and NIR light have strong evidence to support their anti-wrinkle and pro-collagen effects—stronger, in fact, than a huge array of common skincare and supplement ingredients marketed for those purposes.

SLOW HAIR LOSS AND REGROW HAIR

Red and NIR light has been shown to help mitigate certain types of hair loss in both men and women. Three separate meta-analyses have reported that red and NIR light can slow hair loss and increase hair density in healthy adults and those with alopecia areata or androgenetic alopecia.[19–21] The benefits increased with longer daily treatment duration (from 10 to 30 minutes) and increased overall dose (from 1 to 6 J/cm²). In one clinical trial in men and women with androgenetic alopecia, use of a 660-nm LED providing 3.5 mW/cm² for 19 minutes (4 J/cm²) tripled hair density compared to a sham device and increased mean hair diameter by 60 percent.[22]

Many other studies have reported similar benefits. Red-light therapy (655 nm) used every second day for 16 weeks (45 mW/cm² for 25 minutes per session providing 67 J/cm²) increased hair growth by 37 percent compared to a sham treatment in women with androgenetic alopecia.[23] PBM has also been proven to regrow hair in men with hair loss in several studies.[24–27]

Hair Growth Cycle

Anagen
Active growth phase
(3-6 years)

Catagen
Transition phase
(1-2 weeks)

Telogen
Resting phase
(5-6 weeks)

Return to Anagen

To go into detail of the mechanisms, hair growth takes place in several phases:

- Anagen—growth phase of the hair shaft within the follicle

- Catagen—transitional phase during which the hair follicle moves upward toward the skin pore
- Telogen—resting phase during which the dermal papillae fully separate from the hair follicle
- Exogen—final stage of the hair growth cycle, when hair strands are shed from the hair follicles
- After 5 to 6 weeks, the dermal papillae move to meet the hair follicles again and the hair matrix starts forming more hair—that is, returns to the anagen phase.
- Red and NIR light have been shown to help transition hair from the telogen phase back to the anagen phase and prolong the anagen/ growth phase. It can also increase the rate of growth in the anagen phase while preventing premature catagen phases.
- These effects may be mediated by increases in certain growth factors, by changes in inflammation, or by improved mitochondrial function in the cells in that area or in NO levels and blood circulation to the follicle, or by some combination of all these factors.
- In short, it helps hair follicles remain in the growth phase, grow more, and re-enter the growth phase more rapidly (instead of dying off). The end result is less hair loss and more hair growth.

Slow Hair Loss and Regrow Hair

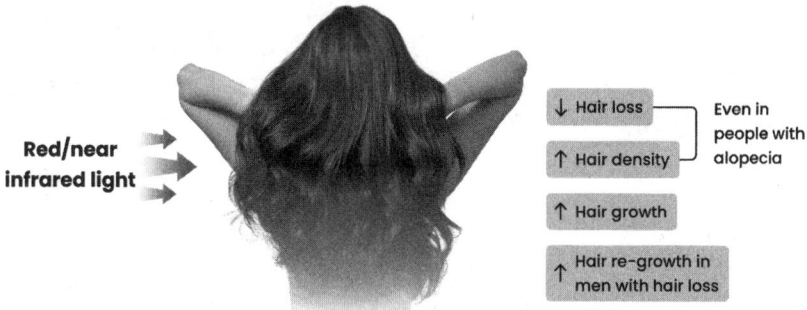

Red/near infrared light

↓ Hair loss
↑ Hair density — Even in people with alopecia
↑ Hair growth
↑ Hair re-growth in men with hair loss

REDUCE CELLULITE

Cellulite is a problem caused by a combination of unhealthy collagen and elastin in the skin layers, combined with excess fat accumulation in the fat cells in that area.

The health of the extracellular matrix likely also plays a role.

Red and NIR light actually combat cellulite in three ways:

1. Bolstering production of collagen and elastin (and supporting the health of the extracellular matrix—the fibrous support structure around the cells)
2. Supporting blood circulation and blood vessel health in the area
3. Causing fat cells to release their fat contents into the blood where they may be burned off

In one study of middle-aged women, combining 650-nm red light and 915-nm NIR light with massage (100 mW/cm² for 15 minutes, providing 90 J/cm²) produced **an astounding 71 percent reduction in cellulite!**[28] Another study using the same wavelengths of red and NIR light found that the treatment reduced cellulite in four of every five women after 4 to 6 weeks.[29]

Reduce Cellulite

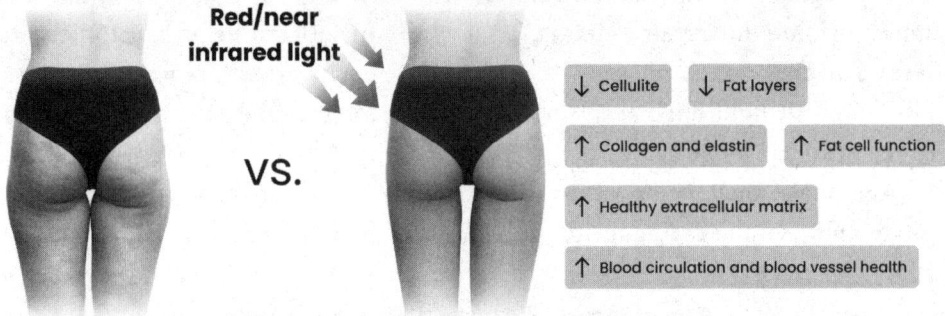

Red/near infrared light

VS.

↓ Cellulite   ↓ Fat layers

↑ Collagen and elastin   ↑ Fat cell function

↑ Healthy extracellular matrix

↑ Blood circulation and blood vessel health

In fact, this is one of the only scientifically proven ways to reduce cellulite, and maybe the most powerful. (Note: Most creams and other products sold to reduce cellulite have little to no scientific evidence of effectiveness.)

SPEED WOUND HEALING

One of the original findings of the NASA research that put red light therapy on the map was its powerful effect on wound healing. In fact, red and NIR light have been found to help close wounds—even those resistant to healing—far faster and with less scarring.[30, 31]

In hospitalized patients with traumatic soft-tissue injuries associated with bone fractures, PBM not only cut the time required for wound healing by 44 percent compared to a sham treatment (13 vs. 23 days), but it also reduced the occurrence of infection from 57 to 15 percent and reduced the pain experienced by the patients.[32]

In elderly adults suffering from diabetic foot ulcers, use of an at-home 808-nm

NIR light device for 8 minutes every day (17 mW/cm² providing 9 J/cm²) achieved 97-percent wound closure after 12 weeks, compared to just 47 percent in the control group.[33] In fact, 70 percent of patients using NIR light therapy achieved greater than 90-percent wound closure, compared to just 10 percent of patients in the control group.

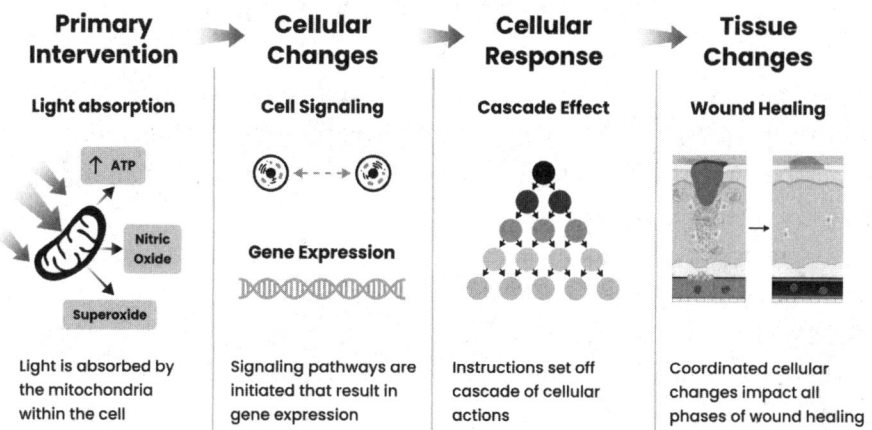

Primary Intervention	**Cellular Changes**	**Cellular Response**	**Tissue Changes**
Light absorption	Cell Signaling	Cascade Effect	Wound Healing
Light is absorbed by the mitochondria within the cell	Signaling pathways are initiated that result in gene expression	Instructions set off cascade of cellular actions	Coordinated cellular changes impact all phases of wound healing

Numerous studies have also found benefits from red and NIR light used in the mouth as part of the healing process for gingival and dental surgery, which we'll talk about later on.

PBM improves wound healing largely by increasing circulation and the formation of new capillaries, along with stimulating stem cells and progenitor cells. Increased circulation and the formation of new capillaries means that the wounded tissue receives more oxygen and nutrients that it needs to initiate and maintain the healing process. PBM accomplishes this in several ways:

- Cleaning up dead and damaged skin cells (phagocytosis)

- Increasing ATP in skin cells, giving them more energy to heal themselves
- Increasing the production of fibroblasts[34]
- Increasing blood flow, supplying the wound with more oxygen and nutrients needed for repair
- Stimulating stem cells and progenitor cells
- Reducing chronic inflammation, which inhibits wound healing
- Stimulating the production of collagen and the health of the extracellular matrix
- Stimulating lymph activity
- Stimulating the formation of new connective tissue and capillaries on the surface of the wound[10, 30, 35–38]

It's also worth noting that PBM not only hastens the healing process but also can simultaneously reduce symptoms like pain and swelling, which can make life a lot more tolerable.[39]

COMBAT FIBROMYALGIA AND CHRONIC FATIGUE, AND INCREASE ENERGY LEVELS

Studies show that red and NIR light therapy is effective at restoring energy and vitality in persons suffering from fibromyalgia. Because this light is so effective at reducing inflammation, it is proving effective at treating fibromyalgia, which is partly caused by inflammation in the brain stem/hypothalamus region.[40, 41] This same effect would likely also benefit chronic fatigue syndrome and long COVID (which share many symptoms with fibromyalgia), although this has not yet been verified.

Multiple studies have found that PBM offers profound benefits for those suffering from fibromyalgia, including:

- Enhanced quality of life
- Decreased pain
- Decreased muscle spasms
- Decreased morning stiffness
- Decreased total number of tender points

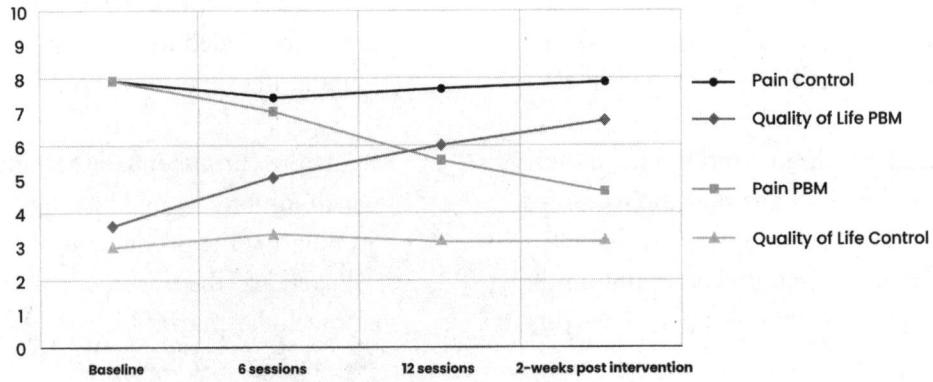

Changes in Pain and Quality of Life in Fibromyalgia Patients Using a 10-Point Scale

Research suggests that the light-therapy method is a safe and effective treatment for fibromyalgia.[40, 42–43] Two studies published in 2022 and 2023 have found that whole-body treatment with 650-nm red light and 850-nm NIR light (28 mW/cm² for 20 minutes providing 25 J/cm²) cut pain in half, doubled the quality of life, and nearly tripled leisure physical activity compared to a control group.[44, 45]

Once you understand the pathways by which PBM works its magic on the human body, it makes sense that it would benefit chronic fatigue conditions and increase energy levels. Much research over the last 5 years suggests that **mitochondrial dysfunction, impaired brain function, and inflammation are at the core of chronic fatigue.**[46–50]

As explained throughout this book, hundreds of studies now show that **PBM has huge benefits on mitochondrial and brain function, and that it powerfully decreases inflammation.** So even though only a few studies have directly tested this application, based on a simple understanding of the mechanisms at play and the science that is already known, it is perfectly reasonable to suppose that PBM has the potential for helping people struggling with chronic fatigue.

I've used PBM with clients for over 10 years now, and I've seen over and over again that red and NIR light therapy is very often one of the biggest factors in their recovery from chronic fatigue.

Combat Fibromyalgia and Chronic Fatigue and Increase Energy Levels

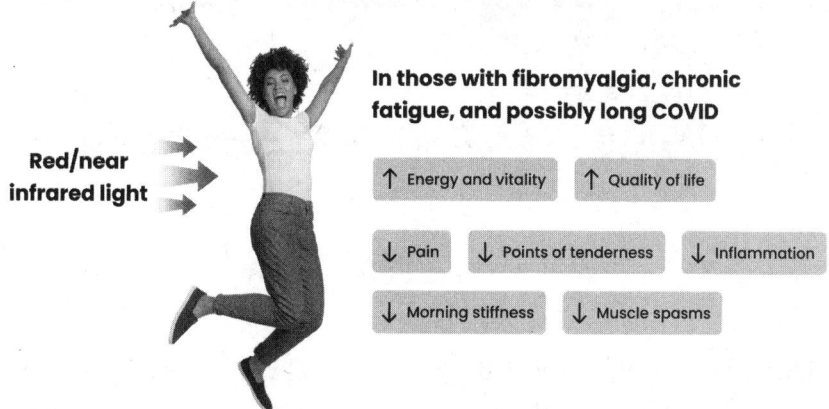

Red/near infrared light

In those with fibromyalgia, chronic fatigue, and possibly long COVID

↑ Energy and vitality   ↑ Quality of life

↓ Pain   ↓ Points of tenderness   ↓ Inflammation

↓ Morning stiffness   ↓ Muscle spasms

FIGHT HASHIMOTO'S HYPOTHYROIDISM

Several studies have shown profound benefits of PBM for autoimmune hypothyroidism. It is one of very few treatments shown to potentially reverse (or at least greatly slow the progression of) autoimmune hypothyroidism.

Essentially, Hashimoto's thyroiditis is defined by immune infiltration of the thyroid gland as an autoimmune attack against thyroglobulin, which leads to the production of thyroid peroxidase auto-antibodies (TPO) that damage thyroid cells. Several studies have now shown that PBM applied to the thyroid gland is able to reduce levels of inflammatory cytokines and free radicals while simultaneously increasing antioxidant molecules and growth factors that help regenerate injured tissue—all leading to improved thyroid function.[51]

The most recent clinical trial gave a group of women with Hashimoto's disease a supplement containing vitamin D and selenium.[52] A subgroup additionally received treatment with an 820-nm laser (1,600 mW/cm² for 20 seconds providing 32 J/cm² to each of eight spots on the thyroid gland) twice per week for 3 weeks. Those using NIR light therapy had reduced TSH levels by 65 percent and increased free T4 and T3 levels by 38 percent 6 months after the treatment ended. Moreover, TPO antibodies had dropped by an astounding 85 percent. This clearly demonstrates an enduring effect of NIR light therapy.

Fight Hashimoto's Hypothyroidism

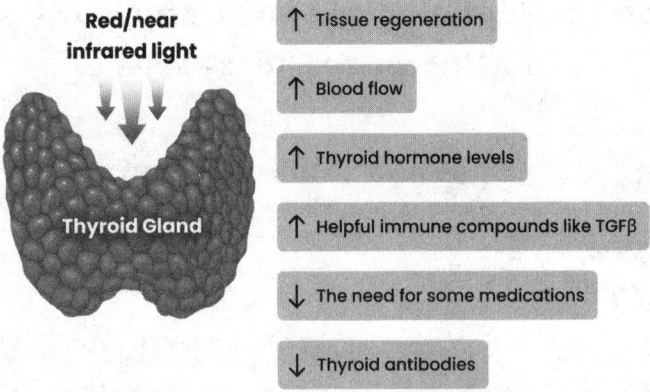

Red/near infrared light

Thyroid Gland

↑ Tissue regeneration

↑ Blood flow

↑ Thyroid hormone levels

↑ Helpful immune compounds like TGFβ

↓ The need for some medications

↓ Thyroid antibodies

Another clinical trial in 2020 reported that 850-nm NIR light therapy twice per day for 3 days (1,430 mW/cm² for 20 seconds providing 28.6 J/cm² to each of eight points on the thyroid gland) increased T3 by 50 percent compared to control and reduced thyroid antibodies by 70 percent, all despite cutting the thyroid medication dose in half.

A 2013 randomized, placebo-controlled study in hypothyroid patients demonstrated that in people who received NIR light therapy, thyroid function dramatically improved and, remarkably, that thyroid antibody (TPOAb) levels were greatly reduced.[53] **Amazingly, 47 percent of patients were able to stop medication completely!** Moreover, the researchers followed up 9 months after treatment and found that the effects were still evident. They even published a 6-year follow-up, which reported that even at 6 years, some of the benefits still remained, but that continuing periodic sessions were recommended to maintain all benefits.[54]

A 2010 study found that red light therapy helped 38 percent of study participants reduce their hypothyroid medication dose, with **a whopping 17 percent being able to stop taking the medication altogether.**[55]

A 1997 study done in Russia included some data on people with autoimmune hypothyroidism who underwent thyroid surgery. They found that red and NIR light therapy improved thyroid hormone levels enough that the patients required, on average, half as much thyroid hormone medication afterward.[56]

A 2003 study done in Ukraine showed that red light therapy could decrease thyroid medication needs by 50 to 75 percent in people with postsurgical hypothyroidism.[57]

A 2010 Russian dissertation study applied red light therapy to the thyroid glands of a group of people with hypothyroidism and found that 17 percent of them could completely get off thyroid medication and 38 percent could decrease the dose by 25 to 50 µg.[58]

A 2014 study applied 10 sessions of light therapy to 347 people with subclinical hypothyroidism. At baseline, the average thyroid stimulating hormone (TSH) was 9.1 mIU/L. (Note: Higher TSH is a sign of hypothyroidism.) After 10 sessions of light therapy, the TSH was normalized in 337 (97 percent) of the patients. Their TSH averaged 2.2 mIU/L after just 10 PBM treatments.[59]

While more research is still needed, the existing research is very consistent that PBM has profound beneficial effects on thyroid function. It appears to improve thyroid hormone output, increase blood vessel formation (and thus blood flow) in the thyroid gland, and decrease the progression of the condition through beneficial changes in thyroid gland health and immune system modulation. The pronounced anti-inflammatory effects of PBM make it beneficial in any condition where the body's immune system attacks one of the body's own organs.

CANCER SUPPORTIVE CARE

Since red/NIR light tends to enhance energy production in whatever cells it's shined on, it was speculated many years ago that it might actually enhance cancer growth. However, more recent evidence has suggested that low-dose PBM (5 J/cm² twice daily) doesn't affect melanoma tumors,[60] whereas high doses (640+ J/cm²) may actually reduce melanoma proliferation and increase cell death.[61] Dr. Hamblin has spoken extensively about research showing that using the light on other areas of the body (not directly on the cancerous growth) may improve overall outcomes in some people with cancer.

For example, a 2004 phase 1 trial in patients with advanced neoplasia demonstrated that PBM was safe for clinical use and improved performance status and quality of life.[62] Anti-tumor activity was observed in 88.23 percent of patients and remained unchanged in a 10-year follow-up.

These early results from this 2004 trial, combined with a growing body of research, demonstrate that PBM could exert strong anti-tumor effects.[63–65] These indications are consistent with multiple experimental and clinical reports suggesting that PBM exerts anti-cancer and anti-tumor effects.[66–69]

Light therapy may also help decrease the side effects of chemotherapy and radiation therapy.

The TRANSDERMIS trial of breast cancer patients reported that NIR light treatment (808 and 905 nm at 168 mW/cm² for 7 to 10 minutes providing 4 J/cm²) twice weekly for 6 weeks prevented the development of severe acute skin reactions and dermatitis caused by conventional radiotherapy, and improved quality of life.[70, 71]

Using the same NIR treatment protocol, the DERMISHEAD trial of head and neck cancer patients reported that adverse events caused by radiation and chemotherapy were cut in half.[72] The LABRA trial of breast cancer patients found an 18 percent reduction in the incidence of severe radiation-induced dermatitis,[73] and the NEUROLASER trial of breast cancer patients reported a reduction in the severity of chemotherapy-induced peripheral neuropathy and improved quality of life.[74]

In another study, PBM in the mouth was used as an adjunct to conventional cancer therapy. The light attenuated chemotherapy-induced taste loss and prevented weight loss, while improving quality of life and reducing the incidence of cachexia, anorexia, diarrhea, oral mucositis, and vomiting.[75] Using both red and NIR light together was more effective than either wavelength alone.[76]

Lastly, a systematic review with meta-analysis of six studies including head and neck cancer patients reported that the use of PBM increased salivary flow and minimized radiation-induced hyposalivation.[76]

Interestingly, very recently, researchers have identified a type of molecule aptly called a "jackhammer," which responds to NIR light by vibrating within the membranes of cancer cells.[77] The result? Complete eradication of human melanoma cells after 12 J/cm² of 80 mW/cm² NIR light for 2.5 minutes. So there seems to be great potential to leverage red and NIR light (perhaps in combination with specific molecules, as is done in "photodynamic therapy") in cancer care.

WARNING: This information is for educational purposes only. Do not attempt to self-diagnose or self-treat cancer with red and NIR light therapy. If you have cancer or any medical condition, consult your doctor before trying any treatments.

INCREASE BONE HEALING

Studies on animals and humans have found that PBM greatly aids in healing bone lesions, including breaks, fractures, and defects.[78] ATP production is interrupted in broken bones, and cells begin to die from lack of energy. PBM has been shown to:

- Stimulate energy production in bone cells
- Increase bone-related growth factors
- Enhance blood-vessel formation and blood flow to the affected area
- Modulate inflammation
- Enhance the attachment and production of collagen and procollagen and stimulate stem and progenitor cells—all of which accelerate the bone-repair process[79, 80]
- Increase active range of motion and grip strength
- Improve rehabilitation
- Promote remineralization and bone remodeling

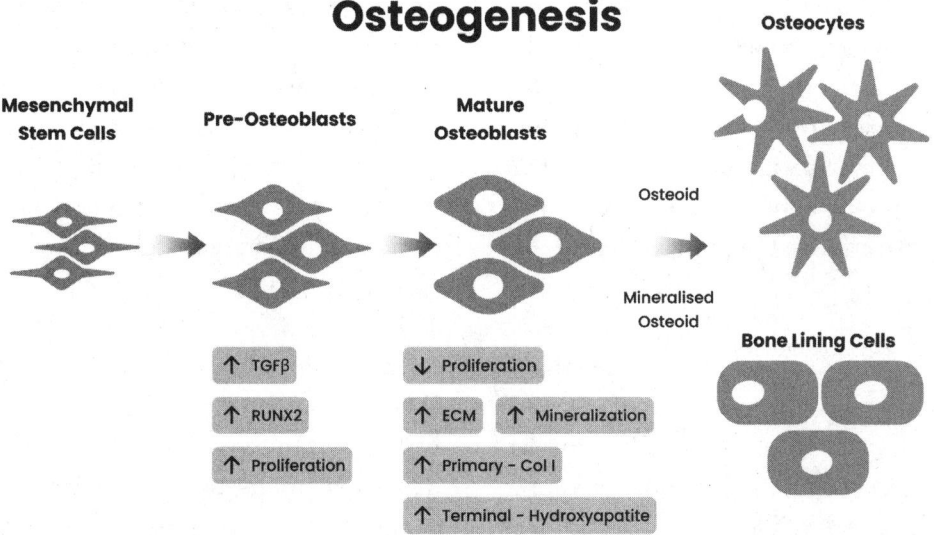

Osteogenesis

Overall, the bone irradiated with red/NIR wavelengths shows increased formation of new bone and collagen deposition.[81] PBM is becoming very popular in all sports where breaks, sprains, and fractures are frequent—from horse racing to football.

Increase Bone Healing

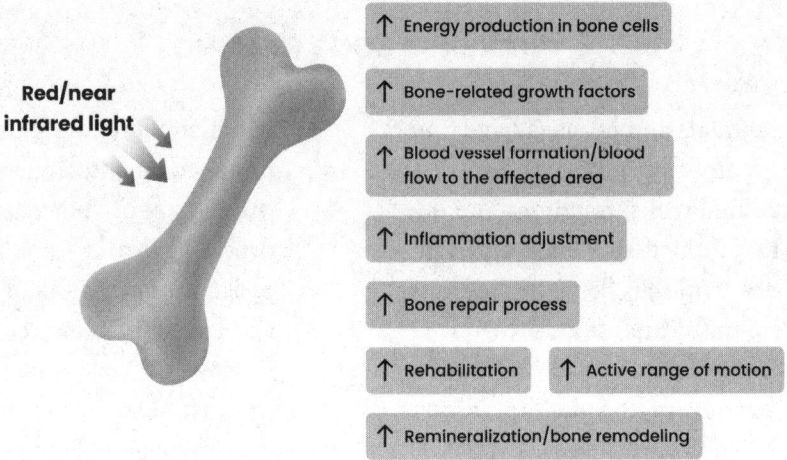

Red/near infrared light

↑ Energy production in bone cells

↑ Bone-related growth factors

↑ Blood vessel formation/blood flow to the affected area

↑ Inflammation adjustment

↑ Bone repair process

↑ Rehabilitation   ↑ Active range of motion

↑ Remineralization/bone remodeling

In a recent double-blind randomized controlled trial, using red and NIR light delivered through a cast opening of forearm fractures improved the active range of motion and grip strength while also reducing the loss in grip strength compared to the uninjured arm.[82] It also reduced the level of pain experienced during the night.

A follow-up triple-blind randomized controlled trial by the same authors reported that PBM used after cast removal improved rehabilitation after 8, 12, and 26 weeks of standard home-based exercise therapy while also reducing pain.[83]

These bone-healing effects play out in cases of bone disease, too. For example, people with osteoporosis or osteopenia could benefit from regular PBM application due to its ability to promote mineralization and bone remodeling.

IMPROVE EYE HEALTH

Research into the benefits of PBM for eye health is very promising. Studies on animals show that red light therapy can heal the damage to eyes caused by excessive bright light in the retina. This kind of damage is similar to the damage that occurs in age-related macular degeneration (AMD).[84]

One human study in patients with AMD showed that red light therapy improved vision, and that the improvements were maintained for 3 to 36 months after treatment. It also appeared to improve edema, bleeding, metamorphosia, scotoma, and dyschromatopsia in some patients.[85]

The LIGHTSITE I clinical trial of adults with dry age-related macular degeneration reported that 660-nm red light (65 mW/cm² for 180 seconds) and 850-nm NIR light treatment (8 mW/cm² for 70 seconds) to the eyes three times per week for one month improved visual acuity by 6 percent, as well as contrast sensitivity and quality of life.[86]

Another clinical trial involving adults with macular edema administered 670-nm red light to the eyes twice weekly for 5 weeks, providing either 25, 100, or 200 mW/cm² for 90 seconds.[87] Both higher doses were more effective than the lowest dose for reducing edema, although all doses reversed disease progression.

Note: The eyes are sensitive tissues, and as such, for any self-use of light therapy, I suggest shorter sessions at an increased distance away from the light. I would also suggest opting for lower irradiances like 25 to 75 mW/cm² to be more cautious, even though one study has shown benefits with even higher irradiances. And as always, for any medical conditions, consult your physician rather than attempting self-treatment.

COMBAT DEPRESSION AND ANXIETY

We know that bright light therapy and light boxes have shown great promise in treating seasonal affective disorder and depression. These approaches work when the light is absorbed through the eyes. What about red and NIR light applied to the head?

A recent systematic review of 16 human and animal studies, including four RCTs, concluded that PBM applied to the head could be "strongly recommended" for moderate-grade major depressive disorder and "recommended" for anxiety disorder.[88] NIR wavelength ranges from 800 to 830 nm, power density of 250 mW/cm², and energy density of 60 to 120 J/cm² were the most frequently used parameters. The light is most often applied to the forehead, because there is no hair present to interfere with light absorption.

Another, less recent review of studies on red and NIR light and depression/anxiety disorders concluded that these light therapies offer a promising treatment for major depressive disorder, suicidal ideation, anxiety, and traumatic brain injury.[89]

In the double-blind, sham-controlled ELATED-2 study of people with major depressive disorder, twice-weekly treatment with 823-nm NIR to the forehead

(36 mW/cm² for 30 minutes providing 65 J/cm²) reduced depression scores by 75 percent, compared to just 25 percent in the sham group (placebo effect).[90] Half of the PBM light group reported that their depression went into remission.

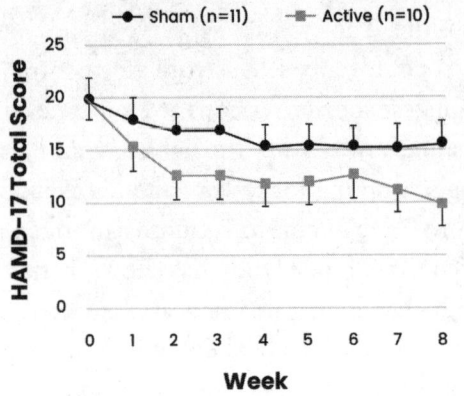

All participants (including those who did not complete the treatment intervention)

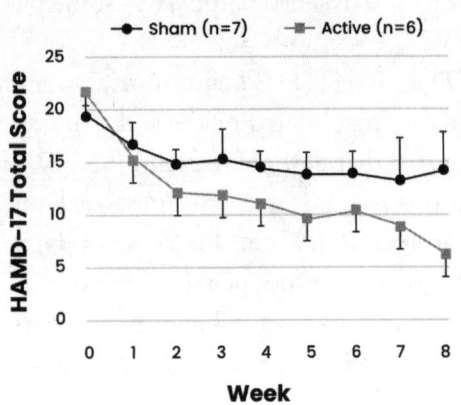

Only participants that completed the study as intended

It's also worth noting that a secondary analysis of the ELATED-2 trial found that both men and women who received PBM treatment improved sexual function by about 75 percent.[91] Libido and sexual arousal were also improved by 80 to 90 percent.

Several studies have found that people with depression have abnormal blood flow in the frontal cortex of the brain.[92] Since PBM improves blood flow and circulation to the brain, it is reasonable to believe that this could be part of the mechanism at play.[93]

A 2009 study **recruited 10 patients with a history of major depression and anxiety** (including PTSD and drug abuse) and administered 4 weeks of PBM treatments to the forehead. Remarkably, by the end of the four-week study, six out of 10 patients experienced a remission of their depression, and seven out of 10 patients experienced a remission of their anxiety.[94]

Another clinical trial included adults with moderate-to-severe anxiety and depression who were treated with 945-nm NIR light on the frontal sinus region (110 mW/cm² for 85 seconds providing 9.25 J/cm²) daily for one month.[95] They found that it reduced anxiety and depression by 30 percent compared to a placebo.

In adults with mild-to-moderate generalized anxiety disorder, treatment with 830-nm NIR light to the forehead (30 mW/cm² for 20 minutes providing 36 J/cm²) daily for 8 weeks reduced anxiety by 60 percent.[96]

Combat Depression and Anxiety

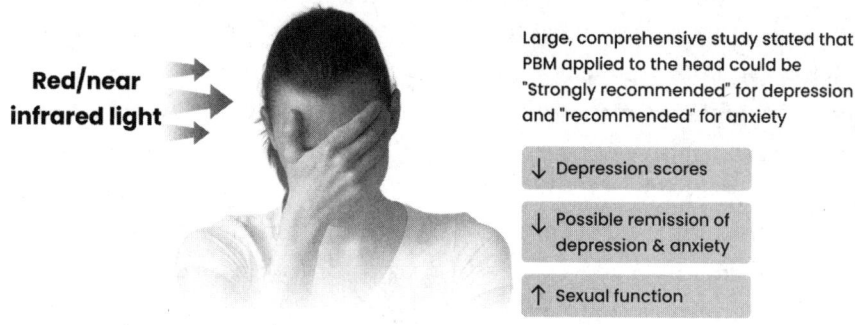

Red/near infrared light

Large, comprehensive study stated that PBM applied to the head could be "Strongly recommended" for depression and "recommended" for anxiety

↓ Depression scores

↓ Possible remission of depression & anxiety

↑ Sexual function

*Near Infrared may be superior to red light for mood disorders / brain injuries

PBM is clearly a powerful tool for combating depression and anxiety, with a growing number of human clinical trials supporting the overwhelmingly positive animal research in this field.[94, 97–104]

Note: When treating the brain, it is likely that NIR will be superior to red light, as it penetrates more deeply. Specifically, research has shown that NIR penetrates the skull better than red light does.[104] We'll discuss in detail later in which scenarios it's better to use red or NIR, but in general, for any brain-related issue, NIR is superior.

IMPROVE COGNITIVE PERFORMANCE

One aspect of human health that red and NIR light almost always improves is cognitive performance. It not only improves metabolic pathways but also enhances the function of the mitochondria in the brain. Since the brain is incredibly rich in mitochondria, this is where people most often notice the effects.

A 2023 systematic review of 35 studies involving humans reported that 29 (83 percent) found improvements in cognitive function after PBM treatments, including all nine studies on participants with subjective memory complaints, mild cognitive impairment, and dementia, as well as seven of eight studies on patients with traumatic brain injury.[105] One of the most common protocols for clinical populations employed devices delivering NIR light (810 nm), an irradiance of 20 to 25 mW/cm², and a fluence of 1 to 10 J/cm².

In studies, researchers have found that transcranial red and NIR light profoundly benefits the brain and cognitive performance.[106] Research has also shown that transcranial NIR light stimulation can increase neurocognitive function in young healthy adults,[107] improve sustained attention and short-term memory retrieval in young adults, and improve memory in older adults with significant memory impairment at risk for cognitive decline.[108]

Even after a single session of 810-nm NIR (20 mW/cm² for 350 seconds providing 7 J/cm²) across the forehead, older adults with mild cognitive impairment experienced a 25-percent increase in cognitive function within one hour following treatment.[109] Another study showed that a single session increased cerebral blood flow alongside improved cognitive function.[110]

A systematic review with meta-analysis of six studies involving healthy young adults reported that NIR light improved cognitive function with a large effect size.[111] Studies used either 1,064-nm lasers or 850-nm LEDs providing 250 to 285 mW/cm² for 2.5 to 8 minutes (60 to 120 J/cm²).

HELP RESOLVE TENDINITIS

One of the most common clinical indications for PBM is to treat injuries and tendinitis. Because red light stimulates collagen production, speeds wound healing, and is highly anti-inflammatory, it has been shown to bring great relief to people suffering from tendinopathy or tendinitis.[112, 113]

A systematic review of the research concluded that PBM has proven highly effective in treating tendon disorders in all 12 of the studies analyzed.[112]

Red Light and Tendon Health

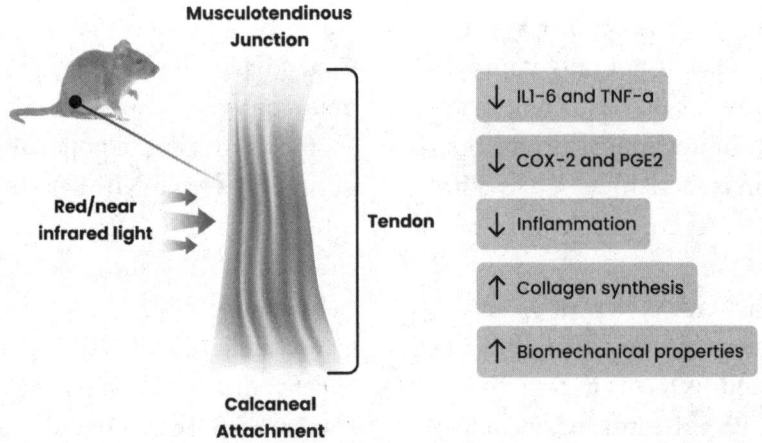

Musculotendinous Junction

Red/near infrared light

Tendon

Calcaneal Attachment

↓ IL1-6 and TNF-a

↓ COX-2 and PGE2

↓ Inflammation

↑ Collagen synthesis

↑ Biomechanical properties

In the first-ever randomized controlled trial of adults with Achilles' tendon rupture, red and NIR light treatment (combined 904-, 858-, and 658-nm PBM delivering 105 mW/cm² for 90 seconds providing 9.5 J/cm²) combined with standard rehabilitation sessions twice weekly for 8 weeks reduced pain when walking.[114]

In another clinical trial of patients with rotator-cuff tendinopathy treated with ultrasound alone or combined with NIR (1,200 mW/cm², 10 seconds) or red light (400 mW/cm², 30 seconds),[115] NIR combined with ultrasound was more effective than ultrasound alone for every tested outcome.

Lastly, a study of people with Achilles' tendinopathy found that applying 810-nm laser with 2,375 mW/cm² power density for 30 seconds in six different places (18 J total dose) led to significant improvements in ankle strength and reduction of pain.[116]

Red light therapy exerts positive effects on tendon disorders by modulating inflammation, improving energy production, and increasing growth of tendon cells, while stimulating collagen production—all of which act to improve tendon healing.[117]

INCREASE FERTILITY

Some research suggests that PBM may be useful for improving fertility, which could make quite an impact for couples trying to conceive.

A growing number of studies have shown that PBM may significantly boost pregnancy rates, even in women who have been unsuccessful with other assisted-reproduction treatments, such as in vitro fertilization. PBM appears to improve fertility by boosting cellular energy production in eggs, profoundly improving their viability.

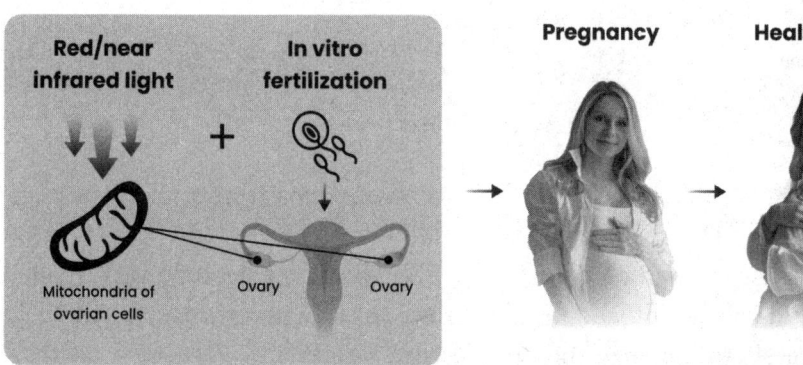

It also improves follicular health, which is highly vulnerable to oxidative stress. One study out of Denmark found that PBM treatment improved pregnancy rates by 68 percent where in vitro fertilization had previously failed.[118]

In Japan, PBM **resulted in pregnancy for 22.3 percent of severely infertile women, with 50.1-percent successful live births.**[119]

It's also worth noting, for mothers who struggle with genitourinary problems from childbirth or menopause, that a growing body of research has shown that intravaginal PBM can help reduce vaginal dryness, improve sexual function, and reduce stress-induced urinary incontinence.[120] In one study using a specific intravaginal device, 84 percent of women reduced their incontinence by more than 50 percent, improved sexual function by 54 percent, and significantly improved pelvic floor muscle strength.[121]

The testicles can also respond to red light, and research shows that PBM can greatly enhance sperm motility, and therefore fertility.[122, 123]

In studies of human sperm, NIR light therapy at 830 nm produced significant improvements in motility.[122] Two other studies found improved sperm motility and other parameters with 655-nm red light (25 mW/cm² for 4 minutes providing 6 J/cm²)[124] and 660-nm red light combined with 810-nm NIR light (39.5 mW/cm² for 50 to 100 seconds providing 2 to 4 J/cm²).[125]

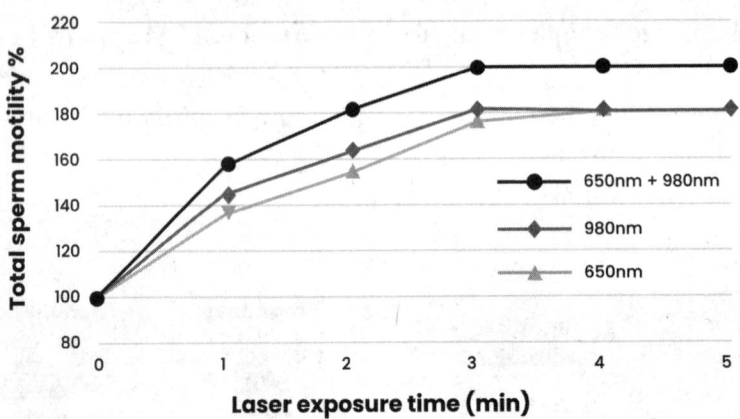

Red Light and Sperm Motility

- 650nm + 980nm
- 980nm
- 650nm

Total sperm motility %

Laser exposure time (min)

Why does PBM enhance sperm motility from outside the body? The tails of spermatozoa contain strings of mitochondria, and because PBM improves mitochondrial function, this increases the sperm's ability to "swim" upstream and enhances sperm viability.

So PBM could be a powerful tool for both men and women trying to conceive.

Increase Fertility

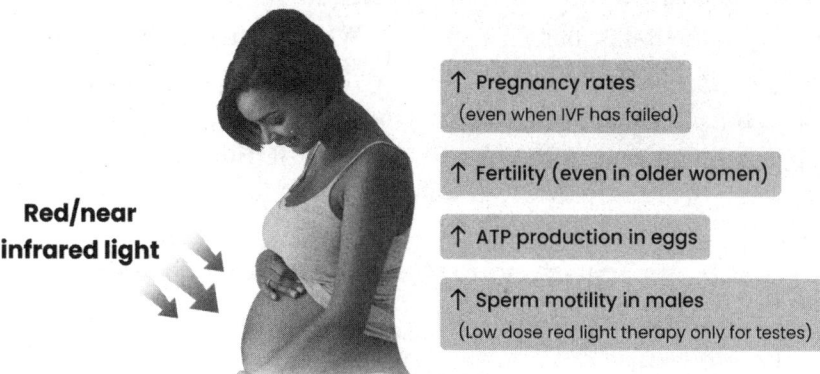

Red/near infrared light

↑ Pregnancy rates
(even when IVF has failed)

↑ Fertility (even in older women)

↑ ATP production in eggs

↑ Sperm motility in males
(Low dose red light therapy only for testes)

One caveat for men: Never use any type of PBM that gets hot, like incandescent heat lamps, near your testicles, as that could damage fragile Leydig cells and sperm cells. In fact, let me make four things very clear about applying light to the testicles:

1. Avoid heating the testicles; heat damages sperm cells and negatively affects the Leydig cells.
2. Avoid blue light on the testes. (Blue light at high doses inhibits the production of ATP—thus decreasing, not promoting, mitochondrial health.)
3. Avoid any infrared heat lamps or infrared bulbs on the testes—these produce far too much heat to be safe.
4. I recommend low-dose red light therapy in general, as the testes may be especially sensitive to overdosing and tissue heating. Don't overdo it—small doses only.

Note: Some people in the red light therapy business and biohacking communities have made claims around the ability of red light therapy to increase testosterone levels. While I was initially excited about this possibility, upon exploring the research that was cited, I have concluded that the evidence is not strong enough to support these claims. The claims are based mostly on one study in rats, which isn't particularly impressive—it only shows an elevation in testosterone briefly on one day, before a return to normal.[126] It also doesn't show testosterone elevation for the group using NIR—only in the group using red light. However, it's worth noting that the study used very high doses (far too high, in my opinion) and it's possible that a more modest dose could lead to benefits for testosterone levels.

However, other studies have failed to show similar benefits,[127] including one study using full-body PBM on water polo athletes.[128] I remain open to the possibility that PBM may increase testosterone levels when used on the testes, but the evidence for it at present (2025) is insufficient. That said, there is some intriguing research on the ability of sun exposure to boost testosterone levels, and that seems a safer bet for now.[129, 130]

While the research on boosting testosterone is not strong, there is an abundance of solid evidence for the ability of PBM to improve fertility.

IMPROVE JOINT HEALTH AND COMBAT ARTHRITIS

Studies have also shown that PBM can help people with osteoarthritis (often just called "arthritis").[131, 132] Even in children with juvenile idiopathic arthritis, NIR therapy improved pain, fatigue perception, and functional status compared to a control group.[133]

It does this through four primary mechanisms:[134, 135]

- Reducing pain
- Decreasing pro-inflammatory and increasing anti-inflammatory signaling molecules
- Increasing blood circulation to the joint area
- Stimulating cellular healing and repair mechanisms in the damaged joint itself

It's worth noting that there have been mixed reports in the literature about the effectiveness of PBM for osteoarthritis. Here's what Dr. Hamblin, Ph.D., wrote in his 2013 review of the scientific literature on this subject:[134]

[PBM] has been used clinically in osteoarthritis for many years but is still considered controversial. Although a Cochrane review reported mixed and conflicting results, a subsequent analysis conducted by Bjordal and colleagues concluded that the Cochrane review conclusion was neither robust nor valid. Further sensitivity analyses with inclusion of valid non-included trials, performance of missing follow-up, and subgroup analyses **revealed consistent and highly significant results in favor of active [PBM] for osteoarthritis.**

A 2022 review of six randomized controlled trials focusing on osteoarthritis of the knee concluded that applying 4 to 8 J of 785 to 860 nm red light or 1 to 3 J of 904-nm NIR light every day significantly reduced pain and disability compared to control groups receiving standard of care.[136]

Given its capacity to decrease inflammation, reduce pain, and support connective tissue growth and regeneration, PBM is likely to be useful for almost any kind of joint problems.

DECREASE DIABETIC ULCERS AND NEUROPATHY

For diabetics, the most positive results gleaned from studies on the effects of PBM are concerned with the healing of foot ulcers. Historically, these are harder to heal due to poor circulation and high glucose levels. Studies in animals and humans reveal that red light therapy restores diabetic patients' normal healing ability by exerting a stimulatory effect on the mitochondria with a resulting increase in adenosine triphosphate (ATP).[137–140]

In elderly adults suffering from diabetic foot ulcers, using an at-home 808-nm NIR light device for 8 minutes every day (17 mW/cm² providing 9 J/cm²) achieved 97 percent wound closure after 12 weeks, compared to just 47 percent in a control group.[33] In fact, 70 percent of patients using NIR light therapy achieved greater than 90-percent wound closure, compared to just 10 percent of patients in the control group.

PBM has also had impressive success in helping patients with painful diabetic neuropathy. Studies have found that PBM also helps to relieve pain, improve nerve function, and increase microcirculation in the feet of diabetic patients.[141–143]

IMPROVE GLYCEMIC CONTROL

There is some evidence that PBM can reduce blood glucose levels, either when used alone or in combination with exercise. In one study, healthy volunteers were exposed to 670-nm LED light onto an 800-cm² region of the upper back for 15 minutes at an intensity of 40 mW/cm² (28,800 J).[144] PBM reduced the degree of blood glucose elevation following glucose intake by 27.7 percent, integrated over the 2 h following the glucose challenge.

Another study recruited 13 men with type 2 diabetes and delivered 850-nm LED light to a variety of muscles (rectus abdominis, external obliques, quadriceps, hamstrings, and several others) bilaterally at different total energy levels (sham, 75, 150, 300, 450, and 600 J).[145] PBM statistically decreased plasma-glucose levels at 15 minutes after application of 75 and 450 J irradiation protocols.

These effects are likely due to how red and NIR light interact with skeletal muscle, the largest "glucose sink" in the body—for example, by stimulating the oxidation of intracellular fatty acids and thereby improving intramuscular insulin signaling.[146] Similar observations have been made with fat tissue, with PBM improving glucose-transporter content of fat cells and thereby allowing for greater energy storage.[147]

IMPROVE ORAL HEALTH

PBM has been shown to have numerous benefits for oral health, and research in this area is booming right now. So far, PBM has been shown to:

- Combat viral and bacterial infections of the mouth (tonsillitis; herpes, including cold sores)[148–150]
- Reduce mouth pain from ulcers or burning mouth syndrome[149]
- Facilitate tooth growth/tooth movement and reduce pain for individuals with corrective braces[151–153]
- Reduce thrush (yeast in the mouth/candidiasis)[154, 155]
- Decrease tooth hypersensitivity[156, 157]
- Help with periodontal disease, gingivitis, and other gum problems[158–162]

Hamblin et al. noted that PBM can be used with a huge variety of dental procedures to improve outcomes and speed healing.[163] For instance, applying 670-nm red light (150 mW for 12 minutes daily for one week) to impacted molars after corrective surgery reduced plaque, probing depth, and bleeding during the first 3 months, and tended to slow the process of root resorption.[164]

Two other studies involving adults undergoing surgery to remove molars, one delivering 3,600 mW/cm² of 808-nm NIR light for 25 seconds (89 J/cm²),[165] and the other delivering 75 mW/cm² of 830-nm NIR light for 45 seconds (3.4 J/cm²),[166] both found that PBM enhanced bone repair, increased new capillary formation in the wound area, and reduced pain and swelling.

Another study of adults undergoing jaw surgery reported that delivering 200 mW/cm² of 980 nm NIR light for 60 seconds (12 J/cm²) before surgery, immediately postoperatively, and on days 1, 3, 7, 14, 21, and 28 postoperatively, improved neurosensory disturbances (general sensitivity, pain, directional discrimination, and heat discrimination) compared to control.[167]

Lastly, a systematic review with meta-analysis of 12 randomized controlled trials involving patients with burning mouth syndrome reported that PBM was superior to placebo for reducing disease severity and associated mood disturbances (anxiety and depression).[168] It also improved quality of life.

Overall, PBM can be a powerful tool for health and healing when applied to the oral tissues.[169]

Improve Oral Health

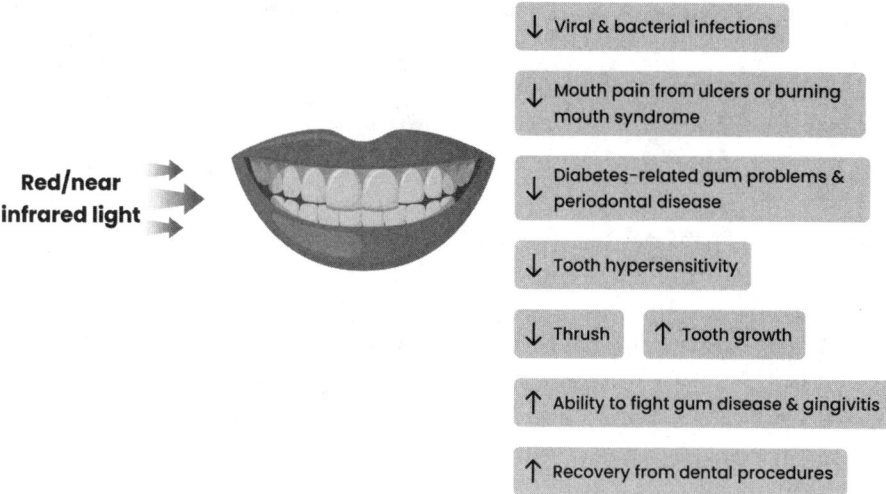

Red/near infrared light

- ↓ Viral & bacterial infections
- ↓ Mouth pain from ulcers or burning mouth syndrome
- ↓ Diabetes-related gum problems & periodontal disease
- ↓ Tooth hypersensitivity
- ↓ Thrush
- ↑ Tooth growth
- ↑ Ability to fight gum disease & gingivitis
- ↑ Recovery from dental procedures

IMPROVE RESPIRATORY HEALTH AND COMBAT RESPIRATORY INFECTIONS

In some studies, PBM has been shown to improve the health of people who suffer from chronic respiratory diseases such as asthma, chronic obstructive pulmonary disease (COPD), bronchiectasis, and inflammatory lung disease,[170–173] as well as patients suffering from chronic obstructive bronchitis.[174]

Red light therapy has also been proven to decrease lung inflammation in rodents after exposure to toxins and common indoor air pollutants, such as formaldehyde.[175]

The ability of red and NIR light therapy to manage respiratory infections has also been shown. The use of 830-nm NIR light on the face reduced the severity of stuffiness in sinuses (chronic rhinosinusitis) by 34 percent after just five sessions.[176]

Throughout the COVID-19 pandemic, there was a growing interest in using red and NIR light as a treatment to help prevent lung inflammation and severe disease outcomes.[177] A meta-analysis of animal studies demonstrated significant reductions in pro-inflammatory signaling molecules following red/infrared light therapy.[178]

One study in COVID patients demonstrated that daily treatment with 940-nm NIR light for one week shortened hospital discharge time and improved a variety of cardiopulmonary function tests compared to a control group receiving standard of care.[179]

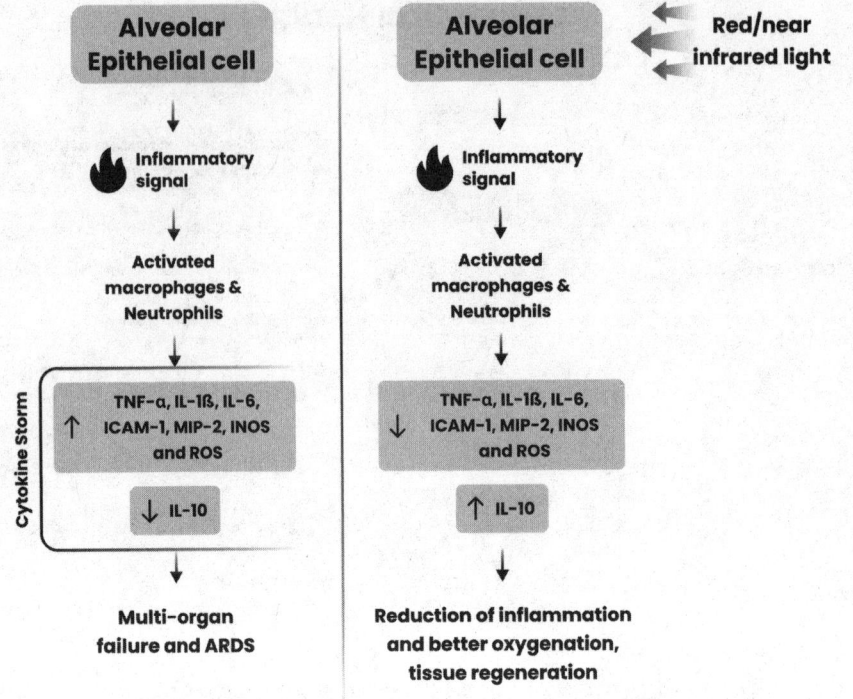

The first double-blind randomized controlled trial was published in 2022.[180] Patients hospitalized with mild-to-moderate COVID-19 received 120 mW/cm² of 620- to 635-nm red light for 6 minutes (providing 45 J/cm²) twice per day for 3 days alongside the standard of care. Red light treatment notably reduced pro-inflammatory signaling molecules that could otherwise give rise to a cytokine storm and respiratory distress.

Another randomized controlled trial divided 199 COVID patients into two groups (136 patients with 0 to 7 days of symptoms at baseline and 63 patients with 8 to 12 days of symptoms), who were randomly assigned to receive PBM plus standard of care or standard of care only. The PBM group self-administered a home-use device (635 nm intranasal and 810 nm chest LEDs) for 20 minutes twice a day for 5 days and, subsequently, once daily for 30 days. Those with 0 to 7 days of symptoms at baseline recovered significantly faster with PBM (18 days vs. 21 days for control).[181]

There's also evidence that PBM can help treat other problems associated with COVID-19, such as lesions in the mouth and loss of smell or taste.[182–184]

Improve Respiratory Health and Combat Respiratory Infections

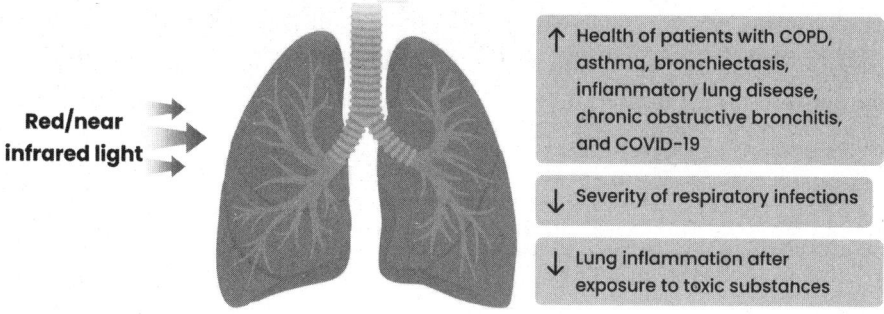

Red/near infrared light →

↑ Health of patients with COPD, asthma, bronchiectasis, inflammatory lung disease, chronic obstructive bronchitis, and COVID-19

↓ Severity of respiratory infections

↓ Lung inflammation after exposure to toxic substances

IMPROVE HEART HEALTH

Most studies on red light therapy for heart health and heart repair after cardiac events and surgery have been carried out on animals. In a 2017 systematic review of the scientific literature, scientists found that animal studies revealed consistently positive effects of red light therapy by reducing infarct size (the size of the damaged area in heart attacks) by up to 76 percent, decreasing inflammation and scarring, and accelerating tissue repair.[185]

In heart tissue studies, PBM works through multiple molecular pathways, including modulation of inflammatory cytokines, signaling molecules, transcription factors, enzymes, and antioxidants.[186] Other studies have noted many other benefits to heart function.[187–192] This may or may not have relevance to humans, however, because in humans, the tissues and bones that lie on top of the heart are

thicker, and it is very plausible that while red light can penetrate directly through the sternum in animals, it likely cannot do so in most humans, unless perhaps using an especially high irradiance device.

One study in humans recruited thirty-two patients each having two or three coronary vessel occlusions (2VD/3VD) who underwent low-level laser therapy post-coronary artery bypass graft, and twenty-eight patients who did not undergo laser therapy were studied as a control group.[193] Diode laser (810 nm, 500 mW) was applied for 3 successive days post-coronary artery bypass graft. The laser probe was placed in direct contact with the skin over the surgical incision (mid-sternum) every 1 cm and over the pericardium (left parasternal, second and third intercostal spaces, and apex). The treatment and control groups were statistically different at the fifth day for white blood cells, neutrophils, and lymphocytes, suggesting anti-inflammatory effects of NIR light.

Other groups have investigated the use of intravascular red laser therapy in humans as an adjunct to coronary artery stent implantation in order to reduce the occurrence of restenosis caused by intimal hyperplasia (the blood vessel narrowing due to thickening of the inner layer of the vessel wall).[194–196] The red laser reduced the expected restenosis rate in patients after coronary stenting in arteries of >2.5 mm.

IMPROVE FUNCTION OF INTERNAL ORGANS

The study of red light therapy to enhance the health of the liver is still in its infancy. Only animal studies have been done so far, and this is another area where the relevance to humans is questionable because of the difficulty in delivering light to the liver, although it may be possible with a high-irradiance device in a person with low body fat. However, in these studies, PBM yielded very positive results for healing cirrhotic liver damage in rodents,[197] as well as in surgical applications, such as to enhance the regeneration of the liver during a liver transplant.[198]

So far, there have been very few studies done on the pancreas using PBM. However, in the animal studies conducted so far, PBM has been shown to enhance islet cell function before transplantation,[199] and stimulate regeneration of islets and pancreatic ducts in experimental models of diabetes.[200] Again, the treatment of internal organs likely will show greater effectiveness in animal models compared to humans, because in humans, light penetration directly to those tissues is much less likely. This is likely to be particularly true for humans in whom large amounts of soft tissue (e.g., body fat) lies atop those internal organs, which would make it impossible for the light to penetrate directly.

DECREASE PAIN

PBM has been shown to be effective at reducing joint pain in virtually all areas of the body.

A number of proposed mechanisms have been shown to be involved in PBM's ability to reduce pain. These include changes in tissue-opioid receptors, changes in substance P, and interference with nerve transmission and pain sensation.[163, 201]

It's worth noting that different stimuli cause different types of pain. Red and NIR light therapy almost certainly does not work equally well for all types, locations, and causes of pain. For that reason, not all studies on various types of pain have shown equal benefits. A 2014 review of the scientific literature noted:[202]

> Studies have demonstrated that [PBM] may have positive effects on symptomology associated with chronic pain; however this finding is not universal. A meta-analysis utilizing 52 effect sizes from 22 articles on [PBM] and pain from Fulop et al. (2010) demonstrated an overall effect size of 0.84. This would be classified as a large effect size and suggests a strong inclination for the use of [PBM] to reduce chronic pain.

Here are several conditions where PBM has proven effective:

- Chronic neck pain[202, 203]
- Knee pain
- Fibromyalgia
- Lower-back pain[204]
- Chronic pain in the elbow, wrist, and fingers[205]
- Chronic joint disorders[206]
- Sacroiliac joint pain[207]
- Chronic tooth pain[208,209]
- Osteoarthritis pain[210]
- Tendinitis and myofascial pain[211]
- Postoperative pain[212, 213]
- Neuropathic pain[214]

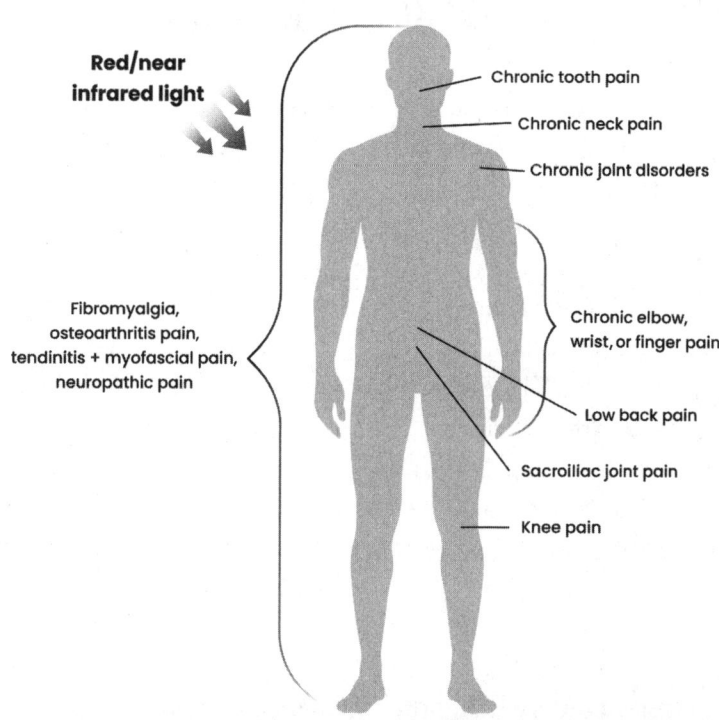

Red/NIR Light May Improve:

Red/near infrared light

Chronic tooth pain

Chronic neck pain

Chronic joint disorders

Fibromyalgia, osteoarthritis pain, tendinitis + myofascial pain, neuropathic pain

Chronic elbow, wrist, or finger pain

Low back pain

Sacroiliac joint pain

Knee pain

There's a wide range of effective doses for pain management, with most studies administering between 1 and 30 J/cm².[215] I would suggest aiming toward the upper end of that range for deeper tissues.

A 2022 review concluded that "low-intensity LASER and LED (PBMT) offers a non-invasive, safe, drug-free, and side-effect-free method for pain relief of both acute and chronic musculoskeletal conditions as well as fibromyalgia".[216]

If we can reduce patients' pain through light, perhaps we don't need to rely so heavily on painkiller drugs. This idea was first proposed in the scientific domain by a dentist, Gerald Ross, who had completely abandoned the use of painkillers in his dental surgery practice, favoring instead the use of PBM postoperatively.[217] Over his 48 years of practice, he found that his patients had such outstanding responses to this approach that they often needed little more than a nonsteroidal anti-inflammatory drug like ibuprofen or acetaminophen for procedures that had once required narcotics.

It's worth noting that many clinicians believe lasers to be superior to LEDs for immediate pain relief (e.g., in musculoskeletal issues). Currently, it's not totally clear why this is, but it may have to do with how the light interacts with pain-sensing neurons.

COMBAT OPIOID ADDICTION

Other researchers have since used red and NIR light to reduce cravings in people addicted to opioids with outstanding results. The idea here is that red and NIR light applied to the head could increase neuroplasticity to repair the abnormal brain pathways that have become established after periods of drug-taking. The earliest randomized placebo-controlled trial in this regard was published in 2020. Adults with significant opioid cravings and a history of opioid-use disorder received two NIR light treatments on the sides of their head (810 nm, 250 mW/cm² for 4 minutes providing 60 J/cm²).[218] Immediately after treatment, cravings were reduced, and this reduction continued for an entire week afterward, reaching a 51 percent reduction. In other words, a single treatment cut opioid cravings in half. On top of that, depression and anxiety were each reduced by 40 percent.

In a larger follow-up randomized placebo-controlled trial using the same treatment protocol, NIR led to a 5-point reduction on a 10-point opioid craving scale, representing a 70 percent reduction from baseline.[219] These effects were consistent regardless of whether the patients were using withdrawal medication or not. Moreover, there were no reported adverse events.

Effects of Active Versus Sham Treatment on Craving

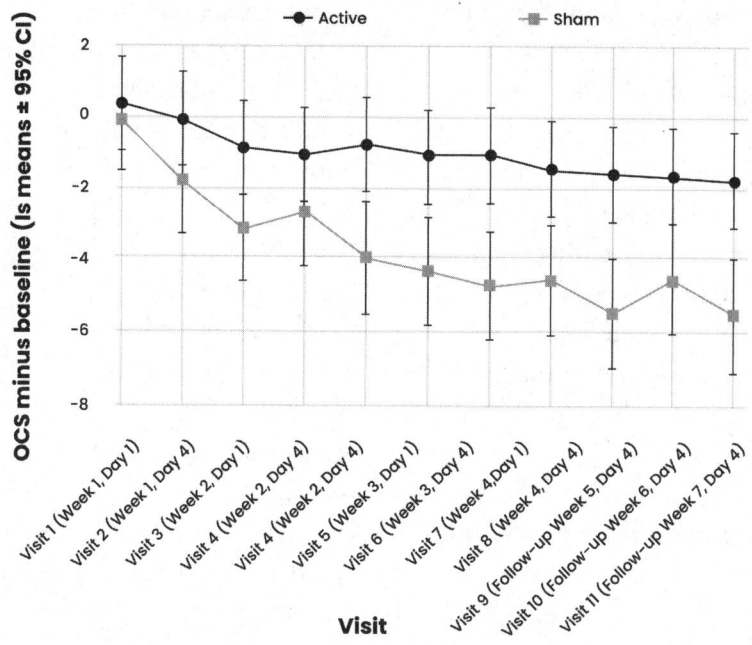

A case series suggested that about 62 percent of patients with opioid-use disorder had consistent favorable responses to NIR treatment, while 19 percent had helpful but not remarkable responses and 19 percent had no noticeable response.[220] In other words, this extremely safe NIR treatment protocol benefited roughly four of every five patients, with three of those

four experiencing remarkable and easily observable benefits.

Not only are red and NIR light therapy incredibly potent for reducing pain across a wide range of painful conditions, but it has now been shown to reduce opioid cravings in those considered to be addicted.

IMPROVE IMMUNITY

In numerous studies, PBM has been shown to benefit the immune system. This benefit may involve either the stimulation of the

immune response in cases of cancer or infection, or the suppression of the immune response in cases of autoimmune diseases.

In animal studies, PBM has a boosting effect on the immune system in immune-deficient animals implanted with malignant tumors, resulting in an increased lifespan.[221]

In human studies, PBM also boosted the immune systems and T cells of preoperative cancer patients without increasing tumor size.[222] (Researchers have expressed hope that these exciting results may lead to a safe treatment for immuno-deficiency diseases in humans.)

In the context of wound healing, PBM has also been shown to have beneficial effects, in part by modulating immune function.[223]

One review of the scientific literature noted:[224]

Immune cells, in particular, appear to be strongly affected by [PBM]. Mast cells, which play a crucial role in the movement of leukocytes, are of considerable importance in inflammation. Specific wavelengths of light are able to trigger mast cell degranulation, which results in the release of the pro-inflammatory cytokine TNF-a from the cells. . . . Lymphocytes become activated and proliferate more rapidly, and epithelial cells become more motile, allowing wound sites to close more quickly. The ability of macrophages to act as phagocytes is also enhanced after the application of [PBM].

Another study found that delivering PBM to the bone marrow could increase the blood platelet count and help resolve situations in which the count has been lowered by chemotherapy or by an autoimmune disease.[225, 226]

It also appears to selectively modulate cell function in some types of infected cells while not affecting healthy uninfected cells in the same way.[227]

In vitro studies using human leukocytes have shown that NIR light can increase the activity of these immune cells. Given that we know red and NIR light penetrates our blood vessels and irradiates our bloodstream, it is reasonable to think that circulating immune cells would be affected.[225, 226]

A fascinating study in mice looked at shining red light on the thymus gland (an important gland in the immune system) and on an area of a back leg. They found that the mice who received the treatment on the thymus gland area (in the center of the chest) had more profound changes in immune-cell function.[228] (They also noted that overdoing the dose could have immunosuppressive effects, which is consistent with what is known in other contexts—you can overdo the dose. We'll talk more about this in chapter 4 on the "biphasic dose response.")

Another remarkable and more recent study from December 2017 looked at the potential for PBM to reverse thymic involution, where the thymus gland "involutes"—they basically shrivel up and become much less functional, which has a negative impact on our immune function.

This study suggests that PBM may be able to slow or even reverse this thymic involution—thus keeping our thymus-gland function and immune function intact as we age.[229] The researchers concluded "This perspective puts forward a hypothesis that PBM [photobiomodulation] can alter thymic involution, improve immune functioning in aged people and even extend lifespan."

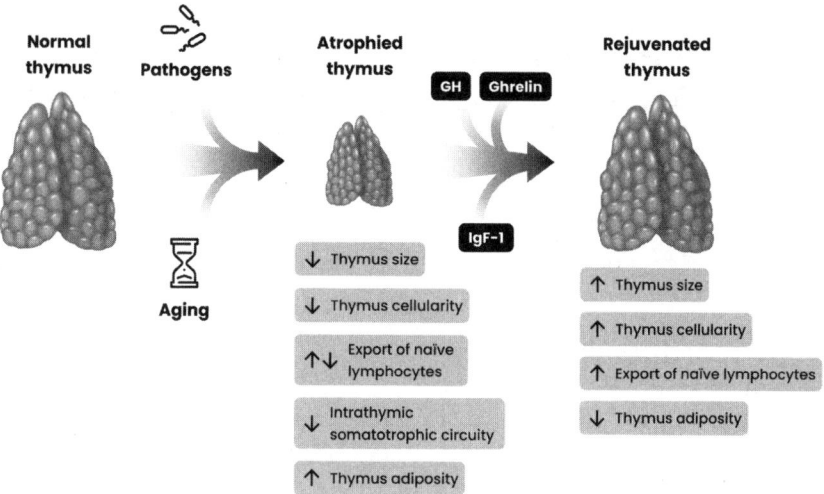

Another fascinating study looked at the influence of PBM on people with treatment-resistant schizophrenia and found symptomatic improvement in a large proportion of people. They also found pronounced improvement in immunological markers.[230]

As discussed in the section on thyroid health, in people with Hashimoto's—a common autoimmune condition responsible for most hypothyroidism—PBM has proven to have remarkably beneficial effects on immune function.[53] Another animal model of multiple sclerosis (an autoimmune condition that degenerates the fatty sheath around nerves that helps nerve conduction) showed that just two treatments over a span of 14 days led to significant improvement with less brain cell death and slowed the progression of the disease.[231] Other animal studies have found similar effects:[232]

> Finally, histological analysis showed that [PBM] blocked neuroinflammation through a reduction of inflammatory cells in the CNS, especially lymphocytes, as well as preventing demyelination in the spinal cord after EAE induction. Together, our results suggest the use of [PBM] as a therapy to treat autoimmune neuroinflammatory responses, such as MS, may be effective.

As you can see, light therapy doesn't just appear to increase immune activity, but may also beneficially modulate immune activity, regardless of whether the patient has underactive or overactive (or otherwise imbalanced) immune activity.

Overall, the body of research looking at immune function in different conditions paints a more complex picture than simply that red and NIR light stimulates or inhibits immune function. While I'm sure we'll find exceptions to this rule as more

studies are done, red and NIR light seems to be an "immune regulator" that supports *optimal* immune function in a wide variety of scenarios and health conditions. It seems to be able to positively affect immune function, regardless of whether someone has a deficient immune response during an infection or has an overly active and imbalanced immune response in auto-immune disease.

HELP HEAL TRAUMATIC BRAIN INJURY AND SPINAL CORD INJURY

Red light therapy can help recovery and enhance cognition in people suffering from traumatic brain injury. Patients who have suffered traumatic brain in-

jury report improved cognition, better sleep, and enhanced recovery from the traumatic experience of their accident.[233]

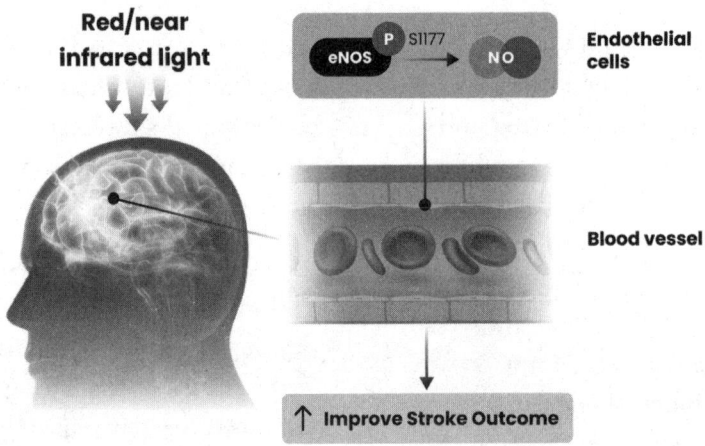

Red/near infrared light

eNOS — P S1177 → NO — Endothelial cells

Blood vessel

↑ Improve Stroke Outcome

A study of veterans with chronic traumatic brain injury reported that delivering 6.4 mW/cm² of red and NIR light to the head for 20 minutes three times per week improved neuropsychological health and

cerebral blood flow for years after the traumatic brain injury incident.[234]

According to a systematic review and meta-analysis of animal experiments, the best results were obtained using wavelengths between 665 and 810 nm, administering the first treatment within 4 hours of the traumatic brain injury, and using three or fewer sessions per day.[235]

In animal research, PBM has shown impressive results in mitigating neurological damage suffered after a stroke. Scientists believe that the therapeutic effects stem largely from increased mitochondrial function (i.e., increased ATP production) in brain cells irradiated with PBM.[236–238]

Spinal cord injuries cause severe damage to the central nervous system and have no effective known restorative therapies. However, PBM has been found to ac-celerate regeneration of injured peripheral nerves and increase the axonal number and distance of nerve axon regrowth, while significantly improving aspects of function toward normal levels. Numerous studies suggest that PBM could be a promising treatment for spinal cord injury.[239–242]

In one study of spinal cord injury patients undergoing physical rehabilitation, NIR light therapy three times per week led to significantly greater EMG signal activity, indicative of spinal nerve function and improved motor response, after one month.[243]

Help Heal Traumatic Brain Injury (TBI) and Spinal Cord Injury

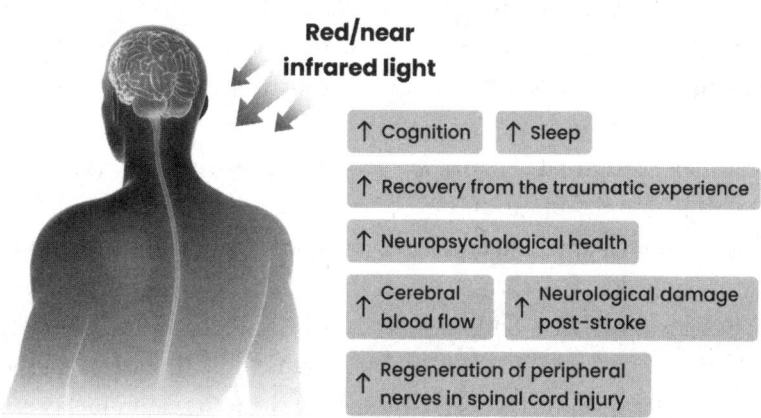

Red/near infrared light

↑ Cognition ↑ Sleep

↑ Recovery from the traumatic experience

↑ Neuropsychological health

↑ Cerebral blood flow ↑ Neurological damage post-stroke

↑ Regeneration of peripheral nerves in spinal cord injury

IMPROVE SLEEP ONSET AND SLEEP QUALITY

Research suggests that red and NIR light can improve sleep, perhaps by affecting melatonin, and maybe through other mechanisms as well. Melatonin is a hormone produced primarily by the pineal gland in the brain, and even most nonscientists are somewhat familiar with melatonin for its role in promoting sleep.

Several studies (mostly out of China) have shown that red and NIR light seems to increase melatonin produced by the body. **The studies found increased melatonin in the blood circulation following PBM, and studies have also found dramatic improvement in sleep in people with insomnia.**[244]

Here is some of the relevant research:

- The first documented use of an intranasal light therapy device to directly affect melatonin levels was conducted by Xu et al. in 2001.[337] They treated 38 subjects that had insomnia with intranasal low-level laser therapy once a day for 10 days. They found that serum melatonin had increased.
- The same group of researchers treated another group of 128 patients with insomnia and found that the polysomnogram (a sleep study that includes data on brain waves as electrical activity) had improved.[338]
- In 2006, Wang et al. reported that they had treated 50 patients with

insomnia with intranasal low-level laser therapy (with similar specifications to Vielight's LED device) for 60 minutes per session.[339] Each session was conducted once a day for between 10 and 14 days. They found that the condition had **improved significantly in 41 (82 percent) of the cases, mild improvement in four (8 percent) of the cases, and no improvement for five (10 percent) of the cases.**

More research is still needed on this topic to clarify what types of devices are ways of applying it (and to what body areas) are most effective for enhancing sleep. However, I've seen hundreds of people with insomnia achieve significant sleep improvements by using red and NIR light therapy before bed, using a wide variety of devices and methods of application.

It's interesting to think that maybe our bodies are wired to benefit from sitting next to a fire for several hours each night, as many of our ancestors did. Perhaps the red and NIR light emitted from the fire actually benefits us and promotes healing systemically, at least partly because of the effect it can have on melatonin production and sleep enhancement.

IMPROVE BRAIN HEALTH AND SLOW PROGRESSION OF ALZHEIMER'S AND PARKINSON'S DISEASES

PBM is having a *profound impact* in areas of medicine that deal with diseases and conditions of the nervous system, including traumatic brain injury, spinal cord injury, peripheral nerve injury, and painful diabetic neuropathy; it has the potential to help with Alzheimer's and Parkinson's diseases and may potentially contribute to delaying and/or halting them if implemented early enough.

PBM has been shown to:[163, 245–248]

- Benefit cognitive performance and memory

- Improve mitochondrial function of brain cells
- Protect neurons
- Improve cellular repair of neurons
- Increase brain-derived neurotrophic factor (BDNF) and nerve growth factor (NGF)
- Decrease brain inflammation (decreased pro-inflammatory cytokines and increased anti-inflammatory cytokines)

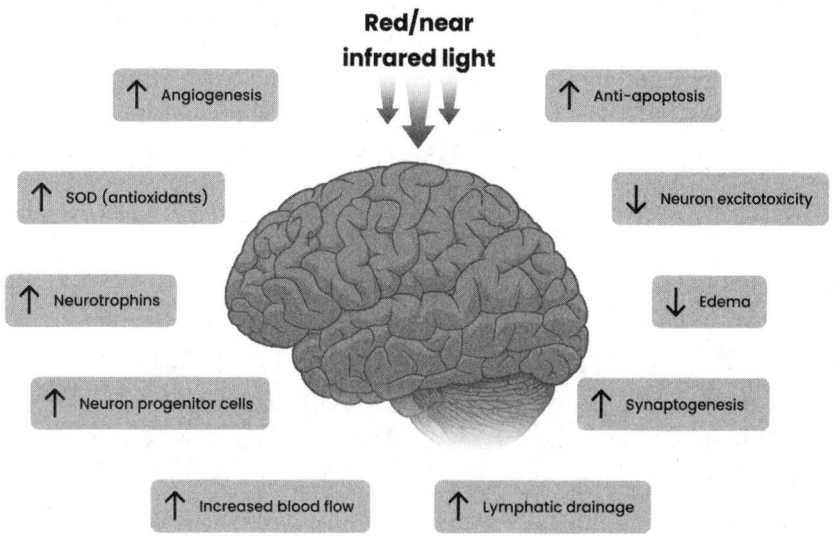

Recent studies have now found that PBM may significantly slow the progression of Alzheimer's and Parkinson's diseases.[249, 249]

One study investigated the effects of using a home LED device in eight elderly dementia patients.[250] The device administered 100 mW/cm² of 810-nm light to the

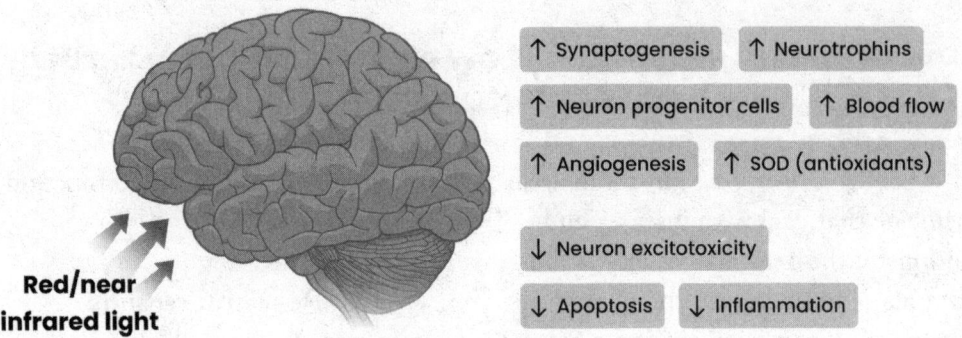

↑ Synaptogenesis   ↑ Neurotrophins

↑ Neuron progenitor cells   ↑ Blood flow

↑ Angiogenesis   ↑ SOD (antioxidants)

↓ Neuron excitotoxicity

↓ Apoptosis   ↓ Inflammation

Red/near infrared light

back of the head, 75 mW/cm² to the fore-head, and 25 mW/cm² into the nose for 20 minutes, three times per week. After 12 weeks, those using the device not only had significantly improved cognitive function and reduced dementia severity; they also showed greater cerebral blood flow and connectivity between brain regions.

Two other studies found similar benefits. One found that a single session of PBM improved cerebral blood flow, cognitive function, memory, and executive function in adults with mild cognitive impairment,[110] while a case series documented notable improvements in overall function, sleep, emotional stability, and mood in adults with mild to moderate cognitive impairment.[251]

Although still in its infancy, scientists are hopeful that PBM may offer a new way to combat Parkinson's and Alzheimer's or halt progression of these conditions if caught early enough. Alzheimer's is, at least in part, caused by mitochondrial damage or dysfunction, which reduces

ATP production and contributes to neuronal death. This process leads to an increase in toxic reactive oxygen species, generating oxidative stress and subsequent neuronal death.[224, 252–254]

A 2022 systematic review of 43 cellular, animal, and human studies found that red and NIR light consistently interfered with Alzheimer's disease pathophysiology, and that 810- to 870-nm NIR light therapy in humans improves brain network connectivity and memory in Alzheimer's patients.[255]

Another review by Dr. Hamblin noted that NIR wavelengths in the 800- to 900-nm range are the most ideal choice, with most of the light entering the brain from the forehead to avoid interference from hair.[256] Most studies typically administer between 10 to 60 J/cm².

Several recent studies have found benefits for Parkinson's disease with these light parameters as well. One study gave patients "bucket" helmets lined with 670-, 810-, and 850-nm red and NIR light devices and reported that symptoms improved by 55 percent over a period of up to 24 months.[257]

In another study, improvements in Parkinson's were seen after just one week of 940-nm NIR light treatment (6 mW/cm² for 30 minutes) combined with hydrogen water.[258]

This is something that you can easily do at home. Parkinson's patients sent home with transcranial and intranasal NIR light devices to be used three times per week reported improvements in most tested parameters after a year of use, including those related to mobility, dynamic balance, cognition, fine motor skills, and static balance.[259] A follow-up study found similar benefits during the COVID pandemic.[260]

Although researchers are still unclear as to the exact way that NIR light induces its neuroprotective effects, they believe it operates by:

1. Activating healing intracellular cascades that result in the survival of target and surrounding cells
2. Spurring neurogenesis (growth and formation of neurons in the brain) for example through increases in BDNF

3. Triggering systemic protective mechanisms

As researchers note,[249]

. . . with the bulk of results still at the preclinical "proof of concept" stage, NIR therapy has the potential to develop into a safe and effective neuroprotective treatment for patients with Alzheimer's and Parkinson's diseases (and presumably other neurodegenerative diseases such as multiple sclerosis and amyotrophic lateral sclerosis). If NIR was applied at early stages of the disease process, for example at first diagnosis, it could potentially slow further progression by protecting neurons from death. Consequently, over time, the greater neuronal survival would lessen the clinical signs and symptoms. Furthermore, NIR therapy—because of its lack of side-effects and neuroprotective potential—is amenable to use in conjunction with other treatments.

In short, NIR light (because it penetrates the skull better than red light), appears to be a promising therapy for neurological conditions and improving brain health.

ENHANCE MUSCLE GAIN, STRENGTH, ENDURANCE, AND EXERCISE RECOVERY

Red and NIR light plus exercise make a potent combination. Not only does PBM

help you recover faster, it seems to amplify everything that happens with exercise—

increased muscle gain, fat loss, performance, strength, and endurance.

Studies show that PBM can powerfully repair muscle tissue and help people perform better. For example, one early study found that applying 240 J/cm² (1,000 mW/cm² for 30 seconds) of 810-nm light to the quadriceps before each of three weekly training sessions doubled the amount of muscle growth and nearly doubled the increase in muscular strength compared to a group training without NIR light application.[261] Other studies by this researcher using a similar protocol have found NIR light to reduce biomarkers of muscle damage and accelerate the recovery of strength after a hard training session.[262, 263]

There is also research (albeit from animal studies) showing that red and NIR light may help prevent the muscle loss that occurs with aging.[264, 265]

Muscle tissue has more mitochondria than almost any other tissue or organ in the human body. Therefore, muscle tissue is particularly responsive to red and NIR light. The muscles are packed with mitochondria because ATP is needed for every muscle twitch and movement, no matter how insignificant. Given what we know about the stimulatory effects of red and NIR light on mitochondria, we can expect that anyone who exercises regularly should benefit from using PBM on their muscles. And that's exactly what we see in the literature.

From Adel Moussa, the author of SuppVersity, a popular fitness blog that reviews scientific research:[266]

When I started this blog a few years ago, I was guilty of believing that supplements would be the most relevant ergogenics [performance enhancers] for anyone who trains, myself. Today, 2,300 articles later, this has changed: don't get me wrong—supplements can be useful, but diet, training and—at least in a few cases—even things like using light emitting diode therapy (LEDT) or low-level laser therapy (LLLT), as it is also called, are much higher on the "things that really work" list.

This is a remarkable quote. Basically, after reviewing thousands of studies examining supplements, Moussa concludes that, in general, PBM provides better effects than the vast majority of supplements. This is significant because there is so much focus and attention on supplements, and far fewer people have heard of PBM.

A 2019 systematic review of more than 50 clinical trials on PBM for exercise performance and post-workout recovery reported that the vast majority of studies showed benefits using a specified range of light dosing.[267] They found that large muscle groups (quadriceps, hamstrings, pectorals) required 120 to 300 joules per treatment, while small muscle groups (biceps, triceps, calves) required 20 to 60 joules per treatment. A range of power intensities can work (mW/cm²), but light exposure needs to last at least 30 seconds per session and cover as much of the muscle as possible. **For acute benefits during exercise, light exposure should take place 5 to 10 minutes before exercise, and 5 to 10 minutes after exercise for post-workout recovery.**

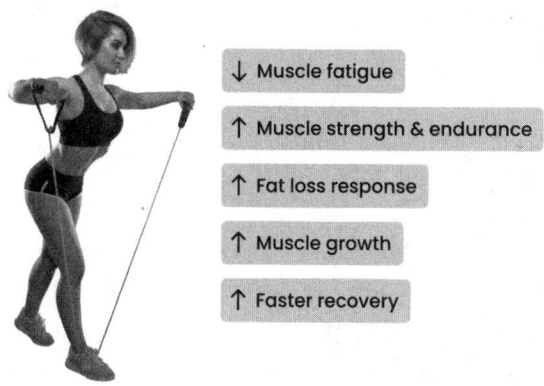

↓ Muscle fatigue

↑ Muscle strength & endurance

↑ Fat loss response

↑ Muscle growth

↑ Faster recovery

For acute benefits **during** exercise, irradiation should take place...

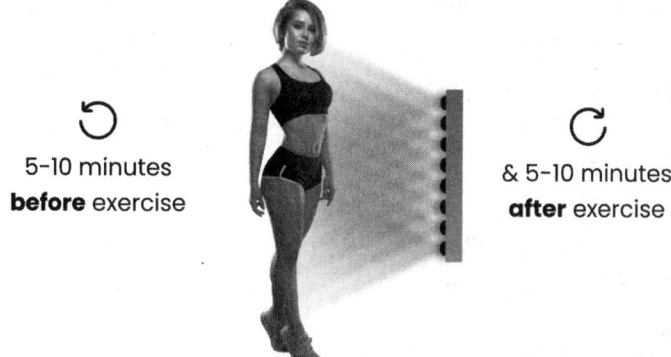

↺
5-10 minutes
before exercise

↻
& 5-10 minutes
after exercise

Through their effect on ATP production and cellular healing mechanisms, red and NIR light helps individuals to recover more quickly from strenuous and resistance exercise and even helps to prevent muscle fatigue *during exercise.*

Studies provide evidence that PBM can help prevent muscle fatigue, enhance muscle strength and endurance, increase the fat loss response from exercise, increase muscle growth responses from exercise, and promote faster recovery.[268–274] Not too shabby for one simple treatment that takes only a few minutes, right?

A 2015 systematic review found consistent benefits for athletic performance with PBM: longer running times before exhaustion, more repetitions while lifting weights, and greater strength, with improvements of 2 to 57 percent.[275]

Several years later, in 2018, they reported an updated analysis that included 39 randomized controlled trials.[276] Once again, it was shown that PBM improved running time until exhaustion, the number of repetitions one could do with a given weight, and overall muscular strength. It was also revealed that red and NIR light reduced signs of muscle damage.

How does PBM affect muscles? What is it actually doing to cause these benefits? It works through several important mechanisms in the body:

- It helps promote the production of internal antioxidants by your cells, which prevents oxidative stress and damage to the muscle tissue (when light is applied before exercise).[269, 270]
- It helps reduce inflammation that will lead to cellular damage (and fatigue) in the muscle tissue as well.[113, 277]
- It protects damaged muscles from secondary damage from further exercise.

- Using the light prior to exercise creates a "preconditioning" effect, which allows the muscle cells to suffer less damage from the exercise, as well as display higher strength/stamina in subsequent exercise following the initial bout of exercise.
- It decreases lactic acid production by muscles.
- It improves mitochondrial function during exercise.
- It increases acetylcholine receptors on muscles (this is the neurotransmitter released from nerve cells that stimulates muscle contraction).
- It increases the production of specific types of heat shock proteins that protect cells from oxidative damage, stress, and apoptosis (cell death).[268]
- It also enhances muscle growth, as well as increasing strength significantly.
- It promotes the development of muscle stem cells, myosatellite cells, which can develop into all the various types of muscles.
- It also has the profound benefit of increasing mitochondrial adaptation and mitochondrial biogenesis (the creation of new mitochondria) following exercise.[271]

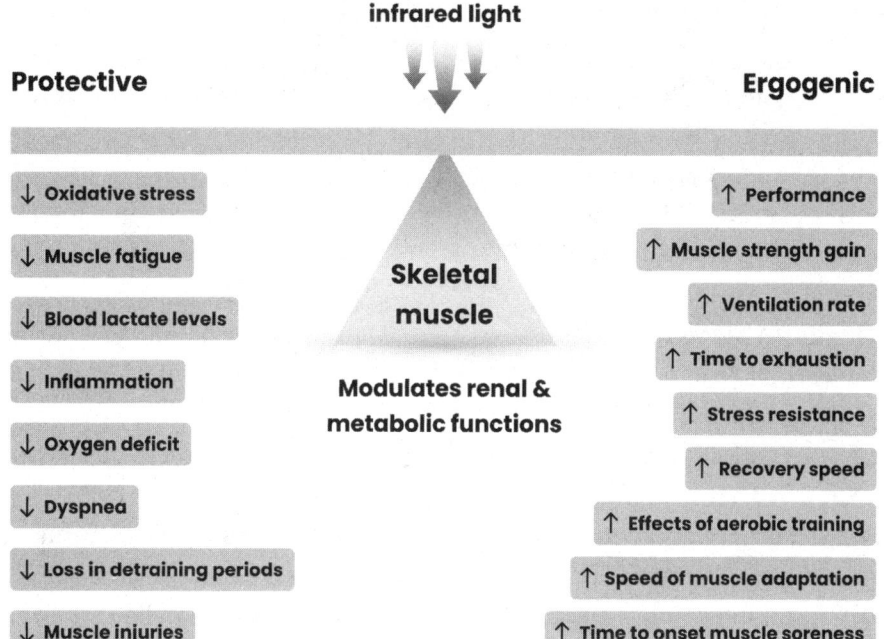

Red/near
infrared light

Protective

Ergogenic

Skeletal
muscle

Modulates renal &
metabolic functions

↓ Oxidative stress

↓ Muscle fatigue

↓ Blood lactate levels

↓ Inflammation

↓ Oxygen deficit

↓ Dyspnea

↓ Loss in detraining periods

↓ Muscle injuries

↑ Performance

↑ Muscle strength gain

↑ Ventilation rate

↑ Time to exhaustion

↑ Stress resistance

↑ Recovery speed

↑ Effects of aerobic training

↑ Speed of muscle adaptation

↑ Time to onset muscle soreness

To get into some of the research on this topic:

- One study looked at the number of repetitions (reps) that 34 athletes were able to perform on a weighted leg extension exercise as well as the amount of lactic acid their muscles produced, comparing placebo treatment (sham PBM) vs. 30, 60, or 90 seconds of real PBM therapy.[272] After receiving 60 or 120 seconds of light therapy, **the number of reps the athletes were able to perform went up by 27 percent.** And in the group that received 120 seconds of light therapy, **their lactic acid levels were significantly lower**—indicating less muscle strain while actually performing better.

  This graph shows the improvement in number of reps performed (blue) with 60 seconds of PBM, and the improvement in both reps performed and lactic acid levels (red) with 120 seconds of light therapy prior to exercise.

- Another study by Vieira et al. examined levels of fatigue in leg muscles after endurance exercise and found that the use of light therapy immediately afterward **significantly reduced fatigue scores** relative to the control group. The researchers concluded "The results suggest that an **endurance training program combined with [PBM] leads to a greater reduction in fatigue than an endurance training program without [PBM].** This is relevant to everyone involved in sport and rehabilitation".[273]

- Leal-Junior et al. performed a review of the relevant research in 2015 to examine the effects of phototherapy on exercise performance and recovery.[275] They compiled data from 13 randomized control trials and examined the number of repetitions and time until exhaustion for muscle performance, as well as markers of exercise-induced muscle damage. **The researchers concluded that preconditioning the muscles with red and NIR light (i.e., using the light prior to exercise) improved muscle performance and accelerated recovery.**

- Another study looked at use of LED PBM in male athletes who performed three intense bouts of exercise on a stationary bike.[278] The **athletes who were given LED light therapy prior to the exercise had significantly lower levels of creatine kinase (a marker for muscle damage)** compared to the sham light therapy (placebo) group.

- A 2016 review of sixteen studies by Nampo et al. looked at research using both laser and LED therapy on exercise capacity and muscle performance of people undergoing exercise compared to placebo/sham treatments.[274] They found an **average improvement of 3.51 reps, a 4-second delay in time to exhaustion (i.e., people were able to exercise longer before exhaustion), increased peak strength, and a significant reduction in lactic acid production.**

- A review of research by Borsa et al. found that studies consistently show that **PBM applied prior to weight training improved performance and decreased muscle damage.**[279]

- Another double-blind study (that means that neither the researchers nor the subjects knew who was getting the real treatment and who was getting the placebo) contained twenty-two non-exercising people who were subjected to exercise on a treadmill until exhaustion.[280] **The group that received the light therapy for 30 seconds before exercise had significantly lower levels of creatine kinase and lactate dehydrogenase— both markers of muscle damage— suggesting that the light therapy decreased the level of muscle damage.**

- Another study compared red and NIR light therapy with LEDs to cold water immersion (e.g., ice baths) as a recovery method after exercise and found that **red and NIR light improved recovery more than ice** baths. The researchers concluded: "We concluded that treating the leg muscles with LEDT five minutes after the Wingate cycle test seemed to inhibit the expected post-exercise increase in blood lactate levels and CK activity. This suggests that LEDT has better potential than 5 minutes of CWIT [cold-water immersion therapy] for improving short-term post-exercise recovery."[281] This is notable for another reason: Ice baths have been found to accelerate recovery, but at the same time, they have been shown to hinder some adaptations to exercise such as muscle growth, **whereas PBM accelerates recovery while also *amplifying* (rather than hindering) adaptations to exercise. So all in all, PBM would appear to be a superior recovery method compared to the typical ice baths that many athletes engage in— certainly in the context of resistance** exercise (where cold inhibits some beneficial adaptations). **It's not known if PBM is superior for recovery in the context of endurance exercise.**

As you can see, PBM also has the ability to increase your strength and endurance adaptations to exercise, decrease muscle damage from your workouts, help you recover faster, and even increase muscle gains. Dr. Hamblin once made this prediction:

Sports medicine will benefit from PBM [photobiomodulation] because both professional and amateur athletes can better recover from intense exercise, and the process also aids training regimens. In the near future, sport agencies must deal with "laser doping" by at least openly discussing it because the aforementioned beneficial effects and the preconditioning achieved by laser and LED irradiation will highly improve athletic performance.[163]

INCREASE FAT LOSS (AND REDUCE "STUBBORN FAT")

How does red light therapy enhance fat loss? While there is still some debate among researchers over the exact mechanisms involved, the research clearly shows that it does work. Red and NIR light therapy is even FDA approved as both an adjunct to liposuction and as a stand-alone body-contouring fat loss method (a standard that requires a high level of evidence).

Here's a quote from one review of the scientific literature on the ability of red and NIR light to help with fat loss:[282]

Within the past decade, [PBM] has also emerged as a new modality for noninvasive body contouring. Research has shown that [PBM] is effective in reducing overall body circumference measurements of specifically treated regions, including the hips, waist, thighs, and upper arms, with recent studies demonstrating the long-term effectiveness of results. The treatment is painless, and there appear to be no adverse events associated with [PBM]. The mechanism of action of [PBM] in body contouring is believed to stem from photoactivation of cytochrome c oxidase within hypertrophic adipocytes, which, in turn, affects intracellular secondary cascades, resulting in the formation of transitory pores within the adipocytes' membrane. The secondary cascades involved may include, but are not limited to, activation of cytosolic lipase and nitric oxide. Newly formed pores release intracellular lipids, which are further metabolized.

In studies, PBM at 635 nm **helped shave 3 to 5 inches off patients' waist and hip circumference by reducing the subcutaneous fat layer after just 4 weeks of use.**[282, 283]

Red and NIR light therapy not only releases the fat into the blood but does so *without* negatively affecting blood-serum lipid profiles.[280]

In a study of 86 individuals using red light therapy at 635 nm for **20 minutes once every 2 days for 2 weeks, study participants lost 2.99 inches across all body parts after 14 days.**[284]

Several other studies have reported similar outcomes, namely that red and NIR light therapy removes inches from the waist, hips, thighs, and upper arms in two to three sessions per week lasting 10 to 30 minutes.[285–287]

A group of twenty women riding stationary bicycles three times per week for 4 weeks while being exposed to NIR lost (on their waist, hips, and thighs) an average of 8 centimeters, or 444 percent more fat (specifically on the waist, hips, and thighs) as compared to 20 women doing the same exercise without NIR.[288]

Studies on "laser liposuction" have also shown that red and NIR light therapy alone can even have significant fat loss benefits: "[PBM] achieved safe and significant girth loss sustained with eight treatments over a four-week period. The girth loss from the waist gave clinically and statistically significant cosmetic improvement."[285]

Red and NIR PBM is thought to contribute to fat loss in two ways:[289]

1. The most widely accepted view is that enhanced mitochondrial energy production increases the activity of enzymes necessary for releasing and breaking down stored body fat, like the enzyme hormone-sensitive lipase.
2. The other, more controversial, idea is that red and NIR light causes fat-cell membranes to develop transitory pores that allow stored fat to "leak" into the surrounding area, where it is removed by the lymph and blood systems.[290]

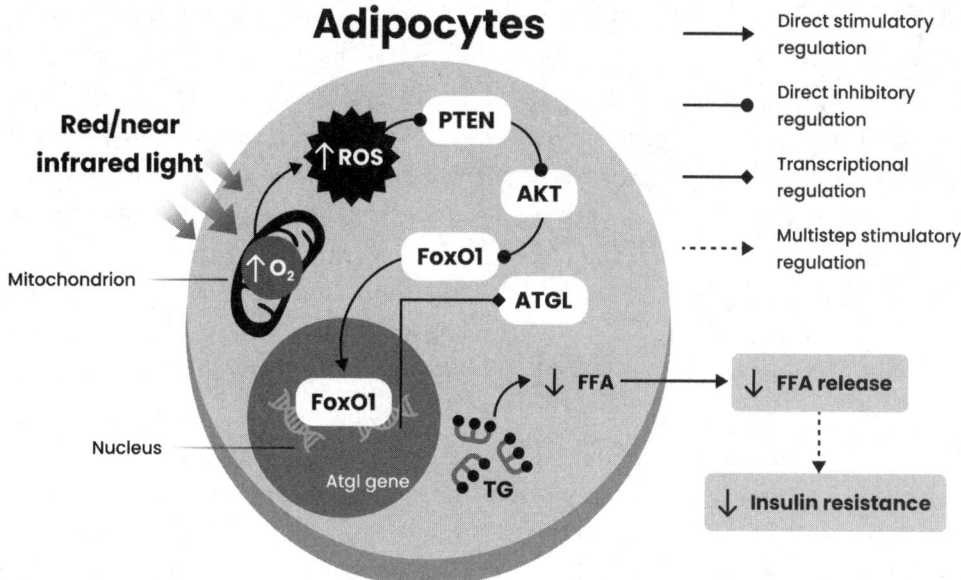

Adipocytes

Red/near infrared light

Mitochondrion

↑ROS

↑O₂

PTEN

AKT

FoxO1

ATGL

Nucleus

FoxO1

Atgl gene

TG

↓ FFA

↓ FFA release

↓ Insulin resistance

→ Direct stimulatory regulation

→• Direct inhibitory regulation

→◆ Transcriptional regulation

⤍ Multistep stimulatory regulation

Though there are clearly many studies that show that PBM can enhance fat loss, I am not a strong advocate of trying to use red and NIR light therapy *alone* to cause fat loss. I believe that red and NIR light therapy really shines (forgive the pun) when it's combined with exercise.

Some research shows that NIR light therapy can nearly *double* fat loss from exercise, as compared to the results of the same exercise alone.[271] **The group using the NIR light therapy in tandem with exercise also saw nearly *double* the improvement in insulin resistance.**

Other studies report that PBM can improve fat cell function and lower inflammation when combined with exercise compared to exercise alone.[291–293]

Light therapy also has some fascinating potential for use on "stubborn fat" areas

and even in the mythical "spot reduction."

For those not familiar with the terms "stubborn fat" and "spot reduction," I'll summarize below:

- Stubborn fat: areas where we store body fat that's hard to get rid of, no matter what we do
- Spot reduction: the idea that you can burn off fat in a specific area by doing exercise that targets that area

For the last several decades, TV infomercials have been selling us various exercise gadgets that are meant to cause fat loss in a specific area. "Use this ab cruncher and you'll shed inches of fat from your waist and stomach!" "This thigh blaster will take inches off your thighs!" This is all based on the idea of spot reduction.

It's crazy to think how many billions of dollars have been spent by consumers in the pursuit of spot reduction—mostly through various exercise devices, wraps that cause temporary water loss, and electrical stimulation devices that activate muscles in a targeted area.

Walk into any gym around the world and you're likely to find lots of men trying to burn off unwanted abdominal fat with 30-minute ab workouts, and women doing all sorts of inner- and outer-thigh exercises and "butt-toning" aerobic classes. Most of us have some area of our body that has a little excess flab, and most people think the solution to this problem is to do exercises for that specific area.

We all tend to store fat in certain areas—generally speaking, men more in the belly/lower back/love handles, and women more in the thighs and hips—so it seems sensible to pursue fat loss from those specific areas.

Indeed, we've been pursuing the goal of spot reduction for well over a century. There were the vibrating belt machines of the early 1900s, countless other machines that looked like they could double as torture devices, and of course, corsets, which have been around forever and seem to be making a comeback. The devices that we've seen come out over the last few decades are really nothing new. They're just the latest gadgets to be created in the century-long pursuit of spot reduction.

So do any of these devices really work?

The simple answer: No. Most of them are based on the general public's lack of understanding that muscle and fat are two separate and distinct tissues, and they confuse the "burning" one feels when working a muscle with the "burning" of body fat from the layer of fat on top of that muscle. Unfortunately, working a muscle in a specific area does not have a significant relationship to how much fat is burned from the adjacent fat layer. Yet, since most people don't understand that, they are gullible when told that working a muscle in a specific area will cause fat loss in that area—or, to use the words of the manufacturers of these products, that the devices will "tone," "shape," "trim," and "sculpt" a specific area of your body.

Interestingly, there have been some studies testing whether spot reduction really exists:

- A 1971 study was conducted on tennis players.[294] Tennis players' right and left arms have been consistently subjected to very different amounts of exercise over several years. Consequently, if spot reduction were a valid concept, one would expect the players' dominant arms to have thinner layers of subcutaneous fat compared to their non-dominant arms. When the researchers measured the thickness of subcutaneous fat at specific points along the players' arms, however, they found no statistically significant difference between the dominant and non-dominant arms.

- A classic 1984 study looked at fat biopsies taken from the abdominal area before and after a 27-day period in which subjects performed progressively greater numbers of sit-ups.[286] Subjects started with 140 sit-ups per day and by the end of the study they were doing 336 sit-ups per day. The group averaged 185 sit-ups a day while a control group did not exercise. Following the study, the fat cells in the abdominal area had not been reduced. There were no significant changes in fat-folds, girth, or total fat content assessed by underwater weighing. **More than 5,000 sit-ups, and zero fat loss from the stomach to show for it. That's pretty damning evidence against spot reduction.**

- In a 2007 study led by the University of Connecticut, 104 participants completed a 12-week supervised resistance-training program in which their non-dominant arm was selectively exercised.[295] MRI assessments of subcutaneous fat before and after the program revealed that fat loss was generalized across the entire body, rather than only occurring in the exercised arm.

- In 2013, an even more impressive study was published.[296] Three times per week for 12 weeks, participants were required to do about 1,000 repetitions of low-resistance activity on a leg-press machine. Here's the cool part: They only did the exercise on *one* leg and left the other one unexercised. The result? **The participants lost 5.1 percent of their body fat on average, but virtually *none* of that loss came from fat tissue in the legs. Most important, there was no difference between the leg that did all of the exercise and the leg that didn't exercise at all!** Where did the fat loss come from? It came from the upper extremities and torso.

- In short, if one can do 36,000 repetitions of an exercise with one leg and none with the other, and it doesn't produce any difference in fat in the two legs, we know that chasing "spot reduction" through "ab crunchers" and "thigh blasters" is a waste of time and money.

So the science is clear: Exercising a muscle does not cause fat loss in the adjacent fat tissue. You don't lose fat from your stomach by doing crunches or from your thighs by using a thigh machine. And for several decades, this is exactly what all respectable fitness professionals have been saying: Spot reduction is a myth!

There are a couple of reasons why this is the case:

1. There's no direct link between the underlying muscle and the adjacent fat. If working a muscle was to burn fat next to it, that fat would have to be connected to the muscle via blood vessels. Because there is no such direct connection, working a muscle has no effect on the burning of the fatty tissue adjacent to it. The exercises may strengthen the muscle responsible for those movements, but they have negligible impact on reducing the amount of fat stored there.

2. Fat is contained in fat cells in the form of triglycerides, and muscle cells cannot directly use triglycerides for energy. The fat must be broken down into glycerol and free fatty acids first; then those enter the bloodstream, where they can be carried to the muscle cells for burning. So the muscle is using up the fatty acids in the bloodstream and doesn't care whether they were released from the area right next to it or from the other side of the body.

The bottom line: Working a muscle does not impact the amount of fat in the areas near the muscle. Whether you lose fat or not comes down to overall energy balance. But you have no control over *where* your body takes that fat from. Your body will lose fat from some areas quicker than from others. This has been the consensus among educated health professionals for the last several decades, and it is what I taught for a decade.

But it may not actually be completely correct. With an understanding of *why* stubborn fat is actually stubborn, perhaps we can impact it after all.

Although most fat loss experts shun the idea of targeting fat loss in specific areas of the body, some suggest that it is possible through an approach that revolves more around burning lots of calories (not just exercising the muscle in a specific area, like the abs or thighs) combined with selectively enhancing blood flow to certain fatty areas of the body.

For example, Dr. Lonnie Lowery (a bodybuilder) and Christian Thibaudeau (a strength coach) have both developed spot-reduction protocols published on a website called T-Nation. Exercise physiologist Lyle McDonald has written a book called *The Stubborn Fat Solution*. That book presented a lot of science-backed information that explains the physiological reasons why some areas are harder to burn fat from than others. Some areas of the body store fat easily and release it poorly, for various physical and biochemical reasons. Other areas don't accumulate fat very easily, and those areas are also the easiest to reduce. That is, when someone is doing things right with their lifestyle such that they are losing body fat, the body burns fat from some areas more readily than from others. So what is going on physiologically here: Why do some areas put on fat so easily and fight so hard to get lean?

Those reasons are outlined by McDonald in his book, but here's a summary:

1. **POOR BLOOD FLOW TO CERTAIN FAT TISSUES.** Certain fatty areas of the body (most commonly, the belly and low-back areas of men, and the thighs and hips of women) receive poorer blood flow than visceral fat (fat in the center of the body around the organs). If there is little blood flow to those fat cells, they are unable to dump their fats into the blood to be burned for energy. It is impossible to lose fat if your body's fat cells cannot dump their contents into the blood, where they have the potential to be burned. Also, when there is low blood circulation to the fat cells, the potential for fat to be burned from those cells is low. Even when you're in a state where you're burning lots of body fat (i.e., on a weight-loss diet), very little of the fat you're burning will come from areas that have poor blood circulation.

2. **MUSCLE CELLS BECOME DESENSITIZED TO INSULIN AND FAT STORES BECOME HYPER-INSULIN SENSITIVE.** This is the body's way of shuttling the calories you eat away from muscle cells (where they are burned) and toward fat cells (where they are stored as fat). The aforementioned gender-specific fatty areas also tend to be more insulin sensitive and generally take up nutrients from the blood most efficiently.

3. **FAT CELLS BECOME RESISTANT TO RELEASING FAT DUE TO THEIR RECEPTORS.** Two types of adrenoceptors (receptors that respond to adrenaline) control the flow of fatty acids into and out of fat cells and the blood flow to the fat cells: Beta receptors are the "good guys" who increase fat burning and fat-tissue blood flow. Alpha-2-receptors do just the opposite: They inhibit fat-burning and fat-tissue blood flow. Stubborn fat areas have a high density of alpha-2 receptors and low density of beta receptors. So not only is there poor blood flow to these fatty areas (making it difficult for the cells to release fats into the blood to be burned), but also, the fat cells are incredibly resistant to releasing any fats into the little blood flow that is present.

McDonald's program to burn off this stubborn body fat is essentially that you do a morning protocol before breakfast whereby you boost adrenaline levels (high-intensity interval training, and taking tyrosine), take some yohimbine to inhibit the alpha receptors on your fat cells, and then do some light exercise. The idea is that this would boost adrenaline and then also allow stubborn fat cells to release more of their fats into the bloodstream. Many people have reported success using this method. (Side note: I tried it, and the yohimbine made me feel so anxious and jittery that I never wanted to do it again. It was like eight cups of coffee and what I can only imagine crack must feel like. But I seem to be particularly sensitive to the negative side effects of stimulants.)

Now, it's important to realize, as McDonald himself points out, that this is *not* true "spot reduction." This is simply for people who are already doing a calorie-restricted diet and *actively losing fat* but still have one area with some fat that won't come off. It is not spot-reducing that specific area—you are burning overall fat, but the only place left to burn it from is that specific area. While oversimplifying the nuances, basically, the idea of this protocol is just to get more blood circulation to those stubborn fat areas and pair that with exercise (burning fat) with the hope that a large portion of the energy you burn would come from fat in the stubborn fat areas rather than in other tissues. With greater blood circulation in those stubborn fat areas, and a bit of coaxing fat cells to release their stored fats, your body will have the opportunity

to release and burn more of the fatty acids stored in those tissues.

Even though this is not spot reduction *per se*, McDonald's examination of all the scientific literature on why certain fat tissues are so hard to burn was instrumental toward figuring out how to get rid of stubborn fat. The most important factors in this regard are how the cellular-receptor profile influences how easily the cell will release its fats into the bloodstream, and even more important, the blood flow to that fatty area. Poor blood flow to an area combined with cells that are resistant to giving up their fats makes fat loss from that area essentially impossible.

Science has now shown that the blood flow to a particular area might be the biggest factor of all in hindering fat loss from that area. Blood flow is critical for fat extraction. Poor blood flow equals poor fat loss. Here's a fun test that you can do to put this into practical terms: Use a forehead thermometer to take the skin temperature of different parts of your body. In particular, test the temperature of your stubborn fat areas. You'll find that these are a *lot* colder than other areas of your body. I've tested this extensively and found that generally, my lower abs/"love handles"/lower-back areas have temperatures that are a full 1 to 2° Fahrenheit lower than other areas of my body. Just prior to writing this, I told my wife about it, and she didn't believe me. She grabbed our thermometer to test it. Sure enough, if she measures in most places on her body, she gets between 97 and 99°F, but on her butt and thighs, it's between 94.7 and 95.7°F. That's 2 to 3 full degrees F lower than anywhere else on her body. This is not a coincidence. Areas where fat is hard to burn are primarily that way due to lack of blood flow to that region, and therefore they are significantly colder. Blood flow to the tissues is a huge factor.

As physiology expert Dr. Keith Frayne notes in Proceedings of the Nutrition Society: "There is evidence that adipose tissue blood flow does not increase sufficiently to allow delivery of all the fatty acids released into the systemic circulation."[297] In other words, fatty acids may indeed be getting released from the cells in our stubborn fat areas, but due to poor circulation to those areas, most of those released fats don't even make it into the bloodstream where they have the potential to be burned, so they end up getting taken right back into the fat cells they originated from, essentially being blocked in that area.

If we can somehow cause all of the blood vessels in a specific fatty area to dilate and be filled with blood, and if we can preferentially stimulate the fat cells in that area to release their glycerol and free fatty acids into the bloodstream, we will have the key to targeting fat loss in specific areas of our bodies.

Here's the key thing to understand: **Most people who have tried to lose fat in a "stubborn fat" area have been trying either to enhance localized fat burning or increase blood flow to a particular region** **through muscle contractions in the muscle next to the fat they want to burn.** As the research described above has shown, relying on muscle contractions in a specific area to burn fat next to that muscle is basically worthless.

But what if there were a truly effective way to get the fat cells in a particular area to be perfused with blood and release their fats into the bloodstream? Something that no one talking about spot reduction has yet thought of?

It turns out that red and NIR light affects both blood circulation to the area it's shined on and also stimulates the release of fatty acids from fat tissue!

Given that red and NIR light stimulates both blood circulation and the release of fatty acids from fat cells, it is reasonable to believe that it may be an effective tool for getting rid of stubborn fat. While more research is needed to confirm this, I actually developed a "stubborn fat protocol" around this several years ago and based on my experimentation with clients over the last few years, I can say with a high degree of confidence that it works extremely well when a person is in a calorie deficit. The basic idea of it is simply to pair an approach to increase blood flow to stubborn fat areas, with PBM specifically on that body area, with zone 2 endurance exercise.

Here's how to do my Stubborn Fat Protocol:

Wake up in the morning in a fasted state.

Get your body (and especially the stubborn fat area) warm. A hot shower or sauna is great. Then put on clothes to stay warm, and maybe even use extra clothing on the stubborn fat areas.

Do some light warm-up exercise (walking, resistance bands, yoga, calisthenics, and the like).

Put on a flexible, battery-powered LED device (like the ones I'll recommend in the Device Selection Guide) on your stubborn fat area. Keep it on during the following exercise for roughly 20 to 40 minutes (depending on the device). As an added bonus, it will also produce some heat in that area to keep more blood circulating there during exercise.

Walk for 30 to 60 minutes at a Zone 2 pace (you should be able to maintain a conversation but feel like you're working). During this period, keep your body warm, especially the stubborn fat area, to maintain optimal blood circulation. You can add a neoprene wrap to create extra heat and circulation.

Optional: After the walk, do 5 to 10 minutes of high-intensity interval training (often referred to as HIIT). Do fast-paced bodyweight exercises like squats, pushups, burpees, jumps, jumping rope, running, or cycling. A simple approach: 20- to 45-second bursts of high-intensity effort with 10 to 30 seconds of rest between bursts.

Ideally, wait at least one hour before eating.

Do this protocol in the mornings during a fat loss phase (i.e., a period when you are actively on a weight-loss regimen and losing fat), and you'll likely notice that you are slimming down in those stubborn fat areas more than you ever have before.

This isn't the only way that you can use red and NIR light therapy to support fat loss. Some studies have shown that using the light in tandem with exercise (before or after) on the muscles used during the workout (as opposed to on fat areas) also leads to increased overall fat loss.

Please note that red and NIR light therapy doesn't actually burn the fat by itself. The mechanism appears to be that it causes the fat cells to release their stored fat into the bloodstream where it can (potentially) be burned for energy. One still must be in a calorie deficit to have actual fat loss. Your overall diet and lifestyle must be conducive to overall net fat loss, or you will just put the fat right back into the fat cells it was released from. Please don't think that light therapy alone will cause fat loss. Think of it as a tool to *amplify* the fat loss effects from diet and exercise. Nevertheless, this technology can be used to greatly accelerate loss of overall body fat, and even "stubborn fat." Overall, the research is clear that red and NIR light can be a powerful tool to support your fat loss efforts.

So with a red and NIR light therapy device of your own, you can potentially achieve significant weight loss and fat reduction in the comfort of your own home.

There's an entire industry built around scaring people out of sun exposure. How many times have you heard that the sun causes skin cancer? Have you ever been scolded by a dermatologist for not using sunscreen or spending too much time in the sun? The idea that regular unprotected sun exposure causes skin cancer, particularly melanoma, in fair-skinned people is pretty much considered common sense at this point.

In a nutshell, this view holds that UV radiation is carcinogenic and contributes to skin cancer through three main mechanisms:[298]

1. UV radiation (mostly UVB) is absorbed by the DNA of melanocytes, basal-layer keratinocytes, and other skin cells, directly damaging it and increasing the likelihood of mutations that give rise to cancer.
2. UV radiation (mostly UVA) leads to the formation of free radicals within the skin, increasing oxidative stress and indirectly damaging DNA.
3. UV radiation inhibits immune surveillance within the skin, which is the process through which our immune system seeks out and destroys cells that have mutations, are at an increased risk of becoming cancerous, or are already cancerous.

In other words, the link between sunlight and skin cancer comes from the ability of UV radiation to damage DNA (directly and indirectly through oxidative stress) and inhibit the ability of our immune system to seek out and destroy cancerous skin cells.

While this conventional view provides a simple and appealing explanation, it falls short of appreciating the complexity of our biology and the sun itself. The truth is that the relationship between sunshine and skin cancer is far more nuanced than many authoritative bodies would have you believe.

Several meta-analyses of studies that connect sun exposure history and habits to melanoma have found that chronic sun exposure is not associated with an increased risk of melanoma, but irregular exposure and severe sunburns are most important.[299–301] However, long-term chronic sun exposure is linked with the formation of basal cell carcinomas.

There are many reasons for this, with one of the most important being the simple fact that sun exposure doesn't intrinsically cause DNA damage. You don't get damaged by exposure; you get damaged by a complex interplay between your inborn resilience to UV radiation, your DNA-repair capacities, and the overall dose of your UV exposure.

This is where PBM comes into play. It's been well-established that red and NIR light has protective action toward our skin, and is able to increase our resilience against UV-induced DNA damage and facilitate repair processes afterward.[302]

For example, when light-skinned adults received regular red-light treatment corresponding to 10 minutes of sun exposure at 10 a.m. in the tropics, their skin became 33 to 80 percent more resistant to the damaging effects of UV radiation.[303] In follow-up work by the lab, it was discovered that NIR had even stronger effects.[302]

Other research has suggested that the benefits of NIR are both long-lasting and cumulative.[304] The protection against UV radiation granted by NIR is noticeable almost immediately and lasts for at least 24 hours, and the extent of protection increases with increasing infrared exposure.

Moreover, thanks to the superior penetrating ability of NIR through the atmosphere, you can easily increase the ratio of infrared to UV radiation that you're exposed to by having most of your sun exposure occur in the morning and evening. Around the equator, this would be before 9:00 a.m. and after 4:00 p.m.

Nature is funny like that. If you were to spend all day outside, you'd naturally precondition your skin with an abundance of red and NIR light in the morning, before the UV radiation intensity picked up, and you'd be hit again in the evening to help kick-start cellular-repair processes.

Of course, you can do that in your home, too, with a PBM device. The studies showing UV protection used red and NIR light therapy 5 days per week for 1 to 3 weeks, with each session providing 60 mW/cm² for 2 minutes and 40 seconds (5 J/cm²).

Regular use of red and NIR light acts very much like sunscreen for your skin, protecting against UV radiation and the potential consequence of getting too much, which is *sunburn*.

BOLSTER GUT HEALTH AND DIVERSIFY THE MICROBIOME

Everyone has battled with an upset stomach, gas, bloating, constipation, or diarrhea at some point in their life. It's not fun, and for some people, it's never-ending.

Irritable bowel syndrome is a chronic functional disorder of the intestinal tract with no known biomarker for diagnosis (e.g., there is no intestinal damage). It's basically a cluster of symptoms like abdominal pain, bloating, and a change in bowel habits (constipation or diarrhea) that comes and goes, with several possible causes.

Inflammatory bowel disease describes a group of disorders where the intestinal tract becomes damaged and inflamed. It's believed to be the result of an immune attack against both the intestinal cells (autoimmune) and the otherwise benign microbes and food particles within the gut (not autoimmune). The two most common types of inflammatory bowel disease are Crohn's disease and ulcerative colitis.

Red and NIR light have been found to play a role in gut health. NIR exposure on the abdomen of mice with inflammatory bowel disease significantly reduced the ex-tent of intestinal damage (lesions) and degree of inflammation, and to be more effective than treatment with a commonly prescribed steroidal anti-inflammatory medication (prednisone).[305]

Studies have also found that abdominal irradiation with NIR light can increase microbial diversity and the proportion of known beneficial bacteria in both mice and humans.[306, 307] Such changes in humans have been observed after several months of using 904-nm NIR light three times per week.[308, 309]

Bolster Gut Health and Diversify the Microbiome

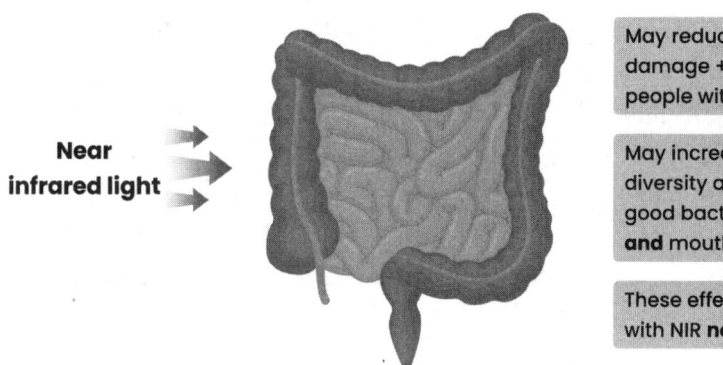

Near infrared light

May reduce intestinal damage + inflammation in people with IBD

May increase microbial diversity and lead to more good bacteria in the gut **and** mouth

These effects were found with NIR **not** red light

This is a brand-new field of research called photobiomics. Researchers have reported benefits to the gut microbiome with NIR but not red light, which makes sense considering the greater penetrative ability of NIR into the body. Having said that, it is unlikely that significant quantities even of NIR light would penetrate into the intestines while shined on the abdomen, though it may be possible in individuals with low body fat and perhaps with direct skin contact and pressure (e.g., pushing the device into the abdomen to compress the tissues). However, even if the light doesn't penetrate directly into the intestines, it's still possible that red and NIR light could alter the microbiome through systemic effects (which we'll discuss shortly). It is not yet clear if the light needs to reach the intestines to have an effect, or whether the benefits are due to the systemic anti-inflammatory effects of light absorbed by superficial layers, going on to affect the host response to the gut bacteria.

On a final note, there's also good data that red and NIR light beneficially affect the microbiome in the mouth.[310] One study found that the light not only increased beneficial bacterial counts but also reduced inflammatory signaling molecules within the mouth.[311]

REDUCE SYMPTOMS OF NEUROPATHY

All of the benefits of red and NIR light for neurons also play out in our peripheral nervous system, which includes all the nerves outside our brains and spinal cords. Whether it's caused by diabetes, injury, medications, or some other reason, many people suffer with pain caused by neuropathy (nerve damage outside the brain and spinal cord).

Essentially, red and NIR light help the nerves heal. In one study, applying 660-nm LED (7.5 mW/cm² for 1 hour) led to significant nerve regeneration following injury, as well as greater antioxidant levels in the surrounding fluid.[312]

Systematic reviews of people with diabetes-induced neuropathy report that red and NIR light (50 to 150 mW/cm² for 5 to 15 minutes two to four times per week) reduces nerve pain and improves nerve conduction velocity (nerve function).[313, 314]

Similarly, an RCT of patients with chemotherapy-induced peripheral neuropathy found that applying NIR light (800 to 970 nm) for 30 minutes three times per week led to a 32-percent reduction in overall neuropathy symptoms after 4 weeks and 52-percent reduction after 8 weeks.[315]

IMPROVE LYMPHATIC FUNCTION

Emerging research highlights the potential of NIR light to enhance lymphatic drainage in the brain. This process is crucial for clearing macromolecules like amyloid-beta, whose accumulation is linked to neurodegenerative diseases such as Alzheimer's. Meningeal lymphatic vessels play a central role in maintaining brain homeostasis by transporting cerebrospinal and interstitial fluids to cervical lymph nodes. Disruptions in this system can exacerbate conditions like Alzheimer's by promoting amyloid-beta deposition.

Since 2018, studies have demonstrated that NIR can significantly improve cerebral lymphatic drainage. For instance, in mouse models of Alzheimer's, NIR (32 J/cm²) not only enhanced amyloid-beta clearance but also increased its transport to peripheral lymph nodes.[316] Other studies have found benefits with just 5 to 10 J/cm² of NIR,[317] and NIR-induced vasodilation was identified as a key mechanism, relaxing lymphatic vessels and increasing their permeability to macromolecules. This relaxation, along with improved mitochondrial ATP production from enhanced blood oxygen saturation, likely boosts lymphatic contractility, accelerating waste clearance.

Further studies revealed PBM's capacity to facilitate the removal of other substances, such as gold nanorods and red blood cells, through the lymphatic vessels, suggesting broader therapeutic applications.[318] By promoting blood-brain barrier permeability and improving lymphatic pumping, NIR offers a promising noninvasive approach to support brain health and potentially delay neurodegenerative disease progression.

HELP YOUR PETS

Literally everything we've discussed about light therapy applies to your pets, too. All of these benefits—for the skin, wound healing, joints, brain health, and more—aren't just for humans. Your pet dog, cat, or hamster can also benefit from PBM.

A 2023 systematic review documented 45 red and NIR light therapy studies involving common domestic animals, most of which involved dogs (the others being cats and horses).[319] These studies found profound benefits for musculoskeletal conditions, skin and wound healing, pain reduction, and neurological conditions, all at doses similar to what you'd use on yourself.

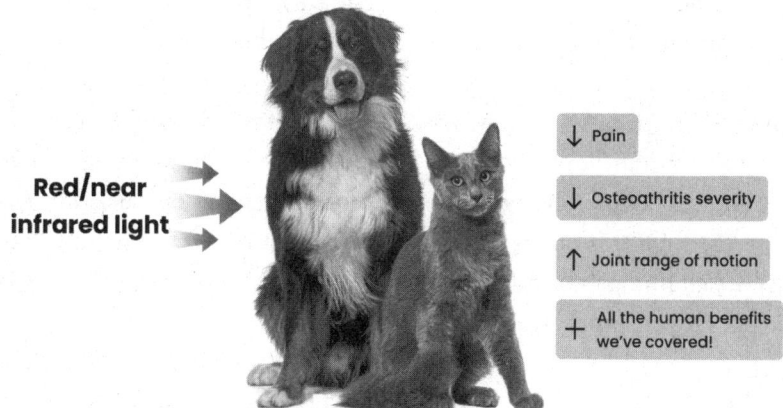

Red/near infrared light

↓ Pain

↓ Osteoathritis severity

↑ Joint range of motion

+ All the human benefits we've covered!

This makes sense, because your pet runs on the same basic mammalian biology that you do. They rely on mitochondria, and they have all the same organs. The differences between us and them are really quite small when it comes to red and NIR light. Much of the laboratory research started in mice and rats, after all!

To illustrate this point, let's look at a randomized controlled trial of dogs with moderate-to-severe osteoarthritis.[320] One of the most difficult things to witness is your best friend having trouble moving around and suffering chronic pain as a result of their aging joints. Just 3 weeks of daily red and NIR light therapy significantly reduced pain, reduced osteoarthritis severity, and improved joint range of motion. Benefits were observed as early as one week after starting.

IMPROVE BRAIN HEALTH AND FIGHT INFECTIONS BY COMBINING PBM WITH METHYLENE BLUE

Methylene blue started off as a textile dye, moved on to be used as a medical staining reagent, was then found to treat malaria, and has since been used to treat a variety of medical conditions.[321, 322] One emerging area of research is its ability to treat diseases of the brain through its potentiation of energy production within mitochondria.

Typically, mitochondria produce energy by having electron donor and acceptor molecules transport electrons through four protein complexes, which then produce a proton gradient to power adenosine triphosphate (ATP) synthase, the enzyme that generates cellular energy. Energy production through this entire electron-transport chain has the side effect of producing free radicals and contributes to oxidative stress.

Methylene blue is able to take an electron from protein complex I and transfer it directly to complex IV, thereby reducing oxidative stress and facilitating energy production even when mitochondrial function is impaired.[323] It also upregulates Nrf2 and the antioxidant response element, further bolstering mitochondrial antioxidant defenses.[324]

Given that red and NIR light increase the activity of complex IV within mitochondria, some researchers have proposed that combining these two modalities would have the best outcomes.[325] Methylene blue transfers electrons directly to the red and NIR light-activated cytochrome C oxidase, giving mitochondrial energy production a one-two punch to increase the efficiency.

The combination of methylene blue and red and NIR light really took off in the field of neurology due to the ability of methylene blue to cross the blood-brain barrier and affect neurons, combined with the transcranial potential of NIR.[326] Both modalities work primarily through their effect on the mitochondria in neurons, which are known to be impaired in the most common neurological diseases:[325]

- Alzheimer's disease
- Traumatic brain injury
- Stroke
- Depression
- Parkinson's disease

Both methylene blue application and PBM have shown promise in the treatment of these neurological conditions, and now research is beginning to investigate how they might work together to be even better than each is individually. In animals, for example, unpredictable chronic stress impaired learning and memory, but treatment with 0.04 mg/kg body weight of methylene blue plus 8 J/cm² of 810-nm NIR reversed these impairments.[327]

There's also been an emerging interest in combining methylene blue with red and NIR light for use against COVID-19 and infectious diseases in general. It's already been established that methylene blue alone ameliorates COVID-19 at virtually every stage of the pathophysiological process:[328]

- Inhibits viral entry into cells
- Reduces viral replication within cells

- Inactivates viruses
- Reduces oxidative stress and inflammation
- Reduces hypoxia

At the same time, as we've already discussed, red and NIR light therapy has shown massive potential for reducing the severity of infection, particularly the exaggerated inflammatory response to COVID-19 known as a cytokine storm.[329]

Recently, these modalities have been combined in a yearlong pilot study to treat COVID-19.[330] Individuals infected with COVID-19 treated themselves with 163 mW/cm² of 660-nm red light in their nose and mouth for 5 minutes after consuming 1 to 2 mg/kg of methylene blue (maximum of 200 mg). The average recovery time was just 4 days and the measured viral loads dropped rapidly. Moreover, most of the participants didn't experience long-term symptoms from the COVID infection (what's been called "long COVID").

Overall, the combination of methylene blue with red and NIR light therapy offers a very promising treatment for any condition in which mitochondrial dysfunction is implicated. This is because they work in a synergistic manner to amplify mitochondrial energy production even in the face of distress. Neurological and immunological conditions have been the pioneering areas of research in this regard, but it's likely that many more will soon follow.

PBM also has the ability to benefit overall health and cellular function throughout the body in a way that supports metabolic health, immune health, cellular energy production, and likely contributes to overall healthspan and longevity.

There are several ways (some only recently discovered, and probably some that are yet to be discovered) by which red and NIR light promote overall whole-organism health, resilience, disease resistance, and help to extend healthspan and potentially lifespan. There are several physiological pathways that stand out as being instrumental to the systemic effects of PBM—the effects on inflammation and immune function, metabolic health, and perhaps especially on releasing stem cells into circulation. Let's take a closer look at each of these.

Inflammation and Immune Function

"Inflamm-aging"—the chronic, low-grade inflammation that increases with age—is now recognized as a fundamental mechanism underlying major killers like heart disease, cancer, Alzheimer's disease, autoimmune conditions, and depression. This inflammatory cascade doesn't just contribute to individual diseases; it accelerates the entire aging process at the cellular level.

Red and NIR light therapy powerfully combats this inflamm-aging process by modulating immune responses and reducing inflammatory cytokines such as IL-1β, IL-6, TNF-α, and NF-κB, while boosting anti-inflammatory mediators like IL-10. Most importantly, as we've discussed, it shifts macrophages from a pro-inflammatory M1 state to an anti-inflammatory M2 state.

Macrophages act as the body's cleanup crew. M1 macrophages rush to injury sites like an emergency response team, attacking invaders and clearing damaged tissue using pro-inflammatory cytokines. However, these weapons are like fire hoses—effective for immediate threats but damaging if left running too long. M2 macrophages then take over, releasing anti-inflammatory cytokines and growth factors that promote repair and regeneration. Without proper M1-to-M2 transition, inflammation becomes chronic and self-sustaining, directly contributing to cellular damage and accelerated aging.

Through mechanisms such as the activation of mitochondrial function, reduced oxidative stress, and modulation of signaling pathways like NF-κB, red and NIR light encourages M2 macrophages to step in sooner.[334] This shift helps prevent the chronic M1 dominance that can lead to ongoing tissue damage and a cycle of unresolved inflammation that accelerates biological aging.

By resolving chronic inflammation, red

and NIR light therapy can help break the cycle of tissue damage and repair, which is especially critical for conditions like arthritis, neuroinflammation, and autoimmune diseases. Also, the therapy's ability to support the repair team (M2) without completely shutting down the demolition crew (M1) ensures that acute inflammatory responses, which are necessary for fighting infections and injuries, remain intact.

This anti-inflammatory effect is remarkably comprehensive, impacting cells and organ systems throughout the body, from joints to major organs like the brain. Studies suggest that red and NIR light therapy may be effective for autoimmune diseases characterized by excessive inflammation, including lupus, rheumatoid arthritis, multiple sclerosis, and Sjogren's syndrome.[231, 335] For example, research has shown that red and NIR light can provide anti-inflammatory effects equivalent to nonsteroidal anti-inflammatory drugs, but without the associated side effects.[201]

This is likely one of the most profound ways that PBM likely translates into improved overall systemic health, reduced risk of disease, extension of healthspan, and potentially adding years to your life.

Melatonin

PBM increases both pineal and non-pineal melatonin levels throughout the body. This light-stimulated melatonin production could explain many of PBM's widespread benefits:

Universal cellular protection: Since virtually all cells contain mitochondria, light-stimulated melatonin provides antioxidant protection throughout the body.

Inflammation control: Melatonin's anti-inflammatory properties could explain PBM's systemic effects.

Longevity effects: Melatonin protects mitochondrial DNA from oxidative damage—a key aging factor.

Metabolic benefits: Melatonin plays a key role in mitochondrial function and metabolic efficiency.

Neuroprotection: Local neuronal melatonin production provides crucial protection against neurodegeneration.

This mechanism makes evolutionary sense—our ancestors received abundant red and NIR light from the sun, which may have been a primary driver of cellular melatonin production. Modern indoor living has largely eliminated this stimulus, creating a potential cellular melatonin deficit that PBM can help restore.

Metabolic Health

Red and NIR light therapy demonstrate significant effects on metabolic health, particularly through improvements in glucose metabolism and insulin sensitivity. As we've already explored, several studies show that PBM enhances glucose uptake into cells and improves insulin sensitivity. While the exact interplay of mechanisms remains under investigation, the clinical outcomes—improved blood sugar control and enhanced insulin sensitivity—are consistently observed.

Beyond glucose metabolism, we've also explored how many studies have demonstrated that PBM can improve body composition, enhancing both lean muscle mass and promoting fat loss. Research has shown that when combined with exercise, PBM can produce more significant reductions in body fat (and amplify improvements in insulin sensitivity) while preserving or even increasing lean muscle mass compared to exercise alone. These body composition improvements—combined with better glucose control and insulin sensitivity—have far-reaching implications for metabolic health. By addressing both blood sugar regulation and body composition, PBM offers a promising approach for managing the interconnected epidemics of obesity, metabolic syndrome, and type 2 diabetes, while reducing the risk of related conditions including heart disease, dementia, and various cancers.

Stem Cells and Cellular Regeneration

PBM's ability to stimulate and mobilize stem cells into circulation potentially represents one of its most profound mechanisms relevant to healthspan and longevity. To understand why PBM's effects on stem cells could be so significant for longevity, it's crucial to understand the central role that stem cell decline plays in biological aging itself. As we age, our stem cell populations progressively diminish in both number and function—a process called stem cell exhaustion, which is recognized as one of the primary hallmarks of aging. Biological aging can be seen as actually revolving around the progressive accumulation of dysfunctional, damaged, and senescent cells throughout our tissues, along with the outright loss of functional cells. In a sense, this cellular deterioration *is* the aging process. Stem cells help combat this accumulation of damaged cells by continuously replacing these problematic cells with fresh, functional ones. The problem is that as stem cell function declines, damaged cells accumulate unchecked while functional cells are lost without replacement.

This decline begins surprisingly early, with stem cell function showing substantial decreases starting around age 30 and accelerating with each decade of life. By our 60s and 70s, we have markedly fewer circulating stem cells and significantly reduced regenerative capacity compared to our youth. Some research has suggested that by the age of 60, we have only about 25 percent of our youthful level of stem cell production. (There is also a shift in the types of stem cells, where for example, with aging, our blood stem cells shift from producing a balanced mix of immune cells to producing more inflammatory cells [myeloid] and fewer infection-fighting cells [lymphoid], which weakens our immune system and increases inflammation.) This dramatic reduction directly correlates with our body's diminished ability to repair tissues, fend off infections, recover from injury, and maintain optimal organ function as we age.

The consequences are far-reaching: slower wound healing, reduced muscle mass and bone density, declining cognitive function, weakened immune responses, and increased susceptibility to age-related diseases. In essence, much of what we experience as "normal aging" is actually the result of our body's repair and regeneration systems becoming progressively less effective due to stem cell depletion.

This is why interventions that can restore or maintain stem cell populations are so promising for extending both healthspan (the period of life spent in good health) and potentially lifespan itself. When stem cells are abundant and functional, tissues can repair damage more effectively, inflammation is better controlled, and the cellular dysfunction that drives aging can be prevented or reversed.

Direct stem cell therapies have shown remarkable potential for treating age-related conditions from heart disease to neurodegeneration. The exciting possibility with PBM is that it might offer a way to continuously stimulate your body's own stem cell production and mobilization, potentially providing ongoing anti-aging benefits.

Given that PBM promotes the activation and release of stem cells into circulation, it's possible that PBM could act in a similar way to actual "stem cell therapy" where millions of stem cells are injected into the body to stimulate healing of damaged cells and injured tissues. Traditional stem cell injections typically involve 10 to 200 million cells per treatment at costs ranging from $5,000 to $50,000 per session, with patients often limited to one to three treatments per year due to cost and medical considerations.

To get a sense of the magnitude of change from PBM, in one human study, applying NIR light (808 nm) to the bone marrow in both tibias increased circulating CD34+ stem cells from 7.8 percent to 29.5 percent of total mononuclear cells in the circulating blood—a nearly 3.8-fold increase. And this wasn't just for a few minutes or hours—the levels peaked 2 to 4 days later and then gradually returned to baseline.[336] (For reference, CD34+ stem cells can differentiate into all types of blood cells—red blood cells, white blood cells, platelets—as well as endothelial cells that line blood vessels, and some other tissue types.) I was curious to translate this into absolute numbers to see how it compares to adding tens of millions of stem cells via direct injection. With some rough math, it's clear that PBM increased CD34+ stem cells by at least several million additional stem cells. Doing this on a regular basis—keeping your circulating stem cells at levels closer to, let's say, 15 million circulating CD34+ stem cells instead of 8 million—logically could have a highly significant impact on the rate of biological aging (the net balance of damage/regeneration) occurring in many organ systems of the body.

(However, an important distinction here is that stem cell therapy generally focuses on mesenchymal stem cells, which differentiate more into muscle, tendon, cartilage, and bone, whereas CD34+ hematopoietic stem cells generally differentiate into red blood cells, white blood cells, and endothelial cells. Though it's important to keep in mind that this is just one study looking specifically at CD34+ cells in circulation, and it's important to note that PBM can also stimulate mesenchymal stem cells and may also trigger their release into circulation.)

While PBM likely produces a much smaller magnitude of stem cell mobilization, and more research is needed about the types of stem cells it helps release into circulation, it offers unique advantages over stem cell injections not only in cost, but through frequency and cumulative effects. Whereas stem cell injections might be done once or perhaps a few times per year, PBM potentially allows for hundreds of treatments per year. Think of it as the difference between massive megadoses of vitamins a few times per year versus consistent daily supplementation.

But there's an important caveat to consider: As we age, our internal stem cell pools become progressively smaller. This means that in older individuals, mobilizing these depleted pools through PBM

may yield diminishing returns compared to younger people. In this context, direct stem cell injections—which introduce large numbers of typically younger, more vigorous cells—may offer unique advantages for older adults whose own stem cell reserves have become compromised. That said, PBM appears to work on multiple levels beyond just mobilization. Research suggests that PBM can actually help maintain and rejuvenate the stem cell pools themselves by improving mitochondrial function, reducing cellular senescence markers, and enhancing the self-renewal capacity of existing stem cells. This means PBM may not just be mobilizing whatever stem cells you have left—it may actually be helping to restore them to a more youthful, functional state.

Also, let's remember that PBM works through dual mechanisms: It both mobilizes stem cells systemically into circulation *and* directly stimulates local stem cells (including mesenchymal stem cells) within the tissues receiving light exposure. This means targeted PBM treatment of specific body areas needing repair can activate local stem cell populations while simultaneously promoting systemic stem cell release. So if you use devices that can cover specific areas of your body that need healing, *and* you pair that with the methods described later in the book to stimulate stem cell release into circulation, PBM creates a comprehensive approach to cellular regeneration that works through both local and systemic mechanisms.

All of this is very speculative, but the key point is that PBM does indeed stimulate measurable increases in stem cells inside your body, and this can result in significant benefits in regenerating injured cells throughout the body.

It's likely that this is a powerful approach for preventing the accumulation of damaged cells and tissues in many systems of the body, and could also be combined with stem cell injections to create a synergistic regenerative protocol much better than either on their own. (Note: There is, in fact, abundant research that red and NIR light synergizes with stem cell injections when they are used together, as many practitioners do.)

Ultimately, the systemic activation of stem cells through PBM may turn out to be one of its most profound contributions to health. It doesn't just treat isolated problems—it engages the body's innate healing systems to promote comprehensive repair and regeneration, making it a powerful tool for overall health and longevity.

CHAPTER SUMMARY

The breadth of benefits of PBM is truly astounding. From facial anti-aging and hair regrowth to arthritis relief and enhanced muscle recovery, from improved body composition and metabolic health to pain management and wound healing, to reduced chronic inflammation, PBM demonstrates therapeutic potential across virtually every system in the body.

Whether you're dealing with chronic pain, seeking to optimize athletic performance, wanting to improve skin appearance, struggling with hair loss, managing inflammatory conditions, or simply looking to enhance overall wellness, PBM offers evidence-based benefits that can meaningfully improve quality of life.

Beyond all the specific treatment goals, the systemic effects we explored—stem cell mobilization, reduced chronic inflammation, enhanced immune function, and improved metabolic health—also suggest that regular PBM use may be one of the most accessible interventions available to enhance healthspan and longevity. PBM doesn't just provide symptomatic relief of various kinds of problems—it supports key biological processes that influence how well you age. While there are no studies directly testing PBM for longevity in humans, the types of improvements we know it creates in overall metabolic and systemic health—improved mitochondrial function, reduced oxidative stress, reduced systemic inflammation, better insulin sensitivity and blood glucose control, improved body composition, and increased circulating stem cells—are well-established in their relationship to disease prevention and longevity.

This means that PBM offers something truly unique in the wellness landscape. It provides tangible benefits you can see and feel in the short term, combined with profound systemic effects that may support optimal health and longevity over the long haul. Your 20-minute session targeting facial skin isn't just a skin-deep treatment that affects how you look; it's also simultaneously working to slow biological aging in your body, by mobilizing stem cells throughout your body, reducing chronic inflammation, optimizing metabolic function, and enhancing immune health. Few other interventions can claim to deliver both immediate, noticeable improvements and comprehensive cellular and metabolic optimization that may influence how well you age and resist disease over decades to come.

CHAPTER FOUR

The Biphasic Dose Response

Biological systems frequently exhibit predictable responses to certain types of stimuli that follow what's known as a biphasic dose response: a situation in which low doses produce some degree of measurable beneficial effects, progressively larger doses may produce better effects, up to a point, and extremely large doses far in excess of that threshold produce reduced benefits or even harmful effects.

The biphasic dose response, often described as the Arndt-Schulz law, has an intriguing history. In the late 1800s, at the University of Greifswald, a pharmacologist named Hugo Schulz was studying how poisons affect yeast cells. His experiments involved exposing yeast cultures to different concentrations of common poisons like bromine, iodine, mercury, and arsenic, then measured their metabolic activity.[1] What he found was surprising: Very low doses of these typically toxic substances actually stimulated yeast metabolism slightly. This went against the

common thinking that poisons were simply harmful at any dose.

Collaborating with Rudolf Arndt, Schulz went on to formulate what became known as the Arndt-Schulz law: Weak stimuli enhance biological activity, stronger stimuli increase it up to an optimal peak, and doses beyond that suppress activity, eventually causing harm. This laid the foundation for what we now call hormesis—the idea how moderate stress can trigger beneficial adaptations in biological organisms that make them stronger and healthier rather than deteriorating their health.

A classic example of hormesis is exercise. When we work out, we impose controlled mechanical and metabolic stress on our muscles. This triggers cellular responses through key pathways like nuclear factor erythroid 2-related factor 2 (Nrf2) and AMPK that enhance metabolic health and make the internal antioxidant system more robust, helping it to fend off free radicals (i.e., protecting the cell from damage from future exposures to free radicals). During recovery, the body doesn't just return to baseline—it overcompensates by building stronger systems, which includes things like increasing mitochondria, boosting protein synthesis, and enhancing antioxidant defenses.

However, if the dose of the hormetic stressor is too large (for example, taking a person who can barely walk a mile and forcing them to run a marathon), it won't result in health benefits—it will only cause damage. The same stressor that was beneficial to health at a lower dose becomes harmful at a very high dosage that exceeds the organism's ability to adapt to that stimulus.

This principle operates through distinct response zones that form a biphasic (two-phase) curve resembling an inverted U-shape. Based on stimulus intensity or dose, the biological system responds in different ways:

1. **SUB-THRESHOLD ZONE:** At very low doses, biological systems show minimal response, as the stimulus intensity fails to overcome intrinsic cellular resistance mechanisms and to adequately provoke a "stress" on the system.

2. **STIMULATION ZONE:** As doses increase, biological functions enhance through activation of cellular signaling cascades, upregulation of protective proteins, and optimization of metabolic pathways.

3. **OPTIMAL ZONE:** Within this narrow window, peak beneficial responses occur through maximized efficiency of cellular processes, optimal protein synthesis, and enhanced energy production.

4. **INHIBITION ZONE:** Beyond optimal levels, increasing doses begin to overwhelm cellular adaptive mechanisms, leading to decreased function through disruption of homeostatic processes.

5. **TOXICITY ZONE:** At excessive doses, cellular damage occurs through mechanisms including oxidative stress, membrane disruption, and protein denaturation.

This response pattern operates across multiple biological scales, from molecular interactions to systemic responses. Like exercise, photobiomodulation (PBM) operates with a biphasic dose response—too little of a dose and nothing happens; too large of a dose and you negate the benefits or potentially cause harm. You have to be in the "Goldilocks Zone" of dosing to get the benefits.

Dr. Hamblin and colleagues describe it like this:[2]

Simply put, it suggests that if insufficient energy is applied, there will be no response (because the minimum threshold has not been met), and if more energy is applied, then a threshold is crossed and biostimulation is achieved. However, when too much energy is applied, then the stimulation disappears and is replaced by bioinhibition.

A comprehensive review by Huang et al. (2009) echoed this idea:[1]

Although the underlying mechanism of [PBM] is still not completely understood, in vitro studies, animal experiments and clinical studies have all tended to indicate that [PBM] delivered at low doses may produce a better result when compared to the same light delivered at high doses.

The biphasic dose response in PBM is typically represented by an inverted U-shaped curve. On this curve:

- The x-axis represents the dose; the dose delivered depends on the intensity as well as the duration of light exposure.
- The y-axis represents the biological response (e.g., tissue healing, growth-factor expression, and other target physiological effects).

The basic idea here is that there exists an optimal range of light exposure that produces the most significant therapeutic benefits. Below this, the dose can be so small that no meaningful benefit occurs, and well above it, harm can occur. So the overall concept looks like this:

- Low doses: When the light exposure is too low and delivered for too short a time, it may be insufficient to stimulate the desired cellular responses.
- Optimal doses: In between the range of too low and too high is the therapeutic window where dosages are optimal to elicit beneficial effects.
- High doses: Excessive light exposure can potentially lead to adverse effects, such as increased inflammation, tissue damage, or cellular death.

Using the skin as an example, according to Hamblin,[3]

Fluences in the range of tens of J/cm^2 are likely to be protective and overall beneficial to the skin, while fluences in the range of hundreds of J/cm^2 are likely to be damaging and overall deleterious to the skin. The same would apply for irradiance parameters.

The basic idea here is that moderate doses of PBM are ideal to stimulate benefits, but it's possible that such a large dose of PBM starts becoming less beneficial, or even harmful. That's the biphasic dose response in a nutshell.

But why exactly does this happen? What's going on at the cellular level that makes very large doses of light potentially harmful? There are a few key mechanisms that help explain this "too much of a good thing" effect:

1. Excessive reactive oxygen species (ROS): Like exercise, PBM generates beneficial ROS in small amounts that trigger antioxidant defenses. However, excessive doses can overwhelm the body's capacity to neutralize free radicals, causing oxidative damage instead of benefits.

2. Cellular overheating: High light doses can raise cellular temperature above optimal levels, activating heat shock proteins that shut down energy production and, at extreme temperatures, deactivate key antioxidant enzymes like catalase and glutathione reductase.

3. Excessive nitric oxide (NO): While beneficial in moderate amounts for blood flow and cellular signaling, excessive NO from very high doses can potentially form peroxynitrite—a toxic free radical—and interfere with mitochondrial energy production.[4]

4. Activation of cell death pathways: Extremely high doses may trigger apoptosis (programmed cell death) rather than

beneficial adaptation, similar to how extreme exercise can cause severe muscle damage.[2, 5]

It is also likely that these pathways are intertwined and it's several of these pathways acting together, rather than just one of them. Nevertheless, the key concept here is that much like overdoing physical activity, you can cause harm if you overdo the dose of PBM.

All of this seems pretty straightforward. However, the issue of the biphasic dose response—while clear and well-established in areas like physical exercise—happens to be one of the most contentious and controversial areas in PBM science. As you're about to see, different experts in the field have very different views about it.

But before diving into the debate, let's take a closer look at the evidence for its existence in PBM.

Numerous studies on PBM in a wide variety of contexts have shown that by overdoing the dose, you negate the benefits or may even cause harm.[4]

THE EVIDENCE SUPPORTING THE BIPHASIC DOSE RESPONSE OF PBM

A number of lines of evidence—particularly from in vitro experiments and animal studies, but also some human evidence—have shown that this biphasic dose response takes place with PBM. Let's briefly examine some of the key evidence

to support the existence of the biphasic dose response.

IN VITRO (CELL CULTURE) STUDIES have shown repeatedly that larger doses of PBM can result in worse responses, or harm, relative to smaller doses (and this research also offers mechanistic insights into the biphasic response at a molecular level):

- **CELL PROLIFERATION:** Fibroblast studies show that proliferation peaks at 2 to 4 J/cm² but declines below baseline at doses >10 J/cm².[6]
- **STEM CELLS:** Doses of 0.5 to 3 J/cm² enhance stem cell proliferation, while slightly higher doses (3 to 6 J/cm²) induce differentiation. Excessive doses (>10 J/cm²) impair both processes.[7]
- **ADENOSINE TRIPHOSPHATE (ATP) PRODUCTION:** Moderate doses increase ATP production by 30 to 50 percent, while higher doses decrease it below baseline, correlating with mitochondrial membrane depolarization.[8]
- **ROS AND NO:** Low doses generate beneficial ROS and NO signaling, but excessive doses overwhelm antioxidant defenses, leading to oxidative stress and disruptions in NO pathways.[9]
- **CELL-DEATH PATHWAYS:** At high doses, PBM may activate apoptotic pathways through mitochondrial stress and excessive ROS generation, similar to overexercising.[10]

ANIMAL MODELS provide further evidence of biphasic dose responses by demonstrating dose-dependent effects across diverse tissues:

- **WOUND HEALING:** Rodent studies show 19 to 24 J/cm² accelerates healing by enhancing collagen deposition and reducing inflammation, while doses above 50 J/cm² delay healing and reduce tissue integrity.[11, 12]
- **MUSCLE PERFORMANCE:** Pre-exercise PBM at 3 to 5 J/cm² enhances muscle contractile force and reduces muscle damage, but doses of greater than 10 J/cm² can impair performance due to excessive ROS.[13, 14]
- **TRAUMATIC BRAIN INJURY:** Administering 18 J/cm² daily for 3 days after a traumatic brain injury improved recovery, whereas 14 days of exposure worsened neurological function.[15]

One study is worth discussing in greater depth. In 2001, Oron and colleagues[16] investigated the effects of PBM on infarct size in rats after inducing myocardial infarction. They applied laser irradiation to the infarcted area at various power densities ranging from 2.5 to 20 mW/cm². The results showed a clear biphasic dose response:

1. At 2.5 mW/cm², there was a 14-percent reduction in infarct size compared to non-irradiated rats.
2. At 6 mW/cm², they observed a significant 62-percent reduction in infarct size.

3. However, at 20 mW/cm², the reduction in infarct size was only 2.8 percent.

This pattern clearly demonstrates the biphasic nature of the dose response in PBM. The irradiance of 6 mW/cm² produced the most substantial benefit, while both lower (2.5 mW/cm²) and higher (20 mW/cm²) irradiances were less effective.

This study also suggests that the difference in effectiveness between optimal and suboptimal doses can be substantial. In this case, the optimal dose (6 mW/cm²) was dramatically more effective than the highest dose (20 mW/cm²) in reducing infarct size. (Keep in mind, this involved opening the chest cavity and applying laser light directly to the heart in living rats—an important detail we'll circle back to when discussing the controversy around the biphasic dose response in PBM.)

CLINICAL EVIDENCE IN HUMANS highlights the practical applications of biphasic dose responses, with a focus on optimizing PBM treatments for various conditions:

- **WOUND HEALING:** Studies on surgical incisions show doses between 19 and 24 J/cm² accelerate healing and reduce scarring. Higher doses (>100 J/cm²) often fail to provide additional benefits, suggesting a plateau effect rather than harm.[11]
- **EXERCISE RECOVERY:** Research on muscle function and recovery following sports or exercise has found benefits with doses of 30 to 50 J/cm², especially when applied immediately following exercise, whereas doses above 150 J/cm² do not confer the same benefits.[17]
- **CHRONIC CONDITIONS:** In osteoarthritis, moderate doses (4 to 6 J/cm²) delivered two to three times per week generally outperform daily high doses or infrequent treatments, emphasizing the importance of timing and frequency in chronic applications.[18]
- **BRAIN HEALTH:** Studies of transcranial light therapy reveal that lower to moderate doses (10 to 100 J/cm²) improve brain blood flow and mood more effectively than higher doses.[19] In another study, transcranial PBM with 10.8 J/cm² improved cognitive function of healthy older adults, but doubling the dose to 21.6 J/cm² negated these improvements.[20]

This body of evidence demonstrates that biphasic dose responses are consistent across various systems and models. While human studies generally show broader therapeutic windows with vastly less evidence of outright negative effects than in vitro experiments, the importance of optimizing PBM dosing for each specific application is clear.

In short, the biphasic dose response is real. From isolated cells to live animals to humans, it's clear that it's possible to apply enough light that it begins to negate the benefits and perhaps even cause harm to tissues.

So why the controversy?

Why Is the Biphasic Dose Response Controversial?

Given all this evidence that shows biphasic dose responses in PBM, you might be wondering why any of this is at all controversial. The short answer is that not all experts agree it's a real concern—at least not in most realistic contexts. Opinions vary widely, and those differences usually fall into three general "camps." Here's a brief general description of the views of each of these camps:

- Camp 1—The biphasic dose response is a big concern in PBM, and many people are commonly overdosing it and negating the benefits, or worse—causing harm.
- Camp 2—The biphasic dose response is a legitimate concern and while it's technically possible to overdo it, the reality is that most people are using it within the safe range.
- Camp 3—The biphasic dose response is not really a major concern for LED-based PBM (as opposed to lasers) and it's pretty hard to cause harm if one is using common devices for reasonable application times. The biphasic dose response is more of a concern with lasers or extreme irradiances and doses.

To be clear, there are experts in all of these camps.

As one example, PBM expert and researcher Dr. Praveen Arany believes that the biphasic dose response is a significant concern and that many people are commonly overdoing the dose. He is particularly concerned about the use of lasers in this regard by untrained persons, but also about the potential for even high-powered LED devices to cause excessive heating of tissues.

When I interviewed him on my podcast, he presented slides from his research in which he indicated that heating the tissues can negate the benefits of the treatment and cause harm to cells. He explained that when certain devices excessively heat the tissues (which may happen with very high-irradiance devices, or devices used inappropriately, particularly lasers)—especially above temperatures of 42°C (108°F) and especially above 45°C (113°F)—that he believes the thermal effects can negate the benefits of PBM and potentially also induce cellular damage at above 45°C (113°F).

Remember, excessive heating of the tissues may induce a biphasic dose response or cellular damage during PBM, and Dr. Arany believes that many people are negating the benefits of PBM or causing harm to tissues through excessive tissue heating.

(Note: The issue of tissue heating from PBM is a big topic, with its own controversial and competing claims. I discuss this topic of tissue heating in depth in the dosing section of this book.)

James Carroll, CEO of Thor Photomedicine, has given presentations that emphasize studies in which higher doses or higher intensities of light have resulted in fewer benefits (or negative effects) relative to much lower doses, and seems to consider there to be a very significant concern with too-high irradiances and too-high doses resulting in negative effects, or at least in less effectiveness.

In contrast, when I spoke with Dr. Hamblin about this, he repeatedly emphasized that he feels the concern over the biphasic dose response is likely greatly overblown for most people using PBM at home with LED devices, because, he argues, most studies that show strong biphasic dose responses are either in vitro experiments or animal studies—and because this kind of research has questionable relevance to in vivo conditions in humans.

Here it is in Dr. Hamblin's words:

Some people are worried about the so-called biphasic dose response. In reality, although you can demonstrate this easily in cell culture, and you can demonstrate it reasonably easily in laboratory animal models, it's very rare that there's been good examples in humans. There have been a few but by and large, no. In humans in general, the more light the better by and large.

Once you start calculating the dose in terms of total energy and you think about what is the total energy in a whole body light bed, which can easily be a million joules of energy to the body. [There are] people who worry about 10 or 100 joules is too much, or even 1,000 joules is too much. You can have a million joules over the whole body and not do any damage at all.

As a point of reference for Dr. Hamblin's views, one 2011 review of the literature on the biphasic dose response presented a great deal of evidence to support the existence of a biphasic dose response phenomenon in PBM from numerous in vitro and animal studies but said in their conclusion:

At present there has been no convincing report of biphasic dose responses occurring in patients [i.e., humans] . . .[4]

However, since that time, a small number of studies in humans have given convincing evidence for biphasic dose responses. Also keep in mind that "absence of evidence does not mean evidence of absence"; the issue could be more that the phenomenon simply hasn't been adequately studied in humans rather than that it has been studied thoroughly, and the evidence has shown it doesn't exist.

Nevertheless, the simple fact is that the vast majority of the evidence for biphasic dose responses from PBM are from in vitro and animal studies, and most studies in humans don't give strong evidence for biphasic dose response effects.

You might ask: Why might there be questionable relevance of in vitro studies (e.g., cells in a petri dish) or animal studies to humans? In other words, why can't we just assume that in vitro and animal studies also apply to humans?

There are several reasons. First, cells in a petri dish exist in a highly artificial environment that fundamentally alters their behavior. These isolated cells lack the complex tissue architecture, extracellular matrix, and intercellular signaling networks present in living organisms. In this simplified state, they often display dramatically different metabolic profiles, stress responses, and gene-expression patterns compared to how cells behave in vivo.

Crucially, in vitro studies often bypass the skin, the body's natural light filtering system. In living organisms, skin serves as a primary protective barrier, and typically more than 60 percent of incident light does not pass through the skin. Of the light that does penetrate, only about 10 percent or less makes it beyond one centimeter of tissue depth. Deep-tissue cells that rarely encounter significant light exposure are naturally more photosensitive than surface cells that routinely face light exposure. When researchers expose these light-naïve cells directly to intense light in a petri dish, they may trigger negative reactions at doses far lower than would be problematic in an intact organism with proper skin and tissue barriers.

In other words, cells in a petri dish often behave very differently than cells in a living human. This creates a fundamental disconnect between in vitro findings and real-world therapeutic applications.

As far as animal studies, while these are certainly far more relevant than in vitro studies, let's consider some important aspects of the physical differences in size and light penetration. The exact same light devices that may deliver light penetration perhaps one or two inches deep in us humans may deliver a huge amount of light deep into a rodent's internal organs and brain—areas where it doesn't reach to any appreciable degree in humans due to the simple differences in physical size.

For example, the thickness of a skull bone or the sternum/ribs in a human may block nearly all the light from a moderately powerful device, and almost no light would penetrate deeply enough to reach the brain or the heart. But the same device applied to a rodent could easily deliver a massive amount of light directly to the heart and brain.

In other words, high-intensity light penetrating 1 to 2 inches deep into a rodent is very different from the same light penetrating 1 to 2 inches deep into a human. In a human, little to no light may reach the internal organs, whereas in a rat, the same light source may blast light essentially almost through (or in some areas, actually through) the entire body from front to back.

This is significant because many of the

internal organs, like the brain or the heart, seem to be extremely sensitive to light photons and much more susceptible to the biphasic dose response.

This is even more exaggerated when researchers open up the bodies of animals and shine light devices directly on an internal organ, with no skin, fat, or connective tissue between the light device and the organ. For example, one of the studies used in James Carroll's presentation about the biphasic dose response was done by directly exposing the hearts of rodents to laser irradiation after inducing a myocardial infarction (heart attack), and it showed that even at the same total dosage, lower- and more moderate-irradiance laser irradiation was more effective than a higher-irradiance laser (specifically, 6 mW/cm^2 was more effective than 20 mW/cm^2).[16] (This is the study I discussed above, in which the chest cavities of rats were opened and their hearts were exteriorized and exposed directly to laser light.) While the results of this study clearly show a biphasic dose response, in which higher irradiance led to far less benefit, the relevance of this to humans, and

specifically to tissues that are not internal organs—where the body has not been cut open to put a laser directly on the organ—is highly questionable. (Such research would be relevant to the use of PBM during open-heart surgery, as it would be important to establish the optimal dosing parameters for lasers applied directly onto the heart.)

Dr. Hamblin makes the important distinction that shining light anywhere on the exterior of the body of a living human (where very little if any of that light would reach internal organs) is not likely to result in biphasic dose responses with reasonable doses—that is, outside of very powerful lights and very high doses—but that if you start opening up the body and shining light directly on internal organs, you're much more likely to invoke biphasic dose responses.

Beyond this, it's also important to understand that the story is actually more complex than just a "biphasic" dose response. Other researchers have put forth the concept of a "multiphasic dose response."

BEYOND THE BIPHASIC DOSE RESPONSE: THE MULTIPHASIC DOSE RESPONSE

Dr. Cronshaw—an authority on PBM dosimetry—challenges the traditional biphasic dose response model in PBM, suggesting instead that the biological response follows a more complex multiphasic pattern.

According to Cronshaw, the dose-response relationship in PBM isn't simply a matter of "Some is good; more is bad." Rather, his observations indicate that as the dose increases, tissues may move through multiple phases of response, including (as he described it to me):

- An initial stimulatory phase at low doses during which cellular activity increases
- An inhibitory phase as doses increase further
- A higher band of inhibition associated with a temperature rise at and above 42° (108°F)
- An ascending risk of damage at sustained temperatures at or above 45° (113°F)

In Dr. Cronshaw's words:

PBM results in a dose-related response. It's a bit like a medicine where there is a range of doses for differing conditions.

Dr. Cronshaw explained to me that the traditional thinking about the biphasic dose response has become outdated with the development of sophisticated high-energy laser systems designed to treat larger and deeper tissue areas. His research indicates that higher doses are often required for effective pain relief (analgesia), with dosimetry that falls within what was traditionally considered the "inhibitory" range. In an email exchange I had with Dr. Cronshaw, he expressed the following:

The adoption of the original concept as defined by the Arndt-Schulz law of an all or none response has become one of the central pillars of received wisdom in PBM dosimetry. However, this neat philosophy of care has been challenged following the development of a new generation of sophisticated high energy laser systems for PBM to treat larger areas of tissues as well as high power to the skin surface. These types of appliances have been designed to treat pain and damaged tissues in deeper tissues, for example, in laser-assisted sports injury rehabilitation therapies. The latest equipment has multiple wavelength simultaneous delivery high-power lasers with many added user and safety features and represent a radical evolution from the original generation of single wavelength, low power, small optic probe devices.

The published research shows that it takes a higher dose to achieve good pain relief (analgesia). The dosimetry required falls within the range that is recognized to activate protective cellular processes associated with inhibition of cellular activity rather than stimulation. In order to achieve a higher dose delivery to tissues beneath the skin, a much higher dose of 10x or more is required at the surface. There is disagreement within the PBM scientific community on the safety aspects associated with high dosimetry applied to skin. This is literally a "hot topic" between the experts as opinions are polarized concerning the effects of high energy systems as they may heat up tissues and stimulate the production of toxic amounts of ROS.

Based on many published clinical studies, there is a substantial body of evidence supporting the use of higher dosimetry for analgesia. As a result, there is a move away from the idea of a biphasic response which is an all-or-nothing outcome, and instead support is growing to view PBM dose outcome as a multiphase response.

The selective application of energy sufficient to trigger the protective cellular processes results in analgesia and providing the energy is not applied at too high a rate or for too long then the cell can recover once the stressor is removed without harm.

This multiphasic model also helps explain why seemingly contradictory results appear in research studies. What one researcher might identify as an "overdose" causing inhibitory effects might actually be a strategic transition point in the response curve, potentially useful for specific therapeutic goals like pain relief. When I asked Dr. Cronshaw about the safety concerns of this high-dose approach, he responded by saying:

This was one of the core topics of my recently published doctoral thesis in which I extensively reviewed the literature as well as conducted my own research investigations. I found that there are safety aspects to this approach and it is important to apply safe parameters. However the risk factors have now largely been defined. At present there is no evidence based agreement on this important topic . . . The usage of more sophisticated high power laser equipment by appropriately trained therapists has resulted in an increased uptake of this type of device and has not been found over a period of the past decade to be associated with frequent problems.

He also explains that there's a critical distinction here between high-powered lasers used in a clinical setting (which can easily cause damage when used inappropriately by an untrained person) vs. LED PBM devices:

If you use a little too much it can start to feel a bit hot in which case stop and no harm will occur. LEDs and lasers have very different optical properties. As a consumer using a home use PBM LED you are using a device which is inherently much safer to apply than a laser. A typical home use PBM LED is unlikely to cause a problem whereas a laser has to be used with a working knowledge of laser safety issues and taught practical skills. LED PBM devices available for home consumer use do not require the same special training needs and safety precautions essential to the safe utilization of high-power lasers.

His model proposes that there is a considerable buffer zone above the optimal biostimulation dose, where you remain in the safe range before actual cellular damage occurs at much higher doses. His work suggests that PBM dosing should be tailored not just to avoid overdosing, but to strategically target specific phases of the response curve depending on the therapeutic goal—stimulation or inhibition/analgesia.

As you can gather, different experts in the field have different views on how much concern we should have about the biphasic dose response. And it is also context-specific: Different body areas have differing sensitivities to light and different thresholds above which harm may occur. So while there is clearly a point at which irradiance and dosage parameters will be too high (negating the benefits or causing overt harm), there seem to be significant differences of opinion on exactly where these thresholds are. The current body of human evidence is quite limited in this regard, which makes drawing strong conclusions difficult—hence the differing opinions among PBM experts.

WHAT FACTORS CONTRIBUTE TO THE BIPHASIC DOSE RESPONSE?

Let's now examine some of the key factors that play into the likelihood of creating an excessive dose of light that negates the benefit or harms the tissue. In PBM, biphasic dose responses can arise from several distinct (though sometimes overlapping) mechanisms:

Excessive dose or irradiance: The total energy delivered (measured in joules) must remain within an optimal range. There are two aspects: total joules across the entire body, and fluence (J/cm^2) delivered to specific tissue areas. Making matters complex is that the intensity or rate of photon delivery (i.e., irradiance) plays a critical role in outcomes. Insufficient irradiance fails to elicit beneficial responses, while excessive intensity may overwhelm cellular mechanisms. Like walking versus sprinting the same distance, the rate of light delivery significantly impacts biological outcomes.

An extremely high irradiance device (500 mW/cm^2) delivering 25 J/cm^2 may invoke a different biological response than the same 25 J/cm^2 delivered by a 50 to 100 mW/cm^2 device, even though the "dose" is identical on paper. Very high irradiance levels can excessively heat the tissues to a level that negates PBM's benefits and may cause tissue damage. This is particularly relevant to lasers and extremely high-irradiance LED devices (and is something we'll discuss in depth in the coming section). In short, we have good data to show that both excessive irradiances and excessive treatment durations can result in negative effects.

Deep vs. superficial tissues: When targeting deep tissues, optimal dose must be based on energy reaching target tissues, not superficial skin. Light reaching deep tissues may only be 1 to 5 percent of surface intensity. This creates a paradox: Effectively treating deep tissues like joints requires deliberately "overdosing" superficial tissues. For example, treating arthritic joints requires high-irradiance light for extended periods, which may exceed optimal skin doses but ensures sufficient energy reaches the target. This is part of the reason why targeted devices are often preferable over large panels for deep-tissue treatments (if you have to deliver a very high dose to the surface to deliver an effective dose to deep tissues, it's best to do this in the most targeted way possible), and why deep-tissue treatments (which generally involve much larger doses) are more likely to cause biphasic responses than low-irradiance superficial treatments.

Photosensitive tissues: Certain tissues like facial skin, eyes, mouth, and genitalia are highly light-sensitive and better suited to lower irradiances to avoid overexposure.

Treatment frequency: Like exercise, frequency matters significantly. Too infrequent treatments (once every 15 days) lack meaningful impact, while too frequent sessions (three times daily) can impair recovery and adaptation. Studies vary from twice weekly to twice daily, but starting slowly with low doses every few days and building up frequency is generally recommended.

Individual variability: Several factors influence PBM effectiveness:

Tissue depth and composition: Higher body fat levels can significantly reduce light penetration to deeper structures, potentially requiring 20 to 40 percent higher doses in individuals with significant adipose tissue.

Skin pigmentation: Melanin substantially affects light absorption and penetration. Darker skin types may need increased duration, higher irradiance, or longer wavelengths, though higher irradiance should be used cautiously to avoid overheating superficial tissues.

Genetic differences: There may be fundamental genetic differences that make some people very sensitive to red and NIR light and others not sensitive at all. When I asked Dr. Hamblin about this, he replied that he believes there are three general categories of people:

- Hyper-responders to light (light-hypersensitive people) for whom much smaller doses may be ideal, and who may be more prone to overdoing it, and may need to be on the low end of the recommended dosage range.
- Non-responders (people who don't seem to respond much to PBM).
- The middle group (probably the vast majority of people), who respond to PBM in a "normal" or predictable way.

Overall health status: The single most consistent predictor I've seen of negative responses to PBM is poor overall health status. Chronically ill people are much more likely to report negative symptoms (fatigue, headaches) after initial treatments. This likely has to do with individual capacity to tolerate the hormetic aspect of PBM. Like exercise intolerance, very ill individuals may only tolerate low light doses, possibly because they lack adequate buffering capacity for the oxidative stress that PBM generates through hormetic mechanisms. PBM dosing should be personalized based on health status, starting with lower doses for those with chronic conditions and gradually adjusting the dose based on individual response.

These factors give a template for understanding how to achieve optimal therapeutic outcomes while avoiding potential negative effects. The simple truth here is that red and NIR light therapy (particularly when done with LEDs as opposed to lasers) is incredibly safe, and there is little reason for concern if you stay within reasonable dosing parameters (which this book will guide you how to do). It's actually quite easy to stay in the safe and effective range, and it's rather difficult to harm yourself (you'd really have to go out of your way to do something extreme).

Please note that this section is designed to give a brief overview of relevant factors that can lead to a biphasic dose response (ineffective PBM or a negative effect). All of the factors that go into proper dosing of PBM will be discussed in much greater depth—with specific practical recommendations given to optimize your PBM treatments for both safety and efficacy—in the dosing section of this book.

POTENTIAL FOR BENEFIT VS. RISK OF HARM—THE THERAPEUTIC WINDOW

A key concept in PBM is the therapeutic window—the range of dosages that are both effective and safe. Some substances, like heavy metals such as arsenic, mercury, or lead, have an extremely narrow safety window outside which even tiny amounts can cause harm. Others, like vitamin C, have a wide margin of safety: Even large doses are generally mostly harmless. Similarly, stressors like sauna bathing or physical exercise have fairly large beneficial ranges, within which widely varying dosages are likely to result in at least some benefit and are unlikely to cause harm.

While it's certainly still possible to overdo them, the body typically signals through discomfort or pain to help prevent severely overdoing it, and generally, one would need to have the willpower to push deep into extreme subjective discomfort and pain (and not listen to their bodies' signals to stop) to do significant harm.

PBM with LED devices appears to have a similarly wide safety margin. The evidence strongly suggests that in general, PBM has a relatively wide therapeutic window within which various devices, methods of application, irradiances, and dosages are, generally speaking, beneficial and safe. This is particularly true with LED devices as opposed to lasers (high-powered lasers carry far more risk of harm). The reason I say this is that an enormous body of studies using vastly different devices and doses—from pinpoint lasers to whole-body LED pods delivering thousands of times higher total dosages in joules—consistently report benefits, vs. very rare instances of clear adverse effects and even rarer instances of outright cellular damage. For example, a systematic review of PBM in myocardial infarction found "consistently positive effects over a range of wavelengths and application parameters."[20] Similar conclusions appear in most systematic reviews across different applications. The exception to this general rule appears mostly, as Dr. Hamblin points out, in in vitro studies and animal models, and especially where internal organs not designed to receive large amounts of light (and which are likely highly photosensitive) are directly exposed to laser or LED devices through surgical methods.

While some doses certainly may work better than others, the difference is usually about *degree of benefit* rather than risk of harm.

This broad therapeutic window is fortunate, because the current literature, with its diverse array of devices and protocols, hasn't yet established precise dosing guidelines for every treatment goal and device type. We simply don't have the body of scientific research that would allow us to establish a scientific consensus that would let us say, for example, "If you're using the FlexBeam device for your Achilles' tendinitis, here's the exact irradiance you want and here's the exact dosage in J/cm² you should do. And if you want to use it for osteoarthritis in your neck, here's the exact dosage you should do . . ." etc. Such data simply doesn't exist. The good news is that we can be confident that PBM is likely to provide some benefit even if dosing isn't totally optimal, as long as we stay within reasonable parameters (as outlined in the dosing section) for our specific treatment goals.

CHAPTER FIVE

PBM Dosing and Key Factors That Influence Photobiomodulation Treatment Efficacy

Many variables are involved in optimizing red and near-infrared (NIR) light therapy, including wavelength, dose (energy density and total energy), irradiance (also called power density), treatment duration, treatment frequency, and more. While this may seem overwhelming at first, the practical application is quite simple. Ultimately, you're just putting the device on a particular area of your body or a slight distance away from your body and turning it on, typically for somewhere between 2 and 30 minutes.

That said, there are a number of important factors that play enormous roles in determining the efficacy (and safety) of photobiomodulation (PBM) treatments. The most important are:

1. Dose per area and total dose
2. Wavelengths
3. Irradiance
4. Duration of treatment
5. Light convergence and spot size (relating to spacing of light-emitting diodes [LEDs] and wavelengths)
6. Contact vs. distance/noncontact
7. Treatment angle/device conformance to body surfaces
8. Optical properties of the tissues (melanin, water content, blood content, body composition, tissue temperature)
9. Laser vs. LED
10. Pulsing vs. continuous wave
11. Treatment frequency
12. Treatment timing

In the following sections, I'll break down the key factors that influence PBM treatment results and how to optimize them for better outcomes. However, it's important to note that the research on PBM is still evolving. There aren't many comparative studies evaluating different PBM devices, treatment protocols, or parameters like irradiance and laser vs. LED. Most PBM devices on the market have never been tested in randomized controlled trials, and expert opinions on the best treatment approaches often vary significantly.

Because of this, I don't have definitive consensus answers on which specific devices, dosages, or methods work best for every treatment goal. Much of what we collectively understand relies on logical speculation and interpretation of the available evidence. I've done my best to present a balanced view of different expert opinions, even when I don't personally agree with all of them.

Important note: For those who want a simple, practical guide to choosing the right PBM devices for your goals, and simple how-to guidance for using it effectively, you can skip this chapter and go straight to chapter 6. This chapter on dosing presents a lot of technical information that may feel overwhelming if you're just looking for simple practical guidance on which device to get for your particular goals.

On the other hand, if you're interested in a deeper dive into the science and technical complexities of PBM dosing, this section will help tremendously. We'll cover how to optimize treatment parameters for best results, key technical differences between various devices, and how these factors affect treatment efficacy in various contexts. We'll also go over how to dose PBM effectively for various goals like skin health, wound healing, athletic recovery, deep-tissue healing, and anti-aging. Ultimately, depending on what you're trying to accomplish, this is the knowledge that can make the difference between getting great results or seeing little to no benefit from your treatments.

Let's begin by defining some key terms:

DOSING: THE BIG PICTURE

Before diving into the specifics of PBM dosing, let's step back and look at the big picture. At its core, PBM is simple: You place a device on your body or put your body in front of a light panel, and the light does the work.

However, getting results isn't just about using any PBM device. The right dosing, device design, and application method make all the difference. If you're using the wrong device for your goal or applying it incorrectly, you may not get the benefits you're expecting. That's why the details matter.

In this chapter, we'll go deep into the factors that determine PBM effectiveness. But first, let's keep it simple by supplying a few of the big-picture fundamentals that you need to understand before selecting a device and determining the right dose.

LIGHT PARAMETER	MEASUREMENT UNIT	NOTES
Wavelength	Nanometers (nm)	This describes the part of the electromagnetic spectrum. Red and NIR light wavelengths used for PBM are generally in the 600 to 1,100 nm range. The most beneficial NIR wavelengths are 780 to 1,070 nm, with the most researched being 800 to 850. The most beneficial red light wavelengths are 630 to 680 nm.
Dose	Joules per centimeter-squared (J/cm^2) and total joules	The overall amount of light reaching a given area, and the total amount of light delivered to the entire body. Determined from power intensity and time of exposure.
Irradiance	Milliwatts per centimeter squared (mW/cm^2)	The power output of the light source per unit of area.
Distance	Centimeters (cm) or inches (in)	The measure of the distance between the light source and the target tissue. As distance increases, the power intensity and penetration ability can decrease. Skin contact can offer superior penetration, though some devices are designed to be used slightly away from the skin to maximize penetration from light-convergence effects.
Duration	Seconds (s) or minutes (min)	The time of light exposure.
Treatment frequency	Hours (hr) or days (d)	The time between light exposure sessions.
Pulse structure	Continuous or pulsed	The light is emitted as a steady stream or in pulses. Two out of three parameters need to be specified (frequency in Hz, pulse duration in msec, and duty cycle in percent).
Spectral beam profile	Gaussian or Flat Top	The power distribution across the width of the beam can vary. Typically with a Gaussian laser, 68 percent of the power is in the middle third of the beam. There are special optics called Flat Top, which even out the power distribution across the laser beam.

See the a table with some of the key information you'll need to understand how to select the right type of device for your goals and how to dose it correctly for those goals. Think of it as a simple general template for how to effectively and safely use PBM for almost any possible use you could think up.

The basic idea is that you want to think about what tissue you're trying to treat, and then you can zero in on what optimal irradiance, dosage, wavelengths, and devices will be for that goal. The simple template looks like this:

It's important to note that this simple table doesn't fully capture all of the fac-

TISSUE TYPE	DOSE	IRRADIANCE	WAVELENGTHS	TYPE OF DEVICE AND METHOD APPLICATION
SUPERFICIAL TISSUES (skin, eyes, body fat and cellulite, hands, feet, mouth, thyroid)	3 to 15 J/cm²	10 to 50 mW/cm²	Prioritize red (630 to 660 nm)	Targeted device that contours to that area and is designed for that specific purpose (e.g., facial masks or pad-style devices), or potentially, full-body panels used with lower irradiances (or farther distances away). Skin contact can be used, but even more important is a device that provides uniform coverage of the superficial tissue.
DEEP TISSUES (joints, brain, muscle/tendon, bone, fat, circulatory system, respiratory system, gut, glands, and internal organs)	20 to 60 J/cm²	50 to 120 mW/cm²	Prioritize NIR (810, 830, 850, and 1,064 nm)	Targeted device designed to be applied directly to that specific area with appropriate irradiance and wavelengths (e.g., joint-specific devices) are ideal. Panels can also be used in some cases. Skin contact or high degrees of light convergence are optimal to facilitate deep penetration.

tors and nuances that have relevance to effective use of PBM devices (which we're going to discuss), but it is a very useful simple template to understand the big picture of how to do PBM. We're about to make sense of all this, and I'll provide a detailed guide to selecting the right device for your goals as well. But I recommend coming back to this simple big-picture table frequently to ensure that you're on the right track.

Rest assured, it's okay if none of this information makes any sense at the moment. This chapter takes you through all of it (and much more) in much greater detail, for those who want to understand it.

Let me also be clear that these are general guidelines that apply with most body parts and most types of treatments for most people. Exceptions exist, and the scientific literature shows a wide range of dosing parameters, devices, and application methods. This is an evolving field with emerging technology, and there isn't one definitive approach. There's still a lot we don't know, and it's likely that our understanding of optimal dosing and device selection will evolve as new research emerges. So think of all of this less as set-in-stone, well-defined rules, and more as guidelines based on our current understanding.

DOSE PER AREA AND TOTAL WHOLE-BODY DOSE

The "dose" of a PBM treatment is itself a surprisingly complex and controversial subject, even among PBM researchers.

Why should such a simple concept like the "dose" of light be so complex? PBM dosing isn't as simple as taking a fixed amount of light like a vitamin supplement (e.g., taking 100 mg vs. 2,000 mg of vitamin C). Light therapy is complicated by a huge array of factors that influence how a particular "dose" of light interacts with human physiology.

Fundamentally, there are two basic ways to measure the "dose" of light you deliver to your body with PBM devices:

1. Fluence/energy density (J/cm^2): This is the dose of light delivered to a particular site on the body, measured per cm^2.
2. Total joules: This is the total amount of light energy delivered (in joules) across all areas treated.

Think of this in terms of a weight workout in the gym. There are the numbers of sets and reps for each body part (like your biceps, pecs, or quads), *and* there's the total work done in the workout. Was it just a brief workout of three sets of 10 reps for just the biceps and nothing else, or was it an exhausting hour-long high-intensity workout in which every muscle was pushed to its limits? Those would produce very different effects.

Both measures are important, and there are contexts in which one or the other metric may give you the more relevant data. To extend this exercise analogy, if you only cared about how big your biceps are, you might only be concerned with how many bicep curls were done, but if you care about the systemic health and longevity benefits of exercise, you need to care about many more aspects of the exercise regimen than just the biceps exercises. A similar concept holds true in PBM, as you'll see shortly—there are contexts where we may care more about a localized effect in a specific area of the body, or creating a whole-body systemic effect.

The key point is that PBM treatment is best understood by using *both* measures of the dose, and what you should focus on and optimize for is context- and goal-dependent.

Let's address both of these measures of the dose in greater depth.

Fluence/Energy Density

Fluence, or energy density, refers to the amount of light energy delivered per unit area—measured in joules per square centimeter (J/cm^2). Think of it like measuring rainfall: Just as we track how much rain falls in inches or centimeters, fluence tells us how much light energy reaches a given area of tissue. This is key because cells need an optimal dose of light—too little won't trigger benefits, and too much may reduce or negate results.

The formula for calculating fluence is:

$$\text{Energy Density (J/cm}^2\text{)} = \text{Time (seconds)} \times [\text{Power (W)} \div \text{Area (cm}^2\text{)}]$$

For example, if a 30-watt device is used for 5 minutes (300 seconds) over a 250 cm² area:

$$\text{Energy Density} = 300 \text{ seconds} \times (30 \text{ watts} \div 250 \text{ cm}^2) = 36 \text{ J/cm}^2$$

When it comes to the fluence, the key principle to understand is that there is an optimal dosing window for the target tissue. Both too little and too much of a dose are problematic.

So then what is the optimal dose in J/cm²? That remains a contentious question that different research groups and PBM experts have somewhat differing views on. Unfortunately, this is still a basic area in PBM where there is no scientific consensus or body of evidence that allows us to definitively determine the optimal dosing parameters. Let's discuss some of the reasons why it's contentious.

First, there is actually a major problem with the studies themselves, because they often don't accurately report key data about the light sources used in their studies, or don't report certain important metrics at all. For example, one review paper titled "The dark art of light measurement" found widespread problems in the research with inaccurate reporting of wavelength, light intensity, and other key aspects of dosing.[2]

Another problem is that a great deal of the research on optimal dosing parameters has been done with in vitro models (e.g., cells in a petri dish). For reasons we discussed in the section on the biphasic dose response, this is a deeply flawed model for understanding proper dosing in a living human being.

Further, as you'll soon see when we explore the many factors that influence PBM treatment efficacy in this section, this issue of the "dose" in J/cm² is further hugely influenced by the irradiance of the light source and whether a given dose was delivered very slowly or very rapidly (with a lower- or higher-irradiance device). The following quote from Zein et al.[1] gives a brief overview of that issue:

The photon intensity i.e., irradiance (W/cm² or spectral irradiance), must be adequate. Using higher intensity, the photon energy will be transformed to excessive heat in the target tissue and, using lower intensity, photons absorption will be insufficient to achieve the goal. The dose also must be adequate (J/cm²). Using low irradiance and prolonging the irradiation time to achieve the ideal fluence or dose will not give an adequate final result. . . . There is no fixed value of dose or fluence that always produces a positive PBM effect. Even within different studies on the same animal models, there can be contradictory findings.

While you can see from this discussion that dosing in PBM is very complex and contentious, we can still establish practical guidelines. Drawing from the substantial body of evidence I've analyzed and insights from leading PBM experts I've worked with to create this guide, we can define effective and safe target dose ranges for superficial and deep-tissue treatments.

First, for big picture context, it's worth considering that humans evolved receiving substantial daily light doses from the sun—with typical irradiance around 100 to 140 mW/cm² around noon, on a clear sunny day (depending on your geographic location). To put this in perspective: Just 15 minutes in bright sunlight at noon (at 100 mW/cm²) delivers about 90 J/cm² total light energy across all wavelengths, or approximately 27 J/cm² specifically in the red and NIR range (since about 30 percent of sunlight falls within these wavelengths). Similarly, an hour of sun exposure delivers around 360 J/cm² total, with roughly 108 J/cm² in the red and NIR range. Even a 5-minute sun exposure at noon provides about 30 J/cm² total, with about 9 J/cm² in therapeutic red and NIR wavelengths. Our ancestors likely received hundreds of thousands to millions

of total joules of light energy across their bodies during daily activities. While PBM therapy using specific wavelengths is distinct from sunlight exposure, this gives some evolutionary context of how human tissue responds to various doses of light. It is logical to assume that our biology evolved to handle and potentially benefit from substantial amounts of light energy, including significant doses in the therapeutic red and NIR range.

Looking to research on PBM specifically, in perhaps the most comprehensive review on PBM dosing parameters, Zein, Selting, and Hamblin[1] note:

Photobiomodulation (PBM) therapy, previously known as low-level laser therapy, was discovered more than 50 years ago, yet there is still no agreement on the parameters and protocols for its clinical application. Some groups have recommended the use of a power density less than 100 mW/cm² and an energy density of 4 to 10 J/cm² at the level of the target tissue. Others recommend as much as 50 J/cm² at the tissue surface. The wide range of parameters that can be applied (wavelength, energy, fluence, power, irradiance, pulse mode, treatment duration, and repetition) in some cases has led to contradictory results.

These conclusions broadly align with the previously cited review of the literature on PBM dosing from Zein et al.[1] And in Dr. Steven Parker's and Dr. Mark

Cronshaw's 2022 review[3] of dosing parameters in dentistry, they stated:

> Dosimetry at a level of 2–8 J/cm² at target cellular level has been accepted to represent the optimum range for the stimulatory benefits associated with photobiomodulation therapies. However, it has been proposed that a higher bracket of 10–30 J/cm² at target tissue level may represent a good and effective range for analgesia, accompanied by at-distance regional anti-inflammatory effects.

The given specifications "at the target cellular level" and "at the target tissue level" are critically important. Deep tissues require a much larger dose, because the dose in this case is calculated based on the surface dose rather than what is actually delivered to the deep tissues you're trying to affect. As we'll see shortly, for many reasons we'll discuss, only a small portion of the light present at the surface of the skin actually reaches those deep tissues (and the deeper the tissues are, the less light will reach them, and thus the more that the overall dose needs to be adjusted upwards to compensate for that).

Putting all this together, the overall body of research and expert opinion guides us to the following general dosing ranges:

- For superficial tissues (e.g., skin, joints, wounds) → 3 to 15 J/cm²

- For deeper tissues (e.g., muscles, nerves, organs) → 20 to 60 J/cm² (This is the surface dose, not what the deep tissue actually receives.)

Don't worry if you're feeling a bit overwhelmed by all the technical details. While this may seem complicated, it will be translated into simple practical recommendations. To give you a sense of how simple this will become, to reach these dosing targets generally means that for skin issues (or issues near the surface of the body), you might use most typical devices for somewhere around 3 to 30 minutes (depending on the light intensity, or irradiance, of the device you're using), and for deeper tissues, you might shoot for either longer treatment times, if using a device of equivalent power, or similar treatment times with a more powerful device.

This gives us our general target dose of light to shoot for, according to our general goal of that treatment. From here, there are still a number of other factors that will greatly influence one's results beyond simply being—on paper—in the right dosing range of J/cm².

Total Joules

Total dose refers to the complete amount of energy delivered to the body during a treatment session. This is measured in joules (J) and includes all treatment points and the entire treatment time. If we continue with the rainfall analogy used earlier, fluence (J/cm²) is like measuring rainfall in inches over a square meter, while total dose is like measuring the total volume of water that fell over an entire city. It doesn't tell us how much any particular area received, but rather the total energy delivered across all treatment areas combined—that is, the total dose of light to the entire body. So, we wouldn't measure it in "inches" but rather liters or gallons or tons.

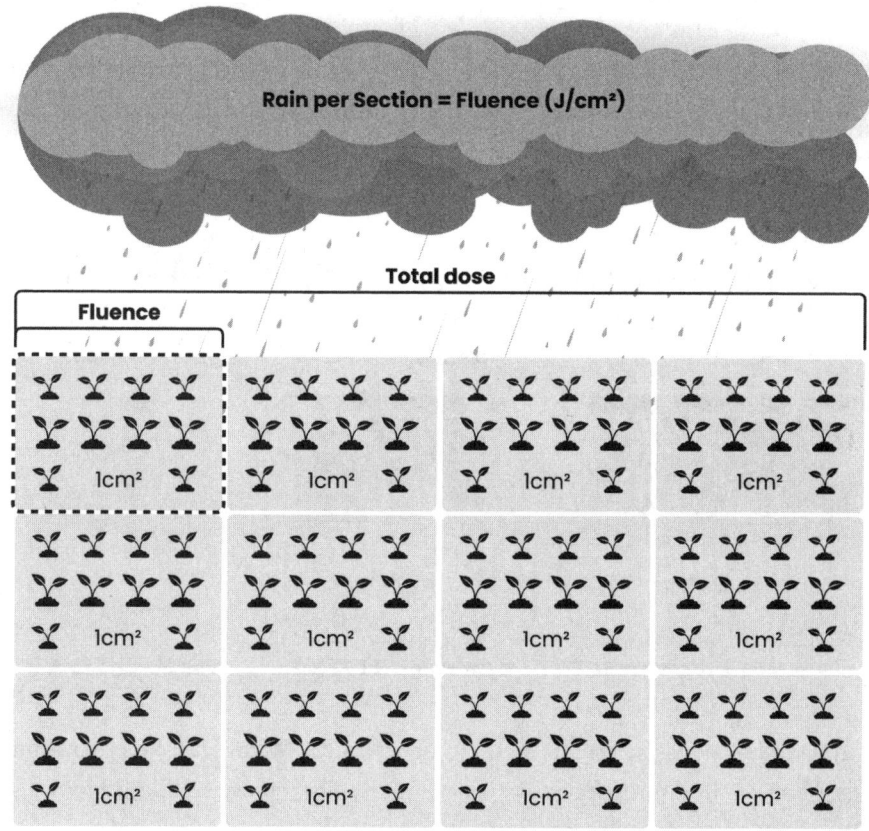

Rain per Section = Fluence (J/cm²)

Total dose

Fluence

Rain gauge = total rain collected   **Total dose** = fluence x area (J)

For example, if you're treating an injury:

- Energy density might be 6 J/cm² at each specific area of the body treated (like 1.5 inches of rain per spot).
- Total dose might be 5,000 J (e.g., 1,000,000 gallons of total rainfall over the whole area you're measuring).

Both measurements matter because:

1. Each treated area needs the right energy density for cellular response in that local area.

2. The body as a whole, needs to receive an appropriate total amount of energy to maximize the systemic response.

Both measurements are essential because while each treated area needs sufficient energy density for local cellular response, the body also requires an appropriate total energy dose to optimize systemic effects. The total joules measurement becomes particularly crucial when treating larger areas or multiple sites, and for trying to maximize systemic benefits (not only an effect on a specific body site).

Given the significant role of systemic effects in PBM therapy, monitoring the total energy dose (J) delivered to the body has emerged as a critical treatment parameter, with some experts such as Dr. Hamblin suggesting it may be even more important than the dose delivered to a particular area in J/cm².

Identical Energy Density, Different Total Energy

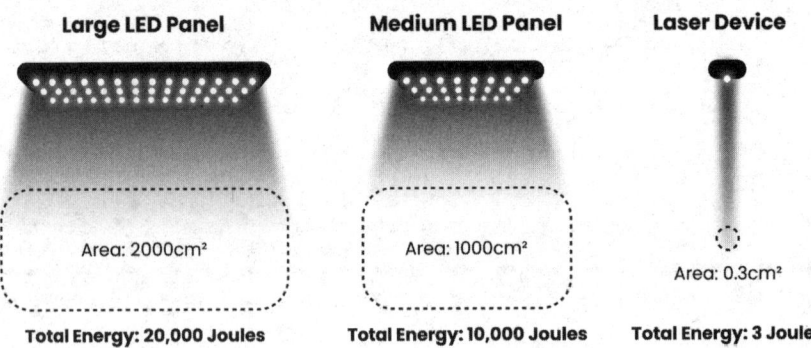

Large LED Panel	**Medium LED Panel**	**Laser Device**
Area: 2000cm²	Area: 1000cm²	Area: 0.3cm²
Total Energy: 20,000 Joules	**Total Energy: 10,000 Joules**	**Total Energy: 3 Joules**

This is one reason why experts like Dr. Hamblin emphasize the importance of considering total dose. In a conversation I had with him, he spoke about the difference in total joules between using a smaller, more targeted PBM device like a flexible pad vs. a large panel:

It's all a matter of absorbing joules. Because a panel emits so many photons, you can absorb a lot of joules relatively easily. From a flexible pad, you're probably not going to get more than 5,000 joules in a session. With a big panel you could get 50,000 joules or 100,000 joules.

So the size of the device (more accurately, the amount of body surface area treated), along with the irradiance and session duration, all hugely influence the total energy delivered.

How do we actually determine how many joules were delivered to the body?

The way to calculate total dose is to take our dose in J/cm² and multiply it by our total area of body coverage in cm².

To calculate total dose, you multiply the energy density (J/cm²) by the area of the body being treated (in cm²).

For reference, total body surface area typically ranges from 16,000 to 20,000 cm², depending on a person's size. You can estimate your total body surface area with the following formula:

Body Surface Area (cm²) = 10,000 × the square root of (Weight × Height / 3131)

For example, if I am 68 inches tall and weigh 200 lbs, my estimated body surface area is 20,840 cm².

We can then use the rule of nines to estimate how much of our body area we are exposing to red and NIR light. Basically, your head, chest, abdomen, upper back, lower back, front leg, back leg, and entire arm each make up 9 percent of your body surface area. The remaining 1 percent belongs to your groin.

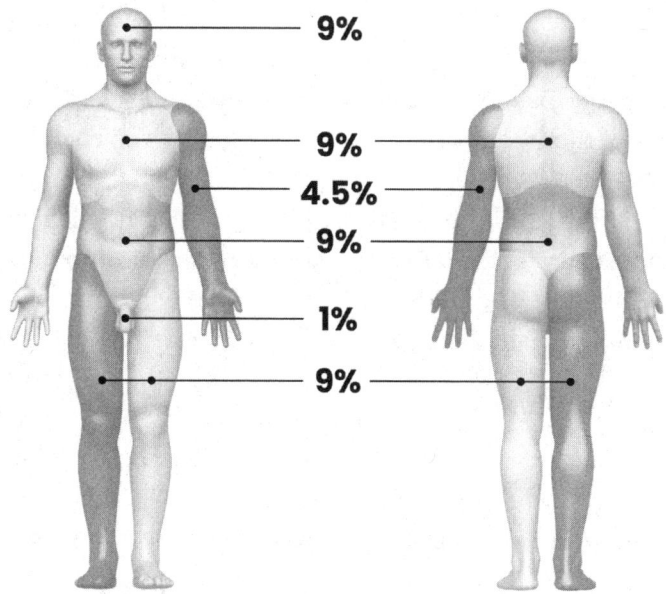

So if a full-body light pod delivers 20 J/cm² across 20,000 cm², that's 400,000 total joules. In contrast, a small handheld device applying 40 J/cm² to a 100 cm² area delivers only 4,000 total joules. This is a hundredfold difference in energy delivered, so you can see why looking at the dose in terms of J/cm² vs. total joules is so significant.

Dr. Hamblin argues that total joules is actually a more important measurement than energy density alone. As he put it, "I never really get too hung up about joules per square centimeter with the human body. What really matters is the total number of joules."

This view (shared by many) comes out of the belief that the systemic effects of PBM are the dominant factor in results.

So what is the ideal dosing of total joules to maximize systemic effects?

We don't have a great body of evidence to go on where different total dosages (and ways of delivering them) have been rigorously compared in terms of effectiveness for different therapeutic goals. From the perspective of systemic effects, it's likely that a few hundred joules is the minimum amount of energy that will have a beneficial systemic effect. A few thousand joules is likely to be more in the optimal range, and this range extends all the way up to hundreds of thousands of joules.

What's considered "too much" remains unclear, but evidence suggests that large total doses are generally safe and well-tolerated. Here's what Dr. Hamblin said about this:

> Once you start calculating the dose in terms of total energy and you think about what is the total energy in a whole-body light bed, which can easily be a million joules of energy to the body. People who worry about 10 or 100 joules is too much, or even 1,000 joules is too much . . . [but] you can have a million joules over the whole body and not do any damage at all.

For context, lying on the beach at the equator at midday, you will easily absorb a million joules of energy in less than an hour.

Full-body light therapy devices (like large panels or whole-body pods) can deliver significantly higher total doses due to their large treatment area and longer session times. A large LED panel or full-body pod might deliver light over 1 to 2 square meters of body surface, with treatment times of 10 to 20 minutes, resulting in total doses of 15,000 to 100,000 joules (or even reaching 500,000 joules or more with full body pods) in a typical session. In contrast, a smaller device that goes on a particular body part might deliver a total dose of somewhere in the thousands of joules, and a highly targeted device like a laser with a very small beam (even with very high irradiance) will generally deliver a low number of total joules (perhaps in the hundreds), even as it delivers a high fluence (J/cm^2) to that specific tissue.

Still, it's important to understand that total dose is not the only factor that matters. Energy density (J/cm^2) at the target tissue remains critical, especially for localized treatments. In practice, this means your PBM approach should be guided by your treatment goals:

- If you're treating a specific issue—like facial skin, joint pain, or a localized wound/injury in a small specific area of the body—energy density on that specific area in J/cm^2 is the key variable.
- For broader wellness goals, chronic inflammation, or systemic conditions,

total energy delivered to the body becomes more important.

However, given the body's interconnected nature, both measurements remain relevant in most cases. Even when treating a specific area, leveraging systemic effects through an appropriate total dose can enhance therapeutic outcomes. (Again, many PBM experts now believe the systemic effects—largely a function of total joules—may be the most critical factor in many contexts.) This dual approach—optimizing both local and total dose—is typically recommended for maximum benefit. But it's important to keep in mind that because of these differences, a particular PBM device might be highly effective for one goal but less useful for another. For example, a small handheld device may work well for a sore knee, but it won't be ideal for full-body systemic effects. On the other hand, a full-body panel or pod may be excellent for whole-body benefits but may not offer the precision or convenience needed for highly targeted applications. We'll explore these differences further in this chapter and in chapter 6, where we'll discuss ideal devices for specific treatment goals.

WAVELENGTHS

Understanding how different wavelengths of light interact with human tissue is fundamental for effective PBM. The wavelength of light, more than any other factor, determines its depth of penetration and the specific biological structures it can influence.[4] There is a dramatic difference in how various wavelengths—such as ultraviolet (UV), blue, red, NIR, and far-infrared—penetrate and interact with tissue.

In the 2017 book, *Photomedicine—Advances in Clinical Practice*, Calderhead and Tanaka explain it this way:[4]

The first law of photobiology states that absorption must occur before there can be any reaction. This might appear to be self-

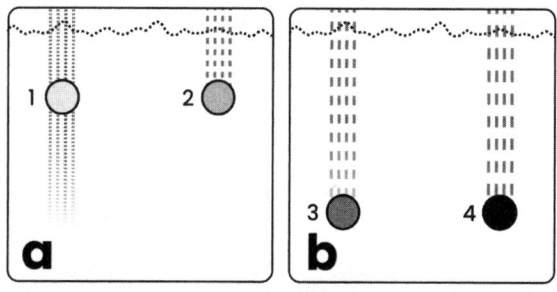

evident, but what actually governs absorption of light in a target, and indeed, what decides the chromophore, or target, for that light? The reader would be excused for thinking it is the output power of the light source, but it is in fact the wavelength. This is particularly critical in phototherapy.

When light contacts living tissue, it encounters a complex biological environment that shapes its journey in fascinating ways. The penetration depth and biological effects of different wavelengths are determined by both what they are and are not absorbed by within our bodies. To understand how this happens, we need to grasp a fundamental concept in PBM called the "optical window," or the phototherapeutic window.

Think back to a common childhood experiment: shining a flashlight through your hand. (You can even do it now to help jog your memory.) You'll notice a reddish glow on the other side. Why is it reddish rather than the same color as the original flashlight beam? And why not blue or green? This simple observation demonstrates the optical window: Certain wavelengths of light can pass through tissue more easily than others can. This selective penetration occurs because different components in our tissues interact with light in distinct ways, creating essentially a sophisticated biological filtering system.

Light behaves differently as it travels through tissue based on its wavelength. Shorter wavelengths (like blue and green light) experience more scattering and absorption near the surface, greatly limiting their penetration. Longer wavelengths (like red and NIR) can penetrate more deeply. Interestingly, even longer wavelengths (mid- and far-infrared) again show limited penetration beneath the skin. These differences in behavior stem from how various tissue components interact with specific wavelengths of light.

When light enters tissue, it encounters several key barriers that affect its penetration:

1. **MELANIN (SKIN PIGMENT):** Melanin absorbs shorter wavelengths (UV, blue, and green light) strongly, limiting their penetration to the epidermis and superficial dermis. This is why blue and green light are most effective for surface-level treatments, such as targeting acne or pigmentation disorders, but have little effect on deeper tissues.

2. **HEMOGLOBIN (BLOOD):** Hemoglobin, both oxygenated and deoxygenated, absorbs light at specific peaks, particularly in the visible spectrum below 600 nm. These absorption characteristics make it challenging for shorter wavelengths to reach deeper targets.

3. **WATER (TISSUE CONTENT):** At wavelengths beyond 1,000 nm

(infrared light), water becomes the dominant absorber. This sharply limits penetration depth at these longer wavelengths, as most of the light energy is absorbed near the surface.

4. **SCATTERING EFFECTS:** Tissue components scatter light, which alters its path rather than absorbing it.

Shorter wavelengths (e.g., blue, green, and red) scatter more than NIR light does, further restricting their penetration depth. NIR wavelengths, which scatter less, achieve deeper penetration into tissues. (Scattering is also strongly affected by the type of tissue, for example, skin, fat, bone, or muscle.)

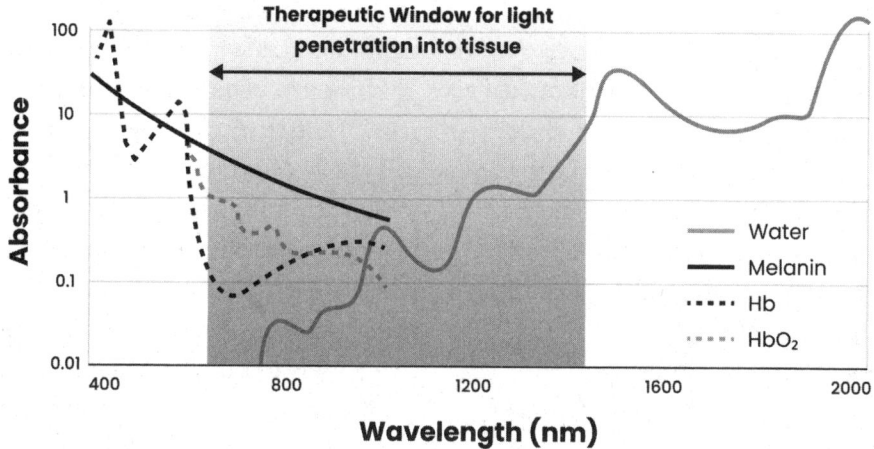

To understand the optical window, imagine three major gatekeepers that control light's passage through tissue: melanin, hemoglobin, and water.

In shorter wavelengths like ultraviolet (UV) and visible blue/green light (below 600 nm), melanin and hemoglobin act as strong barriers. They absorb much of this light, stopping it from penetrating deeply into tissues. Think of them as "security guards" blocking short-wavelength light at the surface.

At longer wavelengths, beyond 1,000 nm (infrared light), water becomes the pri-

mary barrier. Water molecules in our tissues absorb these wavelengths heavily, preventing deep penetration. This acts like a third security guard that blocks long-wavelength light.

Between these extremes—in the range of red and NIR light (~600–1,000 nm)—something unique happens. The security guards don't absorb this range of the spectrum nearly as well. This creates a "window" where light can penetrate tissues more freely.

This window exists because of how these different biological molecules interact with light at various wavelengths. So the first key point is that red and NIR light penetrate into biological tissue much more deeply than other wavelengths do. This deeper penetration, combined with the biological effects of these wavelengths, makes red and NIR light uniquely powerful for therapeutic use—which is a large part of the reason that for many people, "PBM" is basically synonymous with "red light therapy" or red and NIR light therapy.

Understanding this optical window isn't just a physics lesson; it has real implications for which tissues light can affect and which biological processes are triggered. Different wavelengths activate different mechanisms in the body, leading to different physiological effects.

Looking at penetration depth alone, we see a clear pattern: The shorter the wavelength, the lower the penetration is, and vice versa (up to a point). Ultraviolet light (200 to 400 nm) penetrates less than a millimeter into tissue. Blue light (400 to 450 nm) reaches 1 to 2 mm, while green light (500 to 570 nm) extends slightly further to 2 to 3 mm. Red light (~600 to 700≈nm) achieves significantly better penetration and is commonly claimed to penetrate to 3 to 5 mm of depth. NIR light (~780 to 1,000 nm) penetrates deepest, reaching 5 to 10 mm. Beyond that, as you get into mid- and far-infrared, penetration decreases again. (We'll see shortly that these numbers are actually wildly incorrect for red and NIR light, but they are approximately aligned with common statements of penetration depth of light.)

This creates a fascinating cascade of possibilities and limitations for each wavelength range. Obviously, if light can't penetrate significantly beyond the first 1 millimeter of skin, it can't have direct effects on any structures (e.g., joints, muscles, fat, organs) beneath the skin. So, just understanding this one layer of the story already explains a lot about how light interacts with biological tissue.

However, penetration depth tells only part of the story. The depth a wavelength can reach determines which biological structures/compounds it can *potentially* interact with. But the other part of the story is what specific effects and mechanisms are triggered by the wavelengths (which has to do with what structures, compounds, and molecules actually absorb those wavelengths of light), and that certain mechanisms are uniquely triggered by specific wavelengths and not by others.

Think of light like a key that needs to reach a specific lock to work its magic. How deep the light travels determines which "locks" it can potentially reach in your body, but that's only half the story. The other half is about which specific locks actually respond to that particular type of light.

UV light is like a shallow-reaching key that barely gets past your skin's surface—less than a millimeter deep. Even with this limited reach, it finds a very specific lock: the 7-dehydrocholesterol molecule that helps create vitamin D. It's also recognized by your DNA, triggering protective repair mechanisms (though too much can damage that DNA instead). And melanin in your skin grabs onto UV light like a sponge, which is why you tan or burn in the sun.

Blue light travels a bit deeper—about 1 to 2 millimeters into your skin. This light finds different locks: It's absorbed by substances like porphyrins in acne-causing bacteria, essentially creating tiny explosions that kill these microbes. It also triggers nitric oxide (NO) production that dilates your blood vessels and interacts with special receptors in your eyes that help set your internal body clock.

Green light goes 1 to 3 millimeters deep and finds yet another set of locks—specific pain pathways and channels in your nerves and perhaps other mechanisms. That's why it can help with migraines and chronic pain in ways other colors can't.

Red and NIR light are the deep divers, reaching several centimeters below your skin. These wavelengths unlock specific responses we've described in depth in the mechanisms and benefits sections—affecting pathways in the mitochondria, activating repair mechanisms, mobilizing stem cells, triggering collagen production, etc.—effects that other wavelengths simply can't reach and/or don't activate as well.

So while depth determines what light can potentially reach, it's the specific "lock-and-key" relationship between certain wavelengths and molecules in your body that creates such different effects. That's why red light won't trigger vitamin D production even though it reaches deeper than UV, and why blue light works on acne when green and yellow light doesn't.

With this broader context in mind, we can now shift focus more specifically to comparing red and NIR light. While they are both part of the "optical window," they also have important differences in

Relative Penetration of Different Wavelengths into the Skin

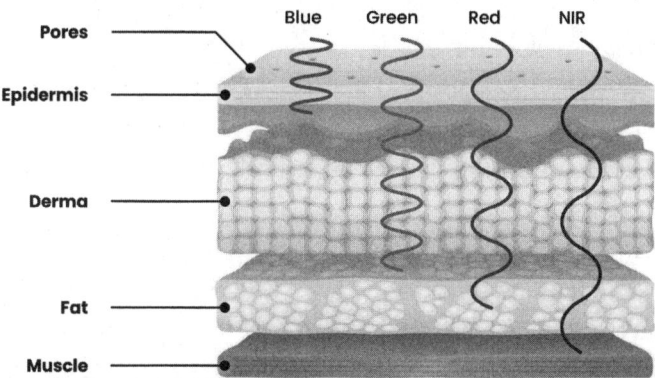

penetration, absorption, and effects that are worth exploring in greater detail.

Red and NIR Wavelength Selection Based on Target Tissue: Red for Skin and NIR for Deep Tissues?

Red and NIR light are often distinguished from one another by how deeply they penetrate the body and what kinds of tissues they are best suited to treat. NIR light penetrates more deeply than red light, so it's commonly considered ideal for reaching deep tissues such as muscles, joints, and the brain. In contrast, red light is typically associated with surface-level treatments like skin rejuvenation and wound healing. As we've discussed at length in chapter 3 on the benefits of PBM and other sections of this book, this general distinction is supported by both the physics of light-tissue interaction and a solid body of scientific evidence.

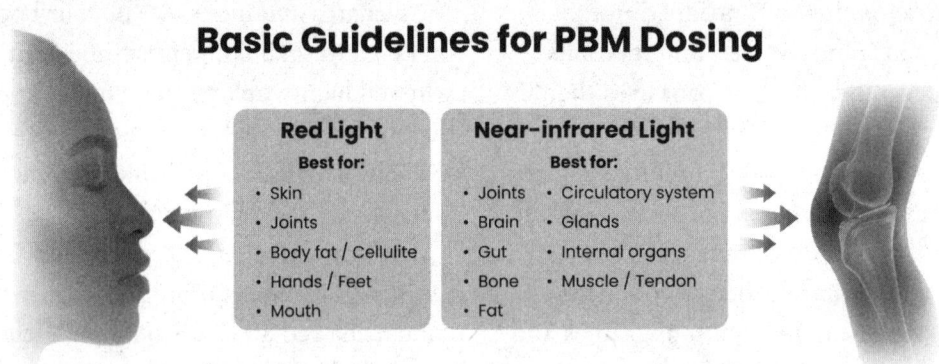

Basic Guidelines for PBM Dosing

Red Light	Near-infrared Light	
Best for:	Best for:	
• Skin	• Joints	• Circulatory system
• Joints	• Brain	• Glands
• Body fat / Cellulite	• Gut	• Internal organs
• Hands / Feet	• Bone	• Muscle / Tendon
• Mouth	• Fat	

We know, for example, that red light wavelengths have proven especially effective for improving skin health by targeting superficial tissues. They stimulate fibroblasts, enhance blood flow in the dermis, and support collagen production. These actions help reduce wrinkles, smooth skin texture, and accelerate healing.[5–7]

Likewise, we've also discussed many studies that show that NIR wavelengths encounter less scattering and absorption in superficial layers, allowing them to reach deeper structures such as skeletal muscle, connective tissues, and even the brain. An abundance of evidence shows that NIR light is effective in treating a wide variety of deep tissues, like muscles, joints, bone, and to the brain through the skull.[8–16]

The key point here is that overall, there is a compelling case to be made based on both logic and evidence that red light is ideal for superficial treatments and NIR is ideal for effecting change in deeper tissues.

However, while there is some truth in this idea, the truth isn't quite so simple or black-and-white. The reality of their effects is more nuanced, with significant overlap and potential synergy between the two wavelengths.

Despite the distinctions outlined above, the therapeutic effects of red and NIR light often overlap. Red light, traditionally associated with superficial treatments, has shown surprising efficacy in addressing deeper tissue conditions such as muscle recovery,[17, 18] joint pain,[19] and even neuropathic conditions.[20] Conversely, NIR light, typically thought of as being best for deep tissues, has also proven effective in skin rejuvenation and wound healing.

Several factors help explain this overlap.

1. Red light can penetrate more deeply than commonly claimed, and in many cases, it can deliver effective doses to tissues located well below the skin.
2. Although NIR light is capable of reaching deep tissues, it also interacts with surface tissues and can be effective for those applications, too.
3. The threshold of light energy required to trigger beneficial biological responses may be lower than previously thought, at least in some tissues. Even if red light delivers less energy to deep tissues than NIR does, it may still be enough to activate significant effects in some types of tissues that are very light-sensitive (likely tissues very rich in

mitochondria, like muscles, nervous tissues, and organs).
4. Different chromophores (the parts of molecules in the body that absorb photons of light) within tissues respond to different wavelengths. Red light may activate targets in deep tissues that NIR does not, and vice versa.
5. Biological systems are interconnected. Stimulating surface tissues can initiate signaling cascades—such as release of anti-inflammatory compounds or growth factors—that benefit deeper tissues through cell-to-cell communication, and through whole-body systemic effects.

In short, the reality is complex and there is still much we don't know. But we do know that red light can be effective for deep-tissue treatment, and that NIR light can be beneficial for superficial treatments. There is plenty of overlap in their efficacy in both superficial and deeper tissues.

It may be the case that the most effective approach is to combine or alternate wavelengths, allowing both red and NIR light to contribute their unique benefits across different tissue depths.

The availability of LED devices with both red- and NIR-emitting diodes in the same array makes simultaneous delivery of two wavelengths entirely feasible (it's actually fairly commonplace in PBM devices now). There is some evidence (though currently rather weak) that administering red and NIR light at the same time is better than either wavelength alone with the same parameters (mW/cm² and J/cm²).

While it's true that NIR will likely be more effective for treating very deep tissues, the point is that we should not think about red and NIR in simplistic, all-or-nothing terms—both red and NIR light can be effective for deep tissues, and both can be effective for superficial tissue treatments. What's more, they may be synergistic when combined.

How Deep Does Red and NIR Light Actually Penetrate?

All of this naturally leads us to another crucially important, and surprisingly controversial, question: How deep does red and NIR light actually penetrate into the human body?

Remarkably, there seems to be widespread disagreement and confusion about how deep red and NIR light actually penetrate into the body. For example, if you do a simple Google search online or even browse some scientific papers, they will say that red light barely even makes it past the skin surface. One source claims that red light and NIR light essentially penetrate no deeper than the skin, and put the figure at 2 to 3 mm.

Some papers claim that red light is extinguished 4 to 5 mm beneath the surface,[21] while others suggest even less. For example, one group of researchers say that red wavelengths penetrate 0.5 to 1 mm and that NIR penetrates only about 2 mm before losing 37 percent of its intensity,[1] while other groups estimate red and NIR penetration at around 5 mm.[22]

For reference, the epidermis is between 0.2 to 1.6 mm thick and the dermis (the

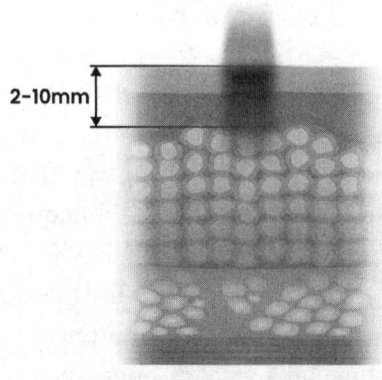

2-10mm

Many claim red/NIR light penetration is only 2-10 mm

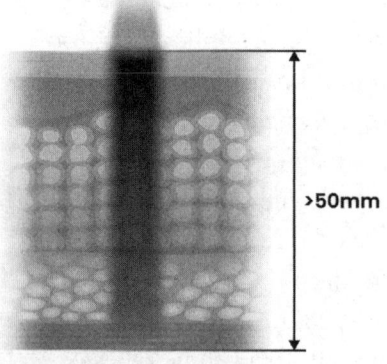

>50mm

Research has shown red/NIR light can penetrate up to 50-100 mm in some cases

Light Penetration into Skin

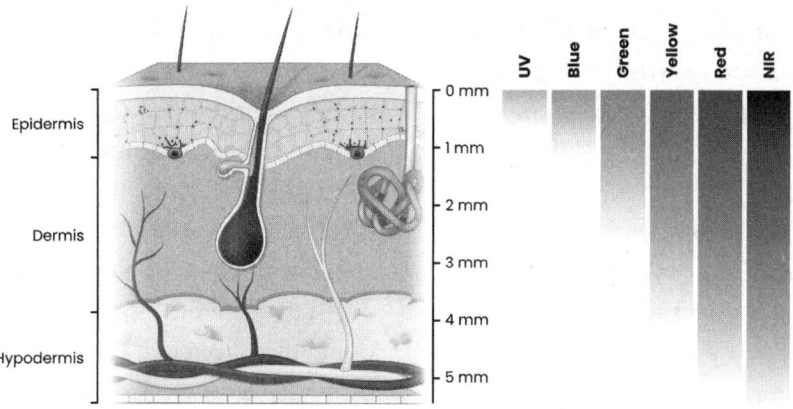

part of the skin just below the surface layer) is about 2 to 4 mm thick (depending on the body area).

These statements about the penetration depth of red and NIR light should be rather shocking, because they imply that red and NIR light basically can't penetrate beneath the skin (epidermis and dermis) almost at all!

So how does this make any sense that red or NIR light could somehow treat muscles and joints, or internal organs, or glands, or bones, or tendons, or something like the brain (where light not only has to penetrate through the skin, but also through a solid layer of bone to deliver any light to the brain) if the light can't even penetrate beneath our skin?

If it were true that red and NIR light were only able to penetrate up to 2 to 5 mm into the body (essentially no further than our skin), it would mean that basi-

cally any effect seen from PBM in deeper tissues beneath the skin (e.g., muscles, tendons, bones, joints, brain, organs, etc.) would have to be due to systemic effects, not from light directly interacting with those tissues.

In other words, it would mean that a large portion of PBM devices on the market claiming to treat muscles, bones, tendons, joints, or the brain are entirely BS!

So what exactly is going on here?

This story gets even stranger, because you can—in the comfort of your own home, in the next 30 seconds—directly observe red light penetrating far beneath the surface of the skin. Go into a dark closet with a powerful red-light device (a flashlight/torch-style device is good because it can be pressed right up against the skin without lighting up the whole room) and shine the light through your fingers or even your whole hand! (It will be best with a powerful red light torch but can even be done with a regular flashlight where only a small portion is in the red wavelengths.) You can visibly see light making it through an entire human hand—not only through the skin, but through another roughly *inch* of tissue (perhaps 15 to 25 mm) and then through the skin on the other side of the hand as well! You can do the same with your ear, or your toes, or a pinch of neck tissue or fat tissue on your belly, or your Achilles tendon or any other area of your body around an inch or less in thickness.

If red light only penetrates 2 to 5mm into our tissue (i.e., never made it beyond the skin), how could we possibly explain images where red light somehow can penetrate visibly through an entire human hand? (By the way, red light doesn't even penetrate as deeply as NIR, so if you could visualize NIR, vastly more light would be traveling through the hand.)[23]

Even more bizarre are photos like this one of Tom Kerber, which although it's not through the skin, shows red light penetrating distances that are several *inches* through human tissue—that is, orders of magnitude greater than the supposed 2 to 5 mm that some of the studies above claimed.

So we have claims that red light penetrates no more than 2 to 5 mm into the body, and yet, somehow we can visibly observe it, with photo evidence, traveling through >2 to 3 *inches* (perhaps 50 to 70mm) greater than that of tissue in living humans.

How do we make sense of this?

Understanding the Confusion and Contradictory Claims About Red and NIR Light Penetration: The 1/e Method

It is likely that much of the contradictory claims and confusion around penetration depth of the light stems from a conventional measurement approach borrowed from physics—the 1/e method. This mathematical concept, derived from studies of electromagnetic radiation in materials, defines "penetration depth" as the distance at which light intensity drops to approximately 37 percent (1/e) of its initial value.

The 1/e method originated in physics to characterize how quickly different materials attenuate electromagnetic radiation. It provides a standardized way to compare light absorption across different materials and wavelengths (e.g., how deeply X-rays can penetrate into wood, or metal, etc.), which explains its widespread adoption in scientific literature. While this approach works well for physics applications and engineering calculations, it creates enormous misconceptions when applied to the human body.

Here's why: The 1/e measurement essentially draws a somewhat arbitrary line at 37 percent of initial intensity. If we start with 100 "units" of light intensity at the surface, this method only tells us where it drops to 37 units. But this doesn't necessarily tell us anything particularly meaningful as it relates to biological realities. In fact, the deeper we get into the body, the more light sensitive tissues often become (this is especially true with mitochondria-rich tissues like muscles, or the brain). This means biologically meaningful amounts of light often reach far beyond the "penetration depth" as defined by the 1/e method.

To give an example of how this works, the light may be reduced to 37 "units" of the original 100 units by the time it's 3 mm deep, but you may still have 33 units another 3 mm deeper, and 30 units 3 mm deeper than that, and 20 units at 9 mm deeper than that, and you may perhaps still have 5 units of light much deeper than that. And perhaps those tissues at that depth of 30 mm or 40 mm into the tissue only need 3 or 5 units of light energy to trigger biological effects.

With this in mind, we also need to consider that many tissues deep inside the body—particularly mitochondria-rich tissues—are likely vastly more light-sensitive than more superficial tissues, so even though light intensity may be very low as it gets to those deep tissues, the light is interacting with tissues that may be extraordinarily sensitive to even small amounts of light. Here are Dr. Hamblin's thoughts on this:

One point that needs to be considered when evaluating claims about light penetration depth is the following. Because the human skin has evolved to be continuously exposed to sunlight, it is not surprising that the skin is not particularly sensitive to red and NIR light. Skin cells do not contain large numbers of mitochondria in the same way that muscle, brain or liver cells do. Partly this is because skin cells do not require the large amounts of energy to carry out their function, that muscle, brain, or liver cells require to carry out their function. **This means that cells located beneath the skin within muscles, brain or organs could respond to a tiny fraction of the light that is absorbed in the skin without any pronounced effect on skin tissue.** This is analogous to the sensitivity of the eyes to red light. When a red laser beam is shone through a hand or a cheek, the clearly visible red light coming out the other side is only a tiny fraction of the intensity impacting on the surface (probably less than 1 percent), but it still looks bright because our eyes are exquisitely sensitive to red wavelengths.

So in essence, this figure of 2 to 5 mm "penetration depth" defined via the 1/e method didn't really tell us much of anything meaningful about how deep those light photons actually penetrate into our tissue or what biological effects they will ultimately trigger at depths far beyond the 1/e depth.

A crucial factor that complicates this measurement even further is that a large portion of red and NIR light may be *reflected* off the skin's surface before it even enters the tissue.

This is not an insignificant amount of light—the best data we have from the National Institute of Standards and Technology—indicate a roughly 40 percent to nearly 70 percent loss of the light from the surface tissues due to reflectance and remittance losses.[24] Other research finds similar values for white and Asian people, while people with darker skin show a lower reflectance of 30 to 50 percent due to higher absorption by melanin.[25]

Now, in reality, this story is more complex than simple "reflection"—there is another term called "remittance," which describes how light technically enters the surface of the skin but is then "backscattered" by layers beneath the surface. But for our purposes, you can still think of this as basically being "reflected" back out.

Since light must actually be absorbed to produce an effect, in either case—no matter if it's true "reflection" or "remittance," the light is essentially not really entering and being absorbed by tissues inside our body but is the portion of light that *doesn't* enter the body or cause a PBM reaction.

NIST Data: Reflectance Spectrum of Human Skin

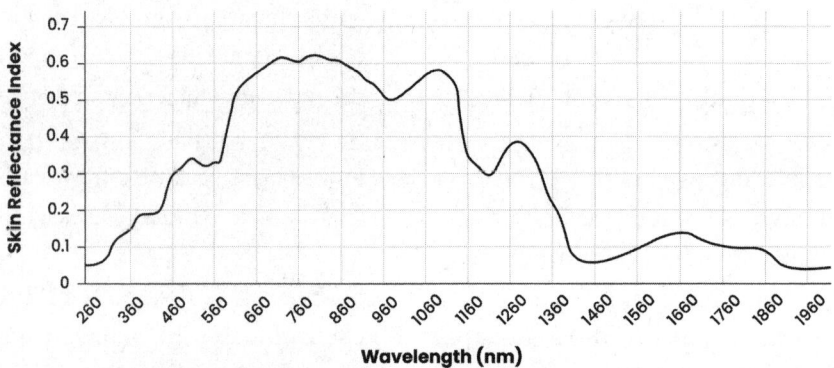

In other words, a huge portion of the light—perhaps 40 to 70 percent—at the surface doesn't really "penetrate" the skin essentially at all! This means that by the time we detect light just below the skin's surface, we might already be approaching that 1/e threshold.

So if we were to strictly apply the 1/e method starting from initial intensity at the surface, we might conclude that red and NIR light have almost no meaningful penetration at all (which is essentially what these claims of "2 to 5 mm of penetration depth" seem to imply).

Now, let's consider the implications of this situation in contrast to non-biological materials. Imagine if we looked at the penetration depth (via the 1/e method) with, for example, X-rays through wood. This would likely be linear—you might expect a very uniform and consistent decrease in the intensity of X-rays present. Let's say it's a decline of 10 percent of the intensity of X-rays for each millimeter into the wood. In this case, the 1/e method may be a perfectly valid and accurate way to understand the depth of penetration of X-rays into that material. But in the case of red and NIR light and the human body, it's a very different situation where we get a radical decrease in the amount of light (perhaps 40 to 70 percent loss of light intensity) in the first few millimeters of skin, but then that remaining portion of light (30 to 60 percent) doesn't continue to be attenuated at the same rate per millimeter (such that it's completely extinguished by the time it's 6 or 8 mm deep), but may travel vastly deeper into the tissues with a much more gradual rate of attenuation once it's beneath the skin. (This is a generalization meant to illustrate the principle, rather than to give exact numbers, because in reality, it also depends on the tissue type—fat, muscle, bone, etc.)

So once we consider that skin reflectance/remittance dramatically lowers the overall amount of light that even makes it beyond the skin, we can see that when studies report that red light penetrates to 2 mm and NIR to 5 mm using the 1/e method, they're actually telling us where the light remains quite strong (at 37 percent of initial intensity). The light continues traveling far beyond these depths, just at

progressively lower intensities. With sufficient initial power, therapeutically relevant amounts of light can potentially reach several *centimeters* deep, far beyond the commonly claimed "penetration depth."

In other words, the "penetration depth" as defined by the 1/e method isn't really a valid or accurate way to measure what is going on in our biology.

A more biologically relevant approach would be to measure penetration depth based on the point where light intensity drops below the therapeutic threshold. This would provide a better understanding of the actual therapeutic reach of different wavelengths. However, the scientific literature continues to use the 1/e method because it's a standard physical measurement, even though it may not accurately represent the biological reality of PBM.

Understanding this distinction helps explain why we often observe therapeutic effects at depths well beyond these commonly cited penetration measurements, and why we can do simple at-home experiments with a flashlight showing that red light can in fact penetrate vastly deeper into the body than just a few millimeters.

What's the bottom line here?

Red and NIR light are not limited to 2 to 5 mm of penetration (as is commonly claimed), but in fact travel vastly deeper into our tissues (depending on the specifics of the light device and tissue type).

Beyond simple at-home experiments, what's the evidence to support the claim that red and NIR light can penetrate far deeper into the body than just a few millimeters?

The Real Evidence On Red and NIR Light Penetration Depth

Fortunately, you don't have to take my word for this claim, because not all studies claim that red/NIR light only penetrates a few millimeters into the body. Some studies that have actually measured red light penetration depth in a rigorous way have shown that it does in fact penetrate deeply into the tissues—not 2 to 5 mm, but *5 centimeters* (50 millimeters) and even beyond! In fact, they showed that with an intense enough light, red light could penetrate up to about 100 mm (roughly 4 *inches* deep)!

For example, one well-designed study showed that even red light (which doesn't penetrate as deeply as NIR) can penetrate tissues up to about 50 mm (10x greater than the claims above) at reasonable light intensities, and even greater depths with higher irradiances.[23] Here's how the researchers described it:

Red-light was produced by a light emitting diode array of various irradiances (15-500 mW/cm²) and measured by a light-probe positioned on the tissue surface opposite to the light emitting diodes. 100 mW/cm² successfully penetrated tissue <50 mm thick; a disproportionate irradiance increase was required to achieve deeper penetration.

The researchers stated: "All hand structures, and most other structures under 50 mm of thickness are readily penetrated by red light."

More specifically, the researchers found the following results in terms of the ability of red light to penetrate through certain body areas:

These observations demonstrate that at irradiances ≤500 mW/cm2, red-light has the capacity to penetrate the entire thickness of the distal upper limb [e.g. the entire wrist] and cranium in all subjects, and the upper arm and ankle joint in half or more subjects.

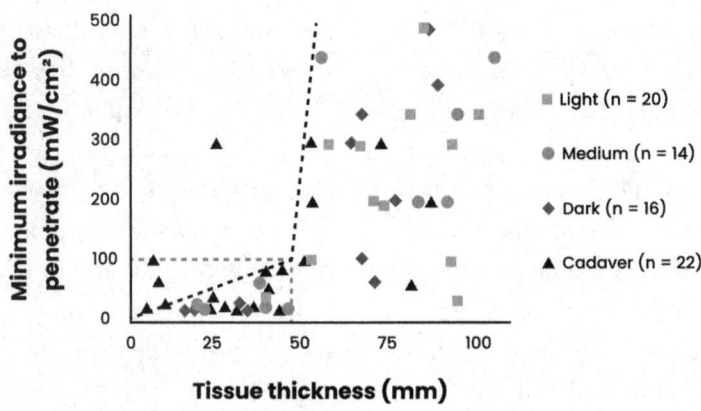

(This graph from the study shows that red light [660 nm] was able to penetrate to depths of tissue to 50 mm and even up to about 100 mm of tissue in some cases, particularly with higher intensities of light.)

So while we can find claims of red and NIR light having a penetration depth of 2 to 5 mm, here we have actual research showing that red light can deliver light through 50 to 100 mm of biological tissue!

In other words, red light isn't something capable of just barely penetrating through the skin, but something capable of penetrating *inches* into the body, traveling through skin, fat, muscle, and even bone. (Importantly, we also need to consider that these results were achieved with 660-nm red light, and NIR light in the range of 800 to 900 nm is capable of vastly deeper penetration than red light, so these results would be even more shocking had they used NIR. Both the penetration depth, and the light intensity seen at a given depth would be much greater with NIR.)

Research from Tom Kerber's team at the University of Buffalo confirmed that even 635-nm red light could penetrate through more than 75 mm of tissue.[26] One caveat with Tom's experiments was that it was done without skin, and as we've discussed, skin does reflect/remit and absorb a large amount of light and will therefore affect these results. On the other hand, another factor is that NIR

light will penetrate far more deeply than 635-nm red light will, so these numbers would be much higher if the same experiments were done with NIR as opposed to 635 nm.

Most remarkably, a brand-new study (as of this writing) in July 2025 has just shown something truly astounding.[104] Glen Jeffery and colleagues at University College London demonstrated that NIR wavelengths from sunlight can actually be measured after passing completely through the human thorax—the chest cavity containing the heart, lungs, and other vital organs—traveling through skin, fat, muscle, connective tissue, bone, organs, and a second layer of skin to emerge detectable on the opposite side of the body.

This finding is truly extraordinary. To be clear, we're not talking about light penetrating to a depth of just a few inches into the body. A portion of light actually transmitted all the way through the human torso and could be measured on the other side! This indicates that living human tissue is vastly more transparent to light than previously known.

Of the sunlight spectrum, as we would expect, they specifically found that wavelengths in the 600-1000nm range were capable of penetrating extraordinarily deeply into human tissue. The study showed that at 850 nm, sunlight with an intensity of 17 mW/cm² was still detectable at 5.6 µW/cm² after passing through the entire chest—representing transmission through what could be 10+ centimeters of mixed biological tissues including skin, fat, bone, muscle, internal organs, and a second layer of skin! Remarkably, this penetration occurred even when subjects wore multiple layers of clothing, which proved nearly 100 times more transparent to 850-nm light than to visible wavelengths.

Now keep in mind that the amount of light that penetrated all the way through the body was extremely minuscule. Though remember that as we get deeper into the body, we encounter more tissues (especially mitochondria-rich tissues) that are far more likely to be sensitive to even tiny amounts of light. So there are certainly still questions about whether light at this low intensity would still be meaningfully bioactive. However, the point is that this study demonstrates that the maximum penetration depth of NIR light extends far beyond what most researchers previously believed possible. This research should probably be replicated by another laboratory before we accept it as established fact, but if confirmed, it would radically alter the conventional wisdom about how deeply light penetrates in the human body.

An additional subtle layer to this story is that we need to not just understand the difference between red and NIR in terms of maximal "penetration depth" but also in terms of how high an irradiance is reaching a certain depth of tissue. For example, while NIR may penetrate 30 percent or 50 percent deeper than red light (let's say to 6 cm instead of 4 cm, just to make up numbers), this way of conceptualizing it doesn't capture the whole story. The reason why is that if we look at how much light penetrates to a depth of 4 cm, NIR may have an irradiance at that depth that's 10x or 20x higher than red wavelengths at the same depth.

To make up numbers, let's imagine we have a red-light device at 100 mW/cm^2 and a NIR device at the same 100 mW/cm^2 irradiance. And let's say, at 4 cm of depth, only 0.5 mW/cm^2 of red light is detectable, but 5 mW/cm^2 of NIR are reaching that depth. (Based on Tom Kerber's data that I've seen him show in real-time testing, these numbers may be realistic.)

So again, it's not just that NIR penetrates to deeper tissues than red does—it's that even at a depth that both red and NIR can technically reach, NIR light of the equivalent starting irradiance may deliver 10-fold or 20-fold more light photons to a given depth of tissue per unit time, because a much higher portion of the surface light will make it to that depth of tissue. (And this may make the difference between a significant effect and no effect.)

Part of the confusion about penetration depth is likely due to the fact that it is heavily influenced by many different factors, and that, depending on the specific light device you use and how you apply it, it may lead to dramatically different results in penetration depth of the light. For example, one research group describes their own experiments by saying that depending on the parameters used, it was the difference between light being completely extinguished at 2 mm (not even penetrating through the skin) vs. penetrating through skin and the skull and delivering biologically relevant amounts of light to even 3 *centimeters* of depth.[27] That's the difference of 2 mm vs. 30 mm of penetration, based on the device and parameters used.

(Note that there are several other factors we'll discuss shortly that also impact on penetration depth—irradiance, spot size/light coverage, laser vs. LED,

and other aspects of the device used and how it's applied, and more. We'll explore more of these influencing factors—including irradiance, spot size, and method of application—in the upcoming sections.)

The key point: Contrary to common claims about red light only penetrating 1 to 5 mm into the body, with a well-designed device used in the right way, red light can penetrate more than 50 millimeters into the body, and NIR can penetrate even deeper. And emerging evidence is now suggesting that at least very small amounts of light can even penetrate distances through human tissue previously regarded as inconceivable.

IRRADIANCE: ITS ROLE IN LIGHT PENETRATION AND BIOLOGICAL EFFECTS

Irradiance, essentially the power or intensity or brightness of the light (measured in milliwatts per square centimeter, or mW/cm^2), plays a critical role in determining both the penetration depth and the biological effects of light therapy.

At first glance, the relationship appears straightforward: the higher the irradiance, the greater the depth of penetration. While this is certainly true to an extent, the story is more complex and nuanced.

Before we get into the role of irradiance in influencing how much light is getting to the deep tissues, it's critical to grasp that

wavelength, not irradiance, is the dominant determinant of light penetration into tissue (as we've already discussed at length).

Think of it this way: The wavelength is like choosing the right vehicle for your terrain, while the intensity is the amount of fuel you put in that vehicle. If you're trying to cross a lake, it doesn't matter how much gas you put in your car—you need a boat. But once you have the right boat, more fuel lets you go farther and faster across that water.

So if you were to compare the penetration depth of red and NIR light vs. blue or UV light, the difference would be enormous. Even with vastly more powerful blue or UV lights, red and NIR wavelengths penetrate far deeper into human tissue. The most powerful UV light imaginable—so strong it would instantly burn your skin—still wouldn't penetrate more than a few millimeters deep. Meanwhile, red and NIR light at that same power level might reach beyond 50 or close to 100 millimeters into tissue.

This vast difference in penetration capability is a fundamental property of the wavelengths themselves—how they physically interact with molecules in your skin, fat, and muscle. So before discussing irradiance, we need to understand that *wavelength* sets the fundamental boundaries for penetration.

Once we've selected a suitable wavelength range (typically red or NIR wavelengths for PBM), *at that point,* irradiance becomes a major factor in how much light actually reaches deeper tissues. So *both* wavelength and irradiance matter.

Think about shining that flashlight through your hand. The color (wavelength) makes the biggest difference in whether you'll see it on the other side, but brightness also matters.

Imagine four different colored flashlights—ultraviolet (UV), blue, green, and red:

With the UV flashlight, no matter how powerful—whether a weak keychain light or an industrial-strength lamp—you won't see anything on the other side. The UV light gets completely absorbed in the first millimeter or two of skin.

With the blue flashlight, a standard intensity shows nothing. An extremely powerful blue light might show the faintest hint through the thinnest parts of your fingers, but that's it.

The green flashlight performs slightly better. With normal brightness, you still won't see it through your hand. With a very high-powered green light, you might see a dim glow through thin parts, but most of your hand will block it.

With a red flashlight, even a low-powered one clearly shows a red glow through your fingers and thinner parts of your palm. A powerful red flashlight will show substantially more light—even through thicker parts of your hand.

Finally, though the light will be invisible to naked eyes, a NIR flashlight (used with special goggles) penetrates even better than red light. A moderate-intensity NIR light would shine through your entire hand, and a high-intensity one would pass through with impressive brightness.

The key point: Wavelength is the foundational factor dictating light penetration in biological tissue. But irradiance also certainly plays a role in determining how deeply light penetrates. All things being equal in terms of wavelengths (e.g., red light at 660 nm or NIR at 810 nm), higher-irradiance light sources will increase the light's penetration. (And there's another even more important benefit we'll discuss shortly that is more nuanced than simply the maximal depth of light penetration.)

This isn't just my opinion—ample research has indeed shown that higher irradiances do in fact enhance penetration depth of the light into the tissue.

One of the best studies on this subject described their robust findings from many different tests in this way:[23]

The proportion of structures from live subjects demonstrating complete penetration at 100 mW/cm² was 9% of all structures tested (n = 53), 28% at 300 mW/cm², and 43% at 500 mW/cm². The proportion of cadaver structures demonstrating complete penetration of all structures tested (n = 19 individual structures across 6 cadavers) was 11% at 100 mW/cm² and 26% at both 300 and 500 mW/cm² irradiance. There were an additional 55 structures with thickness between 95 and 150 mm that were tested in the 9 live subjects. These structures included the shoulder, humerus, coronal elbow, hamstring, femur, sagittal and coronal knee, calf, and sagittal ankle. No detectable readings were obtained at 100 and 300 mW/cm² irradiances, however, 5.5% of structures demonstrated red-light penetration at an irradiance of 500 mW/cm². These data indicate: (1) all 3 red-light irradiances reliably penetrate through live tissue structures with thickness of 50 mm or less, (2) increasing the irradiance to 500 mW/cm² increases the penetration, and (3) complete penetration of red-light is negligible in tissues with an optical path greater than 95 mm, even at an irradiance of 500 mW/cm².

The key point is that they clearly demonstrated the basic principle that higher irradiance light sources were able to penetrate more deeply into the tissue. This is an important advantage of higher irradiance: All other factors being equal, we can deliver the light deeper into tissues than is possible with lower irradiance devices.

While this would tend to lead one to conclude that higher irradiances are always going to be better, the reality is more complex than that. There are concerns and downsides with very high irradiances, too, as we'll discuss.

In the body, the effect of higher irradiance on penetration depth only holds true up to a point. For example, while going from 10 mW/cm² to 100 mW/cm² may provide a large increase in the light's penetration depth, going from 100 mW/cm² to 200 mW/cm² may provide only a relatively small additional increase in penetration depth.

It's also worth noting that in the above study, while going all the way up to 300 mW/cm² or even 500 mW/cm² enhanced penetration depth, the researchers noted that above 100 mW/cm², it required a "disproportionate increase in irradiance" to get significantly deeper penetration into the tissue.

In the body, this effect of higher irradiance on penetration depth is only up to a point—for example, while going from 10 mW/cm² to 100 mW/cm² may provide a large increase in penetration depth of the light, going from 100 mW/cm² to 200 mW/cm² may provide only a relatively small additional increase in penetration depth.

In other words, once a certain irradiance is reached, the benefits of high irradiance on light penetration basically max out, and there isn't actually a big difference in penetration depth of the light even if one dramatically increases the irradiance beyond that.

Fortunately, the researchers noted that "A red-light irradiance of 100 mW/cm² is sufficient to penetrate tissues of up to 50 mm in thickness" and they offered the following practical guidance as a result of this experimentation:[23]

Our main finding is that red-light can successfully penetrate up to 50 mm below the skin surface of lean tissues at 100 mW/cm² in all live subjects. We also demonstrated that increasing the red-light irradiance beyond 100 mW/cm² did not greatly improve penetration, and we therefore propose the use of an irradiance of 100 mW/cm² for red-light treatments and future research in tissues of 50 mm thickness or less.

Make a mental note of this, because it may be that 100 mW/cm² represents an approximately optimal irradiance for treating deep tissues, which maximizes penetration depth but doesn't cause the issues that very high irradiances do. (This is why my recommended irradiance ranges stay around this number.)

So again, the basic idea here is that higher irradiances lead to deeper penetration of light into tissue.

However, there's an important benefit of higher vs. lower irradiances than simply that it increases the maximal penetration depth (the deepest level where any photons are detectable). It also determines the intensity of light present at a given tissue depth *before* that maximal depth.

In other words, there are two distinct aspects of light penetration we need to consider:

- Maximal penetration depth: The deepest measurement where any photons (perhaps even a single photon) are still detectable. After this point, all light is completely extinguished.
- Irradiance at various depths prior to the maximal depth: The intensity of light present at depths of tissue before we get to the maximal depth.

Why is this distinction important? Our cells have a biological threshold for responding to light. Our tissues need light to reach a minimum intensity (generally thought to be around 1 to 5 mW/cm²) before they'll react at all. Below this threshold, nothing happens biologically, no matter how long the exposure.

It's similar to starting a fire. A few sparks won't ignite a log, no matter how many you create or how long you try. You need to reach a minimum heat level before combustion can begin. Your cells work the same way—they need enough light intensity to kickstart a response.

You could also think of it like exercise. You can run 3 miles in 20 minutes or walk those same 3 miles in 2 hours. While both activities cover the exact same distance, only running creates enough intensity to trigger meaningful biological adaptations (in your heart, muscles, mitochondria, etc.) that improve your fitness. You have to get above a certain threshold of intensity to trigger a biological effect.

The point is that when using PBM treatments for deep tissues, we must consider not just whether any light reaches the target depth, but whether enough light (i.e., a high enough intensity of the light) arrives to trigger biological effects (in a reasonable time frame).

So higher irradiances aren't primarily about "making light reach deeper" into the tissue—their real value is making sure that tissues at various depths get *enough light* to cross that biological threshold. With low irradiances, the photons might technically reach deeper tissues, but at such low intensity that your cells simply don't respond. Using more power ensures that tissues at various depths receive enough energy to activate the biological mechanisms that create beneficial responses.

In the 2017 book, *Photomedicine—Advances in Clinical Practice*, Calderhead and Tanaka explain it succinctly:[4]

> So, although wavelength is key, if there is insufficient photon intensity from the light source giving low irradiance, or a too high angle of divergence diluting the irradiance, then the photon intensity at the target will not be sufficient to get the optimum reaction.

Think of it like watering a layered garden bed. Wavelength is like the size of water droplets. Longer wavelengths (like red and NIR light) are similar to larger water droplets that can travel deeper through soil layers before being absorbed, while shorter wavelengths (like blue light) are more like a fine mist that gets captured mostly in the top layers.

Irradiance, on the other hand, is like the volume of water applied per unit time. Consider the following two ways of delivering water to the soil, and think about which approach would deliver more water to 24 inches of depth in that soil:

- Scenario 1: You apply just 30 drops of water (low irradiance) to the soil surface over ten seconds.

- Scenario 2: You pour 3 gallons (high irradiance) onto the same soil over the same ten seconds.

In scenario 1, virtually all of that water will be absorbed and bound up by the top layers of soil with virtually none reaching 24 inches deep. In scenario 2, the top layers become saturated and excess water continues downward, with significant amounts of water reaching 24 inches deep. Only the approach in scenario 2 will actually deliver water effectively to the deep roots of a tree. And at each level before that, at 8, 12, 18 inches, and so on, much more water will be present with the approach of scenario 2.

It's not a perfect analogy, but this is the basic idea of how irradiance influences the way that light interacts with biological tissue. When light enters tissue, it encounters multiple layers that progressively weaken its intensity—each centimeter might reduce the light's strength by perhaps 90 percent or more—so to deliver an effective intensity at a given level of depth, you need to have a high enough starting intensity. Using higher irradiances doesn't just mean that light is going "deeper into the body"—it profoundly changes the intensity of light (and thus the biological effects) even at depths prior to that maximal depth of penetration.

Research illustrates this principle. For example, even with powerful laser devices with extremely high–irradiance beams, the irradiance seen in the deep tissues may be quite low. One study put it this way:[28]

The best penetrating wavelengths [are] in the range of 760–850 nm and may achieve a light density of 5mW/cm² at 5 cm deep when the beam power is 1 watt [1,000 mW] and surface density is 5W/cm² [5,000 mW/cm²].

In other words, less than 1 percent of the light present at the surface was detectable at 5 cm of depth into the tissue, even with an extraordinarily powerful laser.

This helps explain why more powerful devices are often necessary for treating deep tissues, even apart from any differences in maximal penetration depth. In other words, even if for example, a 20 mW/cm² and a 100 mW/cm² device technically had the same maximal "penetration depth" (as defined by the maximal depth that *any* photons are detectable) of 5 cm, the higher irradiance device will be delivering much more light (perhaps 400 to 500 percent more) at every level of depth before the light is extinguished. If roughly 90 percent of the light is attenuated for each centimeter it travels through the tissue, it becomes obvious that a low irradiance of light will much more rapidly be attenuated to levels that are less able to induce a biological effect. For example, with a 20 mW/cm² device, light will be attenuated to just 2 mW/cm² after traveling through 1 cm of tissue, and then

0.2 mW/cm² by 2 cm of depth. In other words, the lower the irradiance, the more rapidly the light will be attenuated to intensities that are likely too low to trigger biological responses.

Even with just this layer of the story, it becomes apparent that there are some serious flaws in a huge percentage of PBM devices on the market. While irradiances below 30 mW/cm² may be perfectly adequate (even optimal) for superficial tissues, if you're trying to treat deep tissues, low-irradiance devices are likely to be relatively ineffective, because the irradiance is going to drop off to extremely low (and probably biologically insignificant) levels by the time you go beyond a couple of centimeters deep into the tissue.

Now, you might logically think that the simple way to overcome these factors and deliver biologically relevant doses of light very deep into the body is to use an extremely powerful device. Unfortunately, it's not that simple, because beyond a certain point, very high irradiances also come with drawbacks, particularly involving overheating the tissues.

These factors create a challenging balance: The starting intensity must be high enough to maintain therapeutic levels at the target depth, but not so high that it creates excessive heating of the tissues.

It's also the case that once you go beyond a certain depth, you get to a point where no light device (no matter what wavelengths it uses, and how powerful the device is) is going to deliver biologically significant amounts of light. In my conversations with Dr. Cronshaw, he made the point that even with very powerful devices, it may take hours to deliver a 4 J/cm² dose (sometimes regarded as an ideal target dose) to very deep tissues beyond 5 to 7 cm of depth.

On the other hand, it is also the case that the deeper you go into the body, the more you tend to encounter tissues that are far more sensitive to even relatively low levels of light. Many mitochondria-rich tissues, like those in muscles and the brain, may still respond to extremely low light intensities.[1] Even very low irradiances reaching the right tissues may offer therapeutic benefits, but more research is needed to understand tissue-specific activation levels.

In summary, the deeper your target tissue, the more critical irradiance becomes. A device that's too weak won't deliver meaningful energy to deep tissues. On the other hand, pushing irradiance too high risks creating excessive heat and damaging tissues.

For superficial goals like treating the skin, lower irradiances may be sufficient or even ideal. For deeper work—such as muscle, joint, or brain therapies—irradiance in the 75 to 125 mW/cm² range (and prioritizing NIR wavelengths) often provides the best balance between depth, intensity, and safety.

As we've seen from one of the most

impressive studies done on penetration of light through biological tissues, the researchers found that around 100 mW/cm² of red light is an effective target irradiance for treating tissues up to 5 cm deep. If you go far higher than that in irradiance, further gains in penetration depth are minimal, and issues with overheating tissues begin to emerge at very high irradiances. (We'll discuss the safe irradiance ranges for both red and NIR light shortly.)

Understanding irradiance this way will help you select the right PBM devices for your goals—and avoid many of the common pitfalls of underpowered or poorly designed devices.

When Low Irradiances Have Effects on Deep Tissues

Some researchers and PBM users argue that high irradiance is not always necessary. In fact, certain studies suggest that relatively low irradiances—sometimes as low as 20 to 30 mW/cm²—can still produce significant effects in deep tissues like those of the brain.

For example, a study of veterans with chronic traumatic brain injuries (TBI) reported that delivering 6.4 mW/cm² of red and NIR light to the head for 20 minutes three times per week improved neuropsychological health and cerebral blood flow for years after the TBI.[29] Even after a single session of 810-nm NIR (20 mW/cm² for 350 seconds providing 7 J/cm²) across the forehead, older adults with mild cognitive impairment experienced a 25-percent increase in cognitive function within one hour following treatment.[30]

What's peculiar about much of this research is that some of these studies are showing benefits to brain health using wavelengths and irradiances that shouldn't be powerful enough to deliver almost *any* significant amount of light through the skull directly to the brain. There are even reports of "red light bucket hats" being used for Parkinson's patients with good results, and these merely use inexpensive red light LED strips (which have a very low irradiance) applied several inches away from the head.[31] In other words, these devices shouldn't really be delivering any significant amount of light through the skull into the brain.

So the real question is: How can light improve brain function when little to no light gets through the skull?

While some people interpret this research to mean that the light is somehow getting into the brain (even though it doesn't make sense that it is), there is another more likely explanation.

The big confounding variable in this type of research is, of course, systemic effects. We know from many lines of research that we can derive benefits in certain areas of the body even when light isn't directed onto those specific tissues.

In an interview I did with Dr. Arany, he described this phenomenon:

> There are some really fascinating studies for Parkinson's where, again, this may be a little too geeky for you, but this is like, they take animals, they inject a toxin, and they create tremors in the animal. When they treat the head, the animal gets better. . . . When they did the same experiment by covering the head with silver foil and just treated the body of the animals, the animals still got better, indicating that the precise location may not be the critical factor . . . the systemic effects are very important.

The same phenomenon was also demonstrated in animal research. When scientists directed light on rats' legs and abdomens—nowhere near their brains—they observed remarkable improvements in brain function that matched or exceeded the benefits seen when light was applied directly to the head.[32] This striking finding suggests that red/NIR light's *systemic* effects, rather than the direct interaction of photons with brain tissue, may be the primary driver of its cognitive benefits.

Dr. Hamblin has also noted in multiple interviews (with me and others) that the research that has shown a benefit to brain health using very weak intranasal devices is much more likely to be mediated by systemic effects (irradiating the bloodstream with light) rather than directly delivering light to the brain, since the light would be expected to be far too weak to deliver a meaningful dose to the brain.

So we need to be cautious in interpreting such studies to mean that those low irradiances were just as good as higher irradiances for a certain purpose; it may be that no light from the treatment was delivered to the target tissue at all and that the benefit was mediated through indirect systemic mechanisms.

When looking at research where very weak lights show benefits for deep tissues (particularly areas like the brain where light delivery is difficult), systemic effects are likely at play. These systemic effects represent a major confounding variable in interpreting PBM research, since studies often show effects on deep tissues even when no light was directly delivered there. If we assume light can only work through direct interaction of photons with those specific target cells, we might draw incorrect conclusions about optimal dosing parameters.

In short, while low irradiances may not deliver enough light to stimulate deep tissues directly, they may still work by triggering systemic changes. This doesn't invalidate the need for higher irradiances when you're trying to reach deep targets directly, but it does highlight an important alternative pathway for PBM to create profound physiological benefits even when no light directly interacts with the target tissue.

Is Higher Irradiance Always Better?

While higher irradiances are necessary for reaching deeper tissues, deeper penetration and higher irradiances are not always the optimal choice. In fact, for certain applications, higher irradiances can be counterproductive.

As discussed earlier (in the section on the biphasic dose response), excessively high irradiances can trigger negative effects through two mechanisms:

1. The sheer rate of photon delivery may overwhelm cellular responses.
2. The heat generation from high-power light exposure may cause tissue stress.

So while higher surface irradiance is helpful to deliver therapeutic light levels at depth, lower irradiances (~10 to 50 mW/cm²) are more optimal for:

- Superficial skin treatments (e.g., anti-aging, wound healing, scalp health)
- Full-body treatments (like in a pod)
- Light-sensitive tissues such as:
  - Oral and nasal mucosa
  - Reproductive organs
  - Eyes

For these applications, higher irradiances may be less effective or even counterproductive.

I spoke with Dr. Hamblin about the fact that many people stand in front of panels that emit upwards of 80 mW/cm² irradiances for facial skin anti-aging benefits, and he replied: "I mean, but would you seriously use a whole-body panel to improve your facial surface?" He went on to suggest that the range of 20 to 40 mW/cm² is likely to be optimal for facial skin anti-aging effects.

In short, different devices and settings are appropriate for different goals. Here's how that breaks down:

- For deep tissues, higher irradiances and NIR wavelengths are often required, but one should not go too high to avoid tissue overheating.
- For superficial or light-sensitive tissues, lower irradiances and red light are usually more appropriate and higher irradiances can either be ineffective or counterproductive.
- For systemic effects, large panels or full-body light beds that deliver a high total dose across a large surface area are ideal.

We'll discuss this in greater depth in the next chapter. The key point here is simply to emphasize that it's not about always choosing higher irradiance—it's about choosing the right tool (device and parameters) for your treatment goal.

How High Is Too High? What Is Excessive Irradiance that Results in Tissue Heating or Other Negative Effects?

The issue of tissue heating during PBM deserves particular attention. As a general rule, we can say that the irradiance needs to be at a high enough intensity to elicit a beneficial biological effect, but that we must also be aware that "using higher intensity, the photon energy will be transformed to excessive heat in the target tissue."[1] In other words, as irradiance increases, so does the potential for tissue heating. And a certain amount of tissue heating can cause harm, either by triggering cellular mechanisms that diminish therapeutic benefits of PBM, or potentially by causing actual damage to the cells.

This situation creates a delicate balance between having a high enough irradiance to achieve sufficient penetration depth (and adequate light intensity at that depth to trigger a biological effect) and maintaining optimal tissue response (i.e., avoiding overheating the tissue).

This irradiance issue has led to an important point of controversy among PBM experts and bloggers/device manufacturers, in which different opinions and interpretations of the scientific literature have emerged about what constitute low, optimal, and excessive irradiance, and what are acceptable and excessive heating of tissues.

First, let's examine the issue of heating of the tissues.

One interesting view held by some PBM experts is the notion that PBM must be "non-thermal"—that is, that for light therapy to truly be "photobiomodulation," it must by definition not heat the tissues. By this line of thinking, any heating of the tissues indicates that the treatment is not "true photobiomodulation" and is inherently nonoptimal, or potentially harmful, due to the presence of heating.

This is an interesting and contentious point that has caused widespread confusion.

The reason is that "heating" (i.e., temperature) is not a binary: It is not "heat vs. no heat" but rather, of course, a spectrum. Stated in terms of temperature, light may not raise the temperature at all, or raise it from 98°F to 98.5°F, or to 99°F, or to 101°F, or to extreme temperatures like 107°F or 110°F. Yet the notion that *any degree of heating* is nonoptimal is problematic because many common devices on the market in reasonable irradiances (perhaps 50 to 130 mW/cm²) and many clinical PBM lasers used in PBM clinics will generally cause at least some warming of the tissues (most likely to levels that are perfectly comfortable for most people). In fact, even many pad-style devices with irradiances under 30 mW/cm² may cause heating in the area (likely more from direct transfer of heat from the device itself in contact with the skin, and from a lack of ventilation, than from light being transformed into heat) during the PBM treatment.

If *any* PBM device that warms tissue to any measurable degree is "not true photobiomodulation," it would mean that an enormous portion—the vast majority—of the PBM devices on the market, from panels, to pads, to many lasers used in clinical settings, are somehow "not true photobiomodulation."

So at what point does "photobiomodulation" with red and NIR light become "not photobiomodulation"? Is it when the light source induces a thermal effect that measurably raises the temperature of the tissue by even one degree, or is it when that temperature reaches above a certain threshold?

One answer to this question comes from research done by PBM researcher Dr. Arany. His team's research showed that when the tissues are heated excessively during PBM, it can begin to deactivate internal oxidant scavengers, and above a higher threshold of temperature, overt cellular damage begins to occur.

I had a discussion with Dr. Arany on this issue when I hosted him on my podcast, and he clarified his views. He believes that PBM should be non-thermal, but his position seems to be that some mild warming of the tissues is not likely to be harmful as long as it's below 42°C (107.6°F) (and/or below the threshold of discomfort), but that over 42°C (107.6°F)

would likely negate the benefits of BPM, and at 45°C (113°F), cellular damage will occur. Importantly, he emphasizes that the feeling of being uncomfortably hot is a good indication that problematic heating is occurring.

While I was initially skeptical that it was possible to heat the skin to these temperatures with LED PBM devices (as can be heard in my exchange with Dr. Arany, when I said that I didn't think PBM devices could raise skin temperature as high as in a sauna where the air temperature may be above 200°F, or 93°C), I have now seen and used some PBM devices—including some LED devices, but more often powerful laser devices—heat the skin temperature to above 42°C (107.6°F) or 43°C (109.4°F). And given that some of the newer generations of devices are pushing for higher and higher irradiances (some LED devices are now above 300 mW/cm^2), this is becoming more of a concern, as Dr. Arany pointed out.

Interestingly, this issue of heating isn't only a phenomenon in high irradiance PBM devices. For example, my son injured his knee a day ago as I write this, and I used a neoprene-pad style PBM device on his knee (which has only about a 25 mW/cm^2 irradiance), and he complained that his knee was getting really hot. (Again, this was likely due to heat transfer from the device itself and how the pad limits skin ventilation, rather than the irradiance being excessive—but it heated his skin a lot nonetheless, and to the degree that tissue heating during PBM is problematic, then this also should be considered.)

The notion that PBM must be "non-thermal" has led some to worry that *any* noticeable tissue warming, even when comfortable, or pleasant, could be harmful or disqualify a treatment from being "true photobiomodulation." However, much evidence suggests—along with the views of other PBM experts—that moderate tissue warming (within comfort bounds and below 42°C or 43°C, or 107.6°F to 109°F) during PBM isn't harmful. In fact, according to many PBM experts, it may even be beneficial.

It's crucial to understand that heating exists on a spectrum—there's a wide range of temperature increase before reaching the point of discomfort. Dr. Arany's research didn't show that any degree of heating was harmful, nor did they find a linear relationship where each increment of heating caused proportional harm. Rather, problematic changes began only above this specific threshold.

For context, it's useful to consider sunlight, our primary light-exposure source. Sunbathing significantly warms our tissues while delivering higher irradiances (~100 to 160 mW/cm²) across multiple wavelengths, including blue, ultraviolet, and far-infrared—all of which generate heat, often more than red and NIR light do. Yet if heat-generating light sources were incompatible with photobiomodulation, sunlight itself couldn't qualify as "photo-

biomodulation" (since of course, sun exposure heats our tissues). This restrictive perspective—limiting "true photobiomodulation" to highly specific, low-irradiance manmade devices—contradicts basic evolutionary biology. The photobiomodulation mechanisms in human physiology evolved through millions of years of sun exposure. It seems bizarre to argue that the sun, which drove the evolution of the very mechanisms that modern PBM devices harness, somehow fails to deliver "true photobiomodulation."

We should also question the idea that tissue heating is inherently harmful or problematic. Many lines of evidence show that it clearly isn't. While *excessive* heating can damage tissues (just as excessive exercise can), mild and moderate tissue heating doesn't harm our cells. Humans have evolved sophisticated mechanisms to handle and benefit from natural heat exposure, whether from sunlight, physical activity, or environmental sources—often experiencing all three simultaneously. Our bodies' remarkable heat-adaptation abilities make moderate tissue warming not only tolerable but potentially beneficial, as demonstrated by the profound health benefits of regular sauna bathing. Like many biological processes, the relationship follows a U-curve: Moderate doses promote health, while extremes can be detrimental or ineffective. While hyperthermia differs from PBM, and tissue heating from red and NIR light might theoretically behave differently than heat from saunas, hot baths, or far-infrared devices (topics requiring further research), it's evolutionarily illogical to believe that any slight heating is fundamentally incompatible with PBM, especially given that the sun—our primary evolutionary PBM source—induces tissue heating.

More directly, all over the world, clinicians who use laser PBM devices frequently heat the tissues up to 42°C (107.6°F) or above it for brief periods of time, with only beneficial effects. This is commonplace for practitioners who use clinical lasers.

To be clear, however, it is certainly possible to overheat tissues to the point of cellular damage, which should obviously be avoided. So the real question is: What level of tissue heating is perfectly acceptable, and at what point does it become harmful?

I spoke with Dr. Hamblin on this topic of tissue heating during PBM, about the claims of PBM treatments needing to be "non-thermal" and when I mentioned that some people argue that any irradiances higher than 50 mW/cm² are problematic because they cause heat generation. Here's how that exchange went:

> **DR. HAMBLIN:** It's pretty well known what the relationship between irradiance and tissue heating is. It's wavelength-dependent. Probably the least heating is 810 nm, and you can easily have up to 500 milliwatts per cm². For red light, it's a bit lower, so maybe 200 to 300 mW/cm², you may be beginning to feel it warm.

> **ARI:** . . . I have an LED panel that is under 100 mW/cm². Let's say it's around 65 mW/cm². I have another one that's close to 100 mW/cm². If I press my skin up against it, within 5 minutes, it starts definitely heating up the tissues. Now, it's not overwhelmingly hot, but it's definitely getting warm. I've also experienced a lot of tissue warming even with pad-style devices with low irradiances below 25 mW/cm², even to the point of sweating inside the pad. Why?

> **DR. HAMBLIN:** Probably because the device itself is heating up. It's got fans in it, has it?

> **ARI:** Yes.

> **DR. HAMBLIN:** The fans are not perfect, they will remove a lot of the heat, but not all of it. The heating of the tissue comes from two things. One is the device itself gets hot because the LEDs are only about 30 percent efficient, so 70 percent of the electrical energy goes to heating, anyway. Then the light energy that's absorbed by the tissue is mostly converted to heat. A little bit of photochemistry goes on, but the vast majority is converted to heat anyway. The tissue is constantly cooling itself. It's cooling itself by blood flow, by re-emitting radiation, by evaporation of sweat, there's all sorts of intrinsic methods that the tissue will try and regain its temperature homeostasis. What do you mean by heating? Uncomfortable or just pleasantly warm?

ARI: Yes, pleasantly warm.

DR. HAMBLIN: Pleasantly warm is good, I think.

ARI: You don't suspect that any warming of the tissues is harmful? . . . Some people have made the argument that true photobiomodulation has to not heat the tissues, essentially—that to be "photobiomodulation," it must not heat the tissues.

DR. HAMBLIN: That's rubbish. Pleasantly warm is good. A part of the mechanism is based on nano-heating of biochemical structures in the cells, like ion channels, for instance, heat-sensitive ion channels—that's part of the mechanism. Saying that a pleasant warmth in the tissue is bad, it's just rubbish.

In contrast to the claims that PBM must be "non-thermal," Dr. Hamblin says that some degree of tissue heating is *actually part of the mechanism* of how red and NIR light exert their effects on our physiology.

Later, I spoke with Dr. Cronshaw, an authority on PBM dosimetry and tissue heating. He strongly disagrees with the notion that PBM should be "non-thermal." He uses lasers in his clinic on a daily basis that induce significant tissue heating. Here's how that exchange went:

ARI: There are some people who argue that photobiomodulation is by definition, non-thermal. . . . By this line of argumentation, anytime you're applying photobiomodulation using parameters that are causing, let's say some degree of heating, let's say a one or two or three or four degree rise in the tissue temperatures, therefore, [according to this line of thinking], it means it's not true "photobiomodulation" because it causes a thermal effect. What do you think of this line of argumentation?

DR. CRONSHAW: It's very pure thinking in the sense that trying to splice what photobiomodulation is into a certain pathway, which is related to a photochemical process, as opposed to the more intricate aspects of electromagnetic irradiation on biological tissues. In any chemical reaction, you get heat as a byproduct. You can't have a chemical reaction without there being some spin-off in terms of heat. The 100 percent pure transfer of photonic energy into a photochemical one just doesn't happen.

You always get heat, and heat is very strictly regulated inside the cell. When they're talking about heat, they're talking about measurable heat in terms of tangible temperature increases, which then may be beyond the cell and into the tissues. This is where, indeed, there is a difference between photobiomodulation and its effects and heat. The two things inevitably go together. You always get some heat, even with a 50 mW/cm^2 source. . . . It's biologically nonsense to say that in photobiomodulation, there is no heat. It's impossible. Either that or they belong to a different physical planet to the rest of us. It's just not possible.

. . .

When you're starting to get (tissue temperature) up to round about 39.5° C (103.1°F) through to about 42°C (107.6°F), some very useful things clinically can happen because this coincides with what I would refer to as an analgesia zone . . . The range beyond which you don't want to go is sustained increases of temperature above 45° C (113°F), where after a while, here you're looking at some time, then you can start to see signs of tissue damage because then you're starting to progressively overwhelm the capacity of the tissues to withstand the sustained insults of the temperature. The hotter it is, the shorter the duration the tissues can stand to exposure to heat.

You can have a sip of coffee or tea, which is maybe 55°C (131°F), not quite 60°C (140°F). You don't burn your lips because it's in contact with the tissues for less than a second. It's spread over an area and you don't burn yourself, just like you can lick your finger and touch the hot stove for a moment, without burning yourself. It's the same. There's a trade-off between the temperature rise, the peak temperature that you achieve, and the amount of damage you're going to get.

In other words, Dr. Cronshaw is saying that claiming that PBM is "non-thermal" is largely an argument of trying to define the very *concept* of "photobiomodulation" as being entirely distinct from mechanisms related to tissue heating, and as being comprised of only specific photochemical mechanisms. Imagine someone trying to define "exercise" as only the muscle contractions while insisting that any increase in heart rate or body temperature "isn't really exercise" or even that it's harmful and should actively be avoided—that you should only exercise in ways that don't elevate your body temperature. Of course, exercise and heat generation go together. While we can conceptually separate muscle contractions from heat generation, the physiological reality is that they go together. The same basic principle holds true with light exposure.

After clarifying the issue with Dr. Arany, Dr. Hamblin, and Dr. Cronshaw, I found that while they may talk about it very differently, they actually all seem to generally agree that more moderate warming of the tissues below 42°C (107.6°F) is not likely to be harmful, and that prolonged tissue heating above the point of discomfort is likely to be harmful.

Both Dr. Hamblin and Dr. Cronshaw emphasized repeatedly in my conversations with them that they don't consider tissue heating to be a big concern for a very simple reason: The body has internal mechanisms to let you know when the tissue is being overheated. In other words, the idea is that our subjective perception of heat—whether we experience something as comfortable warmth or uncomfortably hot—is sufficient to avoid harm from excessive tissue heating. Basically, if a device is causing excessive heating of the tissues, we will naturally *feel* this discomfort and have the urge to move the device or turn it off—people are not just going to sit there and damage themselves.

Now, on an intuitive level, this certainly seems logical. But the question is: What if harm from heating the tissues begins to occur *below* the threshold of where humans tend to feel discomfort from heating of the tissues? In other words, it would be a big concern if evidence showed that PBM treatments induce cellular damage at temperatures well below the threshold of perceptible discomfort. In that scenario, we'd need to be extremely cautious about using devices that could induce this imperceptible cellular damage; perhaps we'd need to use a thermometer during PBM treatments to closely monitor skin temperature and thus prevent unknowingly heating the tissues into the range in which we were damaging our cells.

I was curious to look into this to see if there is any hard data that either confirms or refutes Dr. Hamblin's hypothesis on skin temperature and subjective sense of discomfort/pain. While we don't have perfect data specifically testing this in the context of red and NIR light PBM, the broader scientific literature provides fairly clear guidance on human temperature thresholds.

The transition point from pleasant warmth to perhaps very slight discomfort begins to occur around 41 to 42°C (106 to 107.6°F), with a clear transition to the tissue feeling uncomfortably hot at around 43°C (109°F). This temperature range represents the threshold where our thermoreceptors (temperature-sensing nerve endings) signal clear discomfort, but importantly, *before* significant tissue damage occurs.

The overall body of data is still imperfect, but most sources suggest the following key temperature thresholds:

- Around 41 to 42°C (106 to 107.6°F): Tissues feel distinctly warm, potential onset of a slight or moderate feeling of uncomfortable warmth
- 43°C (109°F): Clear discomfort/pain threshold
- 45°C (113°F): Definite pain and clear sensation of burning in the tissues
- Above 48°C (118°F): Risk of burns begins, especially with prolonged exposure

This also lines up perfectly with Dr. Cronshaw's statements, where he said:

... TRPV1, which is an ion gate which opens when it reaches 43°C (109°F). It's both temperature as well as light-sensitive. When that gate opens, you go, "Oh, oh, that's unpleasant, that's hot, I'm moving." When I'm doing my therapeutic PBM laser treatment with more intensive treatments for my patients, and my patient says, "It's getting really quite warm," I know I'm just getting to that threshold. That's a safe threshold because above that level, this is where if I was to keep doing it, they're not going to just sit there and let me overheat them. Patients don't appreciate being barbecued. It just doesn't happen. People pull away and say it's too hot.

After spending an enormous amount of time exploring this issue, it seems, fortunately, that our internal mechanisms do in fact alert us quite effectively when our tissues are being heated excessively: We feel discomfort and have the natural urge to stop the treatment or move the device (to a different body area) *before* we get to the point where tissue damage occurs. In other words, one would really have to force oneself to endure strong discomfort and pain signals from their body—for a prolonged period of time—to cause significant cellular damage with LED PBM devices.

It's worth noting that high-powered *lasers* are uniquely capable of inducing rapid tissue heating and potentially causing cellular damage, which is why these devices are only available to trained clinicians who know how to use them. (Note: Simple "optical scanning"—slowly moving the device around—is typically enough to avoid tissue overheating for clinicians using lasers.)

But again, with LED devices (i.e., basically all at-home PBM devices), our body's own subjective sense of discomfort is perfectly adequate in helping us avoid any harm to our tissues. To be clear, we *should* listen to these internal signals. If we feel an uncomfortable or painful heat, it indicates that tissues are heating beyond the safe threshold, and we should pause or stop the treatment or move the device to a different body area. More proactively, it's probably best to use devices below the irradiances that will induce a level of tissue overheating that causes pain (and following the guidelines in this book will avoid that possibility).

What Level of Irradiance Is Acceptable, and What Level Is Excessive?

Now as we've seen, higher irradiances are helpful in delivering effective doses of light to the deep tissues, but higher irradiances also carry the potential to overheat tissues. Too low of an irradiance and you get less penetration depth and/or too low of light intensity at tissue depths beyond 1 or 2 cm of tissue depth to have significant biological effects. So the goal is to have a high enough irradiance to maximize the effectiveness of the PBM treatment, but not so high that it creates excessive heating of the tissues.

So let's directly address the controversy about what constitutes an optimal vs. excessively high irradiance. While we've already touched on some of the key evidence relating to this, we need greater clarity.

There are various claims about irradiance levels. On one end of the spectrum, some people (particularly manufacturers of LED panels) claim or imply that the highest irradiance is best (and these manufacturers compete to create the highest-irradiance panels). On the other end of the spectrum are people who warn about the dangers of using irradiances as low as 50 mW/cm² because it can cause heating of the tissues (again, based on the premise we just explored that PBM should be "non-thermal").

Let's avoid getting bogged down in the details of all the competing and contradictory claims about irradiance and simply go straight to the evidence. A 2018 review of the body of evidence on effective and safe dosing parameters states:[1]

[T]here exists a lower threshold (perhaps 0.5 mW/cm²) below which the illumination time could be infinite and would be no different from daylight. Similarly, the upper threshold is fixed by the possible photothermal effect if the power density is too large. **The irradiance values, that produce unacceptable heating of the tissue, are governed by the wavelength and are ~750 mW/cm² at 800 to 900 nm, about 300 mW/cm² at 600 to 700 nm, and as low as 100 mW/cm² at 400 to 500 nm.**

The irradiance values that produce unacceptable tissue heating have been studied and discussed by PBM researchers over many years. The literature suggests that the points at which irradiances become excessively high are above about 300 mW/cm² for red wavelengths. For NIR, it is even higher at around 750 mW/cm². In personal communication, Dr. Hamblin said that the number stated above for NIR is too high, and suggested that the threshold should be about 500 mW/cm². Dr. Cronshaw echoed these numbers.

What's the ideal irradiance range that will help us maximize depth of penetration and PBM treatment efficacy for deep tissues, while still being very cautious to avoid overheating the tissues?

We actually have a pretty good answer to this. Let's integrate a key study we previously discussed in the section on penetration depth. In their study of how different irradiances of red light penetrate through various tissues, the researchers noted:[43]

Our main finding is that red-light can successfully penetrate up to 50 mm below the skin surface of lean tissues at 100 mW/cm² in all live subjects. We also demonstrated that increasing the red-light irradiance beyond 100 mW/cm² did not greatly improve penetration, and we therefore propose the use of an irradiance of 100 mW/cm² for red-light treatments and future research in tissues of 50 mm thickness or less.

They found that penetration depth was close to maximal around 100 mW/cm², and that a "disproportionate increase in irradiance" was required to achieve any deeper penetration than the depth achieved at 100 mW/cm². Fortunately, this advice lines up remarkably well with the above guidelines on irradiances that produce unacceptable heating of the tissues (again, about 300 mW/cm² for 600 to 700 nm and about 500 mW/cm² in the 800 to 900 nm range). Given that 100 mW/cm² offers excellent penetration *and is far below* the established safe irradiance thresholds for excessive tissue heating, it likely represents a good general target irradiance to optimize light penetration to deep tissues while not having to worry about overheating the tissues.

However, note that this research (that proposed 100 mW/cm² as an ideal target irradiance) was done on 660-nm red light, and to my knowledge, researchers have not as yet conducted similar research on NIR. We know 800- to 900-nm NIR is less heating to the skin and has a much higher safe irradiance range, so the ideal irradiance for maximizing tissue penetration but avoiding excessive tissue heating is likely to be higher than 100 mW/cm² for NIR wavelengths.

Keep in mind that these numbers are in the context of targeted treatments for **deep tissues** in specific areas of the body. This is *not* a claim that 100 mW/cm² is the ideal number in every PBM treatment context. As discussed in the facial skin section, for example, lower irradiances (under 50 mW/cm²) are generally optimal in superficial tissues, and it's not wise to use higher irradiances on the face. Another scenario where lower irradiances under 50 mW/cm² are likely to be ideal is in whole-body pods, where the entire body is being treated at once. In this scenario, especially if the face is also receiving the light, under 50 mW/cm², and perhaps closer to 20 to 40 mW/cm² is preferable.

PRACTICAL GUIDE TO AVOIDING TISSUE OVERHEATING DURING PBM

Core Principles

- PBM should deliver optimal light doses to target tissues while avoiding excessive tissue heating.

- Higher irradiances help reach deeper tissues, but the higher the irradiance, the more it will potentially raise skin temperature.

- Stay under the established evidence-based guidelines for safe irradiances.
- Mild warming of tissues (below the threshold of discomfort) is acceptable and won't negate benefits; researchers like Dr. Hamblin and Dr. Cronshaw consider some degree of tissue warming to be a *beneficial* rather than harmful part of the PBM treatment, that goes hand in hand with how PBM works.
- Try to keep skin temperatures below 42 or 43°C (107.6 to 109°F), which aligns with the subjective sense of discomfort/overheating.
- Most LED PBM devices won't heat tissues beyond 42°C (107.6°F). However, some newer high-power devices can exceed this threshold.
- Listen to your body—it has built-in mechanisms that alert you to tissue overheating. The temperatures that induce cellular damage align with your body's sensation of excessive heating. Trust biological warning signs: If treatment becomes uncomfortably hot or painful, stop immediately or move the device to a different area of your body. In other words, don't push through painful or uncomfortable heating of your tissues. This simple advice is likely sufficient to avoid harming yourself.

Safe Irradiance Guidelines

EVIDENCE-BASED SAFETY THRESHOLDS:

- 800 to 900 nm range: under 500 mW/cm²
- 600 to 700 nm range: under 200 to 300 mW/cm²

MY RECOMMENDED RANGES:

- **FOR SUPERFICIAL TISSUES:** 10 to 50 mW/cm² (minimal heat management typically needed)
- **FOR DEEP TISSUES:** 50 to 150 mW/cm² (Penetration is nearly maximal around 100 mW/cm² for 660 nm wavelengths, with diminishing returns above this.)

RECOMMENDATION: Please note that I keep my recommended irradiance ranges far below these established thresholds so that I can only err in the direction of excessive safety. It's ideal to stay well below these thresholds and remain closer to approximately 100 mW/cm² for excellent penetration without excessive heating. (Note: This number is for red wavelengths; the threshold is likely to be considerably higher for NIR wavelengths.)

Factors Affecting Tissue Heating

- **DURATION:** If you are using higher-irradiance devices, be aware, that prolonged exposure of a specific area may begin to heat that area as you get to about 5 to 10 minutes. The duration you spend with your tissues at above 42°C (107.6°F) may also be a factor—perhaps 5 minutes at that temperature is harmless, but 20 minutes might cause harm. (We need research to answer these kinds of questions.) As Dr. Cronshaw explained in his examples of drinking hot liquids or touching a hot stove, it's not just a function of the temperature, but the *time* spent at a given temperature.

- **DEVICE HEAT TRANSFER:** A common issue—particularly when using skin contact—is that the device itself heats up and transfers heat into the tissue. This is distinct from the light itself causing heating of the tissue. For example, imagine using a blender for several minutes and putting your hand on the device or even very close to it. The device itself heats up and emits heat that causes tissue heating if it's very close, or on, your skin. People sometimes confuse this type of direct heat transfer with the heating induced by excessively high irradiances of light. This is an issue even with low-irradiance pad-style devices, which often transfer a lot of heat into the tissue due to lack of cooling in the device and lack of skin ventilation (due to the pad being right on the skin). I've used low-irradiance pad devices under 30 mW/cm² that heat up my skin more than devices with irradiances

four or five times higher, that allow for skin ventilation. It's critical to understand that it's not just the *light* that can heat up the tissues via photothermal mechanisms (light photons leading to heat generation once they contact cells), but also direct heat transfer via simple conduction from the device itself. With some devices, particularly with direct skin contact, there is a much larger tissue-heating effect from conduction and limited ventilation than from the light photons being transformed into heat.

- **COVERAGE AREA:** There may also be an important distinction between localized heating of tissues and whole-body temperature. The reason is that large panels and whole-body pods may cause an increase in whole-body temperature, as distinct from heating of tissue on a specific small area of the body. The threshold for feeling uncomfortable or for inducing negative effects from this increase in whole-body temperature may be significantly different from the threshold for harm from localized tissue heating in, for example, your arm or knee.

- **SKIN TYPE:** Darker skin (with higher melanin content) may heat up more than paler skin (particularly with red wavelengths). Therefore, be mindful that depending on your skin type, your skin temperature from a given

PBM device may differ from someone else's.

Heat-Management Strategies

If you do wish to use very high-irradiance devices to treat deep tissues but are concerned about potentially overheating the tissues, here are some strategies to minimize skin heating.

PREVENTIVE STRATEGIES FOR HIGH-IRRADIANCE DEVICES

VENTILATION

- Use fans for continuous airflow over treatment areas to help keep the tissues cooler.
- Ensure good ventilation in the treatment space. (This is particularly important for pad-style devices that limit skin ventilation.)

TEMPERATURE MONITORING

- Since overheating the tissues generally aligns with the subjective sense of discomfort, measuring the recipient's temperature is not typically necessary, but if you're using very high irradiance devices, you can use a thermometer to make sure that the skin temperatures stay below 42 to 43°C (107.6 to 109°F).

PULSING

- Pulsing of the light has long been used in lasers to mitigate heating. By using a device in which the light is rapidly turned off and on multiple times per second, tissue heat has time to dissipate between pulses.

MOVEMENT TECHNIQUES

- With very high-irradiance devices, moving the device ("optical scanning") can be an easy way to minimize tissue heating. (This is commonly done with powerful lasers used in clinics that do PBM.)
- Follow manufacturer movement guidelines (e.g., Chroma's Ironforge device, with an extremely high irradiance, recommends constant movement or "scanning" of the device over the body).

TREATMENT MODIFICATION

- Split a session into two or three shorter sessions with cooling breaks. Or simply use the device for a few minutes on one location, move it to a new spot (which allows the first area to cool), and then cycle back through each area as needed to reach the target dose.

These strategies can be used individually or in combination, depending on your device and treatment needs. The goal is to deliver effective treatment while keeping tissue temperature in a safe and comfortable range.

All of this can potentially be overwhelming, so let's simplify. There's no real need for fear or excessive worry that you'll damage your cells (or ruin the effects of PBM) through warming the tissues. If you are using LED devices (as opposed to lasers), staying within the established safe irradiance ranges (and especially if you're sticking with my far lower recommended ranges), and not pushing through any uncomfortable sensation of excessive heating, you're safe. It's really that simple.

IRRADIANCE AND WAVELENGTH TRADE-OFFS IN DEVICES

As we've seen, to achieve optimal results, both factors—irradiance and wavelength—must align with the treatment objective. So as a general guideline:

- Deeper tissues: High irradiance and NIR wavelengths are more optimal to deliver enough photons to deeper targets like muscles or joints.
- Superficial tissues: Lower or more moderate irradiances and a focus on red wavelengths are more ideal for skin regeneration and anti-aging.

With that in mind, there is another critical issue to understand that ties into both irradiance and wavelengths simultaneously. Many devices are now using multiple wavelengths in their devices—perhaps 660 and 850 nm, or perhaps even four or more wavelengths (e.g., 630, 660, 810, 830, 850, and 1,064 nm).

On paper, this is clearly a beneficial thing—ideally, the more wavelengths used, the more potential you have to have synergistic effects and to reach different depths of tissue. But there is a subtle issue at play here that many people fail to consider: how a total irradiance number is "divided up" between the number of wavelengths in a device.

If irradiance is constant (let's say at 50 mW/cm²), the increase in the number of wavelengths means that each individual wavelength carries a lower irradiance. In other words, the total irradiance is divided up between the number of different wavelengths—so of the 50 mW/cm², perhaps 30 mW/cm² is in the red wavelengths and 15 mW/cm² is in the 800 nm range, and another 5 mW/cm² is in the 1,064 nm range.

So now let's imagine that our goal is to treat deeper tissues like muscles or joints, and we're trying to deliver as much light as possible to a depth of 2 to 5 cm into the tissues. It would be more ideal for this purpose to use wavelengths that have increased ability to penetrate to these depths—that is, more energy in the NIR wavelengths.

So in this case, for the goal of treating deep tissues, using a 50 mW/cm² device where the total irradiance was spread over many wavelengths (i.e., much of it was in the red wavelengths) may very well be less effective than using a device of the same irradiance where *all* of that energy was concentrated in the NIR wavelengths. In other words, having a device with *more* wavelengths is not inherently beneficial, and in this context, may actually lead to poorer results than a device with the same total irradiance concentrated only in the NIR range. It is perfectly conceivable that for a particular goal (i.e., let's say treating an arthritic joint), a device with a single wavelength (let's say 810 nm) would be superior to a device with the same irradiance spread over six or eight different wavelengths where only a small portion of the overall irradiance was in the NIR wavelengths able to penetrate to that depth of tissue.

Conversely, in the case of treating superficial tissues like for skin anti-aging in the face, if you have a device with an optimal irradiance for that purpose (let's say 15 mW/cm^2), and lots of that total energy is concentrated in NIR wavelengths, that means that perhaps too much of it may pass through the superficial tissues and end up in deeper tissues (or not be absorbed by the same chromophores that act to stimulate skin health in the same way as red light wavelengths do). A device that was more of a pure red device (where all of that 15 mW/cm^2 was concentrated at 630 and/or 660 nm) may actually lead to a better result because more of that light will end up being absorbed in the tissues you're trying to target. (Note: It's not either/or and there is certainly still overlap where NIR will absorb in the skin, too,

and stimulate mechanisms that benefit skin health—I'm intentionally simplifying things to make the point clearer.) We also don't have good research that has compared these differences in devices across many different treatment goals, so keep in mind that some of this is logical speculation rather than definitive claims.

Another issue relevant to this is that some companies are simply adding more wavelengths to their devices without scientific evidence to support combining wavelengths in that way. While this may give companies a marketing angle—to claim "our lights have seven wavelengths while competitors only have two or four"—it may, in some cases, actually be worse for the user of the device. One example of this is that some companies have now started putting blue light LEDs into their LED panels. They may do this while citing research on how, for example, blue light combats acne and therefore just generally imply that it is a generally beneficial thing for everyone that blue light is present. To be clear, blue light devices specifically designed for a particular purpose like facial acne treatment or treatment of jaundice in newborns (or a few other specific contexts) can absolutely have benefits for that specific goal, but blue light devices used for these specific purposes is a totally different context than just a random insertion of sparse blue LEDs in a large full-body LED panel designed for general red and NIR PBM. Having a blue light LED here and there in a mostly red and NIR LED panel does not make logical or scientific sense; it's extremely unlikely to provide any meaningful benefit, even for something like combating acne. All it does is simply reduce the overall irradiance being delivered at effective PBM wavelengths in the red and NIR range. Moreover, intense blue light has been linked to *pro-aging* effects in the skin, directly opposing the anti-aging benefits of red light on the skin.[54] This represents a clear example where device design becomes more about marketing than science, and not only that, but where a marketing gimmick could make the device less effective and perhaps even increases the potential that it is counterproductive for one's goals.

As you can see, we have to be careful with the widespread assumption that simply increasing the number of wavelengths of a device makes it better than a device with fewer wavelengths. Be wary of companies simply adding more wavelengths to devices *just based on the vague notion that "more wavelengths are better" or are inherently superior to fewer wavelengths*—that is, without any specific scientific rationale or any actual evidence that supports what they are doing.

What you want is a device with the ideal wavelength(s) for the intended purpose, at the right irradiance for that purpose—not simply more wavelengths for the sake of more wavelengths.

However, keep in mind that this is simply a good general framework to follow, and that in reality, it's more nuanced—red light can also be effective for tissues below the skin's surface, and NIR can also be beneficial for superficial tissues.

KEY POINTS FOR OPTIMIZING IRRADIANCE

Here is an easy-to-use practical framework that can help guide most of your PBM treatment goals.

Based on the body of evidence, we have a fairly good idea of optimal irradiance parameters for different goals.

For skin issues (e.g., anti-aging benefits) and treating other superficial or sensitive tissues, we want a relatively low overall dose on each area of skin, roughly 3 to 20 J/cm² and relatively low irradiance of 10 to 50 mW/cm².

In contrast, for targeted treatment of deeper tissues like muscles, joints, visceral organs, bones, the brain—really anything significantly beneath the surface of the skin—you want a higher irradiance (perhaps between 50 mW/cm² and roughly 150 mW/cm²) to help overcome tissue absorption and scattering effects, which will ensure that a significant amount of light makes it to the deep tissues. NIR is likely more optimal due to its superior penetrative ability (although red light can penetrate quite deeply). The overall dose delivered needs to be higher (from 20 to 60 J/cm², because that is the surface dose, and only a small portion of that will actually make it to the deeper tissues, as we discussed above.

Another nuance here is that in the context of treating large body areas (full-body treatments) using very large LED panels and whole-body pods, particularly where the facial skin is also exposed, one should likely aim for the dosing parameters of superficial tissues (lower to moderate irradiances).

Here's the information in a table. (Note: This is the same information on irradiance and dose contained in the table at the start of this chapter.)

SUPERFICIAL TISSUES (skin, joints, body fat and cellulite, hands, feet, mouth, and full-body treatments)	3 to 20 J/cm²	10 to 50 mW/cm²
DEEP TISSUES (targeted muscle, bone, brain, gut, and visceral organs on smaller body areas)	20 to 60 J/cm²	50 to 120 mW/cm²

RAMPANT MISREPRESENTATION AND LYING IN THE INDUSTRY ABOUT IRRADIANCE

Now, all of this discussion of irradiance is based on one central assumption: that you actually know the irradiance of the device you're using. Unfortunately, this assumption is very often a bad one. And that's despite—or perhaps because of—the fact that many manufacturers of PBM devices actually *tell you* the irradiance levels of their devices.

One of the big current problems in the PBM space is a pervasive issue of misrepresentation of the irradiances by manufacturers of PBM devices.

Irradiance numbers used to be inaccurate because many people (including myself) were using inaccurate instruments—solar-power meters—to measure the irradiance of these panels. We now know that these instruments overestimate the true irradiances of red and NIR PBM devices by 30 to 50 percent.

However, I am now aware of numerous manufacturers who, despite having access to third-party lab data on the true irradiances of their devices, still knowingly misrepresent the irradiances of their devices on their websites. For example, devices advertised as emitting 160 mW/cm² might deliver only 80 mW/cm², or even less. This misrepresentation leads to underdosing or ineffective treatments, especially when consumers rely on inaccurate figures to calculate treatment times.

Why are companies doing this? Largely as a result of market pressures causing manufacturers to compete with one another based on who has the higher irradiance panels. (Regretfully, I also probably contributed to this phenomenon with the first version of my book, because at that time there were a great many underpowered devices on the market, and I was advocating for the devices that had higher irradiances because I believed that these devices would be more effective for treating deeper tissues.) Subsequently, many manufacturers of LED panels came to the market, and a market race to the highest irradiance was created: Companies began to compete with one another, each claiming to have "the highest irradiance panel on the market."

Now, we're in a situation where many of the most popular PBM device manufacturers, who are almost all aware of the true irradiances of their devices, are knowingly misrepresenting those irradiances. Many people are now under the mistaken impression that higher irradiances are always better—that a more powerful light is better for every treatment purpose—and thus, the whole red light panel market has become a competition based on wattage, size, and irradiance. (In reality, going from a large light to a massive light, or from a high-irradiance panel to an extremely high-irradiance panel, is

unlikely to offer any further benefits and may even be worse in some ways, particularly if it is used on the face at irradiances above 80 mW/cm².)

Sadly, this practice of wildly misrepresenting irradiances of panels has become entrenched in the culture of lying now present in the industry. Many companies seem to feel they *must* lie in order to compete with other companies who are lying.

Unfortunately, I have now also seen this dishonesty issue become rampant among pad-style devices as well. Companies are claiming 75 to 130 mW/cm² irradiance figures for pads whose data I have seen, and which I know actually emit roughly only 5 to 20 mW/cm².

In the realm of whole-body pods—devices for which companies are asking $30,000 to $100,000—James Carroll, the CEO of Thor Photomedicine, has shown in one online presentation (found on YouTube with the title "Devil's Advocate: Why I do not believe any of you") that several of these devices perform nowhere near their irradiance claims. In general, their testing found that among LED device manufacturers, the true mean output of the devices was about 31 percent of the manufacturers' claimed output. When it comes to whole-body pods, he mentions one company that claimed that their light bed produced 60 mW/cm² actually delivered only 13 mW/cm², and another company that claimed 100 mW/cm² only produced about 9 mW/cm². These are not trivial differences. As you can see, the representation is often five- or tenfold off the real numbers. (Consider, by the way, that if companies selling premium and ultra-expensive PBM devices for the price of a new car are engaged in these kinds of unethical practices, what might many companies selling much cheaper devices be doing?)

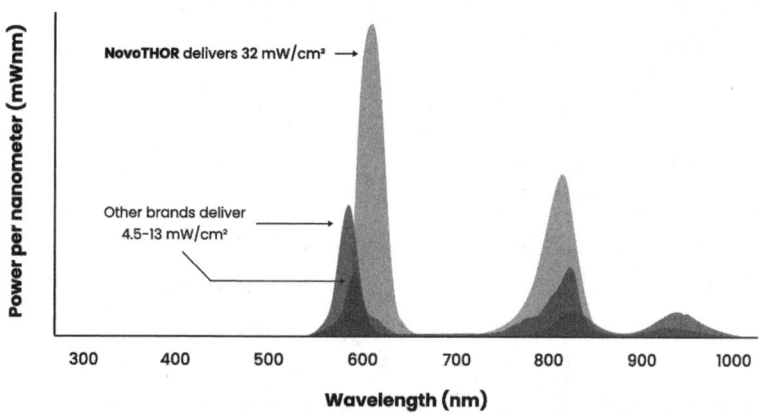

NovoTHOR Irradiance Compared with Other PBM Light Beds

Source: Reproduced from James Carroll, "Devils Advocate: Why I do not believe any of you," YouTube, May 13, 2024.

How does all this matter to you, the end consumer? Well, you're the one who pays the price for all these companies misrepresenting the true irradiances of their devices.

The reason is that we need to know the true irradiance figures of a device to accurately calculate dosing. If we believe that our device is two or three times as powerful than it is—or even ten times as powerful, as I have seen with some manufacturers—we will be wildly off in calculating optimal dosing parameters.

For example, if we believe that our device emits 160 mW/cm² when it actually emits 80 mW/cm², and we calculate our treatment time and dose based on this mistaken irradiance figure, we will underdose by *half*!

A perhaps even bigger problem is caused by device manufacturers' messaging, which often implies that higher irradiance means better results for every treatment goal. If we are led to believe that the highest possible PBM irradiance is the most effective, many people will use excessively high irradiances on body areas such as on the facial skin, which may do more harm than good.

Sadly, these unethical practices have become rampant. This kind of overt lying and misrepresentation of products is an enormous problem for the industry, and it damages the end consumer more than anyone else. Without knowing the true irradiance of the devices we're using, we simply cannot dose the light properly.

On my website (www.redlightdevice guide.com), I've published a list of companies that provide **third-party verified irradiance data** and operate with complete transparency, so you can have confidence that you're dosing your PBM properly.

To ensure that you purchase an effective and trustworthy PBM device, here are some suggestions:

1. **DEMAND TRANSPARENCY:** Before buying, ask manufacturers for third-party lab data that verifies the true irradiance capabilities of their devices. Ethical companies should be transparent and willing to share this information. (I would only accept lab data from a U.S.- or Europe-based lab, like LightLab International in Pennsylvania.)

2. **AVOID MISLEADING CLAIMS:** Be cautious of devices boasting exceptionally high irradiance without providing credible data to back their claims. If a manufacturer is unwilling to share lab-verified figures, consider it a red flag. (Be aware that testing of irradiance with solar-power meters is highly inaccurate, so this form of data

or photos using these kinds of light meters is not valid.)

3. **SUPPORT ETHICAL COMPANIES:** Choose to buy from manufacturers that prioritize honesty and transparency in their marketing. If the company isn't openly sharing third-party data on the true irradiances of their devices, I'd advise avoiding it. Supporting only transparent and ethical companies encourages better practices across the industry. (My major goal with this section of the book is to help clean up these deceptive practices.)

4. **CHECK INDEPENDENT REVIEWS:** Look for reviews from trusted sources that use professional spectrometers to measure irradiance. While this type of data is not perfect (it's not nearly as accurate as third-party lab data from a lab that specializes in measuring light), these types of video reviews measuring light output with a home spectrometer can certainly catch major discrepancies between manufacturer claims and actual light output.

5. **EDUCATE YOURSELF:** Remember, higher irradiance isn't always better. Focus on matching the device's specifications—wavelength, irradiance, and size—to your specific therapeutic goals, rather than being swayed by the mistaken assumption that a larger and higher-wattage/irradiance device is going to be superior for every purpose. Remember that for facial skin, you don't want a

very high irradiance. And for deep tissues, you want a powerful light that can be applied to—perhaps directly on, or at the least distance from, with good anatomical conformance—the target area. Very large and powerful panels are often not ideal for either of these purposes, but they may be best suited for full-body systemic benefits. Though very high irradiances (above 100 mW/cm²) may also not be well-suited for whole-body light treatments, and one may want to aim for about 20 to 80 mW/cm². In short, be mindful of the widespread tendency to assume that the biggest, most powerful, and highest-irradiance panel must be the best choice for every PBM goal.

Make your purchasing decisions count. Choose to support only ethical and transparent companies that provide third-party verified data about their devices' performance. If you detect any lack of transparency, choose to do business with another company. If all of us demand this before making purchases, it will clean up the whole industry very quickly.

DURATION OF TREATMENT

Treatment time is a key factor in achieving therapeutic outcomes, also influenced by the total dose (in J/cm²) and the irradiance (mW/cm²). The relationship between energy dose, irradiance, and treatment time is straightforward.

On paper, duration of treatment for a given body part is largely a byproduct of our total dose and our irradiance.

Time (s) = Energy Density (J/cm²) ÷ Power Density (W/cm²)

For example, to deliver 40 J/cm² using a device with 80 mW/cm² (0.08 W/cm²):

Time = 40 ÷ 0.08 = 500 seconds (about 8 minutes and 20 seconds)

Basically, if we know the irradiance of our device and our target dose, we can simply solve the equation to get the ideal length of time for which we should apply that device.

You can see that time (duration of light exposure) and irradiance are inversely related: the higher the irradiance, the more rapidly you'll reach your target dose. Here are some sample calculations to show you how this works:

- 10 mW/cm² applied for 100 seconds gives 1 J/cm²
- 25 mW/cm² applied for 40 seconds gives 1 J/cm²
- 50 mW/cm² applied for 20 seconds gives 1 J/cm²

- 75 mW/cm² applied for 13.3 seconds gives 1 J/cm²
- 100 mW/cm² applied for 10 seconds gives 1 J/cm²
- 500 mW/cm² applied for 2 seconds gives 1 J/cm²
- 1,000 mW/cm² applied for 1 second gives 1 J/cm²

When it's looked at this way, we can see that, assuming our target dose remains the same, irradiance has an inverse relationship with treatment time: Higher irradiance means that you'd get to your target dose faster, while lower irradiance requires longer exposure to achieve the same total energy dose.

Imagine trying to put out a fire using a squirt gun vs. using a fire hose—the squirt gun may take 75 minutes to put out the amount of water that a fire hose unleashes in 25 seconds.

Simply looking at it mathematically, we can see the duration of treatment purely as a byproduct of what irradiance we're using and our target dose. The temptation from this point of view is to believe that we can achieve the same dose in perhaps half, or 1/10th the time, by simply using a device with a higher irradiance.

Let's say we use the device with an irradiance of 100 mW/cm² for 120 seconds and get to 12 J/cm². If we simply use the 10 mW/cm² device for 1,200 seconds (20 minutes), we can arrive at the same 12 J/cm². In other words, we can use an irradiance 10x higher for 1/10th the time.

Or 1/10th of the irradiance for 10x longer of a duration and arrive at the same total dose.

This is known as the Bunsen-Roscoe law of reciprocity. One group of researchers described it this way:

The Bunsen-Roscoe law (BRL) of reciprocity states that a certain biological effect is directly proportional to the total energy dose irrespective of the administered regime. Dose is the product of intensity and the duration of exposure and thus the time required to deliver a certain dose is influenced by the intensity of the source . . .[33]

In other words, this law states that in PBM, the effect is the result of the total quantity of photons delivered to the target cells, not how quickly or slowly they are delivered. That is, according to this law, the same dose (e.g., 20 J/cm²) delivered in 10 seconds or 20 minutes creates the same result. Using an analogy of rainfall, we can all understand that 5 minutes of intense rainfall might deliver the same amount of water as 45 minutes of light drizzle. So the idea here is that if the total dose is the same, it doesn't matter whether the light arrived slowly or rapidly.

But when it comes to PBM, this law is only partially true.

While on paper—simply doing the math—an extremely high irradiance and a very low irradiance can obviously arrive at an equal total dose if you simply change the duration the devices are used, the

45 minutes of Light Rainfall Provides the Same Amount of Rain as 5 minutes of Intense Rainfall

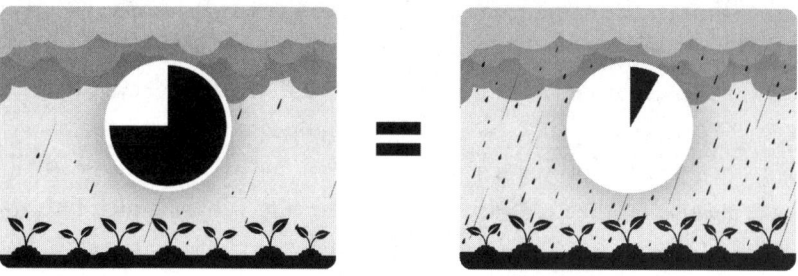

Low irradiance applied for a long time can deliver the same fluence as high irradiance applied for a short time.

same total dose may actually behave very differently in our physiology depending on the irradiance and duration.

To make the point in an extreme way, even though 1,000 mW/cm² for 25 seconds and 10 mW/cm² applied for 42 minutes may mathematically deliver the exact same total amount of photons (~25 J/cm²), these two PBM treatments may lead to wildly different physiological effects. The 1,000 mW/cm² light is likely to create a lot of heat (and perhaps burn the tissue) while not creating much benefit because the target tissue may need a certain duration of exposure to derive benefits. On the other hand, the 10 mW/cm² may not be powerful enough to even deliver a meaningful dose of light to the target depth of tissue and therefore not create any benefit for that reason. Moreover, it may only be the zone in between those—perhaps 40 mW/cm² to 150 mW/cm² applied for 2 to 10 minutes that gives the best effects.

What this means is that the duration of treatment should be treated as its own legitimate variable that influences treatment outcomes, rather than merely a mathematical byproduct of irradiance and target dose.

The reason is that some biological responses require a minimum threshold time for activation, regardless of power density. There is evidence that the time of treatment must be long enough to give the tissue time to respond to the light. For instance, it was shown in a rat model of arthritis that the same dose (30 J/cm²) was effective when delivered in 10 minutes, but it was not effective when the same dose was delivered in only 1 minute.[34]

This is another reason why extremely high irradiances (such as those that cause heating within seconds and must be moved around frequently to combat tissue heating) may actually be much *less effective* than a moderate irradiance device that can be held in place on those tissues for an extended period of time. Again, this may hold true even when the math of dosing is the same—that is, the same total dose is delivered.

One review from 2020 noted:[35]

> Even though when a device provides a high power, it means that the necessary "dose" is reached in less time. However, there is a "dose rate effect," and when the dose is applied very quickly, the beneficial effects diminish.

Many PBM experts have also suggested that it's misleading to look at PBM through this kind of simple math where wildly varying irradiances can all technically lead to the same overall dose, and instead have made the point that a smarter and more effective way to think about ideal dosing parameters is to focus on being in the ideal range of irradiance with an ideal duration of treatment. For example, James Carroll has said:[36]

> *Many researchers also only talk about the total energy delivery, when in fact the rate of delivery is actually more important.*

One 2009 review described it this way:[37]

> Energy (J) or energy density (J/cm²) is often used as an important descriptor of [PBM] dose, but this neglects the fact that

energy has two components, power and time,

$$\text{Energy (J)} = \text{Power (W)} \times \text{Time (s)}$$

and it has been demonstrated that there is not necessarily reciprocity between them; in other words, if the power doubled and the time is halved then the same energy is delivered but a different biological response is often observed.

It is our view [PBM] is best described as two separate sets of parameters:

The medicine (irradiation parameters)
The dose (time)

In other words, at the level of our physiology, it's not only the total water delivered to the bucket that matters, but also how long it took to get there, which plays a role in the effects of the PBM treatment.

There are a couple of reasons why the Bunsen-Roscoe law doesn't hold all that well:

The problem of excessively high irradiance: Too fast of a rate of delivery of photons to the tissues may hinder beneficial biological effects. Think in terms of an evolutionary context: If we get roughly 100 to 140 mW/cm² of light from the sun (roughly 30 percent of which is in the red and NIR spectrum), our physiology may have evolved to be tuned to a "flow rate" of photons roughly comparable to this. It's logical to assume that within this range or perhaps a bit outside of it, we can handle well, but it may be the case that a flow rate of photons five or ten times larger may not play so nicely with our biology. Think of watering a plant—you can use a garden hose with moderate intensity or a fire hose, and you can, on paper, deliver the exact same total amount of water. But if you blast it with a fire hose at full force, it will just spray water everywhere, blast away soil, and potentially damage the plant. (Not a perfect analogy of what likely happens in our physiology, but it's just meant to illustrate that higher power doesn't necessarily mean it's better and may actually be counterproductive.) As we've already discussed, very high irradiances can lead to excessive heat generation—that is, the cells can only absorb a certain amount of photons at a given time and going far above that just creates a lot of heat generation in the tissues. There also may be other mechanisms at play separate from heating, like oxidative stress.

The problem of low irradiance: Another factor that further complicates things is seen on the other end of the irradiance spectrum. As we've seen, higher irradiances allow for deeper penetration of the light. So again, let's imagine a hypothetical scenario of two devices—one at 10 mW/cm^2 and one at 100 mW/cm^2. And let's imagine they both deliver the exact same dose of 12 J/cm^2. On paper, it's the same dose. However, if we were to measure the amount of light delivered 2 to 3 cm deep in the tissue, the higher-irradiance device delivered a significant quantity of light to those tissues, while the low-irradiance device didn't. In fact, given how light is attenuated through the tissue, with a low-irradiance device, you could theoretically leave it on for extremely long periods of time (perhaps an hour or two) and deliver a much higher dose (on paper), but the amount of light reaching those deeper tissues (per unit time) may still be so minute that it's not enough to trigger any biological effect at all. As an analogy, consider someone who slowly walks twenty steps every 10 minutes. At the end of a day, they may have walked a total of three miles. But the physiological effect of this approach will be different than if they *ran* those same 3 miles in 20 minutes. The same total distance was traveled, but *how* it was done influences the nature of the stimulus and ultimately how the physiology responds. The intensity is a critical component of what triggers a biological response.

A common clinical approach is to use moderate irradiances (see the guidelines in the irradiance section) with moderate treatment times (perhaps somewhere between 3 to 30 minutes) to stay within the therapeutic window. In short, there is a balance that needs to be struck between irradiance and treatment duration.

This is why we have guidelines for *both* the target dose delivered to the tissue, *and the optimal range of irradiances* to accomplish that. Following those guidelines will naturally tend to put us in the optimal range for treatment duration.

So basically, we can start with our goal and then aim for a target dose and target irradiance: Refer to the table at the beginning of the chapter for your specific goal and find the target dose and the target irradiance parameters to aim for to achieve that particular treatment goal. From there, you can easily calculate the ideal time you want to apply it for.

Here's the math part of how this works: Again, the dose of exposure equals the irradiance multiplied by the time of exposure.

$$\text{Irradiance (mW/cm}^2) \times \text{Time (seconds)} \times 0.001 = \text{Dose (J/cm}^2)$$

All we are doing is rearranging this equation to solve for time of exposure, but, crucially, doing so within our provided guidelines for dosage and irradiance. We're taking that number we already have for irradiance (in mW/cm²) and our target dose (in J/cm²) and then calculating how long we should apply that light for.

PRACTICAL EXAMPLES

If you're not into doing math, this may feel overwhelming, but it's actually quite simple.

These numbers (that correspond to the recommended irradiance ranges in this book) will come in handy:

- 10 mW/cm² applied for 100 seconds gives 1 J/cm²
- 25 mW/cm² applied for 40 seconds gives 1 J/cm²
- 50 mW/cm² applied for 20 seconds gives 1 J/cm²
- 75 mW/cm² applied for 13.3 seconds gives 1 J/cm²
- 100 mW/cm² applied for 10 seconds gives 1 J/cm²

So now, let's take a specific example.

Example 1: Facial Skin Anti-Aging Treatment

Target Parameters
- Desired dose: 14 J/cm² (within recommended range of 3 to 15 J/cm²)
- Selected irradiance: 25 mW/cm² (within recommended range of 10 to 50 mW/cm²)

Calculating Treatment Time
- At 25 mW/cm², every 40 seconds delivers 1 J/cm²
- For 14 J/cm², multiply 40 seconds × 14
- Total time = 560 seconds (9 minutes and 20 seconds)

- Practical treatment window: Roughly 8 to 12 minutes

Example 2: Deep-Tissue Treatment for Arthritic Knee

Target Parameters

- Desired dose: 45 J/cm² (at the surface)
- Selected irradiance: 100 mW/cm²

Calculating Treatment Time

- At 100 mW/cm², every 10 seconds delivers 1 J/cm²
- For 45 J/cm², multiply 10 seconds × 45
- Total time = 450 seconds (7.5 minutes)
- Practical treatment window: Roughly 6 to 9 minutes

This approach shows how once you select your target dose and irradiance, calculating treatment duration becomes straightforward. Each device's irradiance determines how long it takes to deliver 1 J/cm², and you simply multiply that time by your target dose to get total treatment duration.

As you can see, by following the guidelines of dose (J/cm²) and using a device with an irradiance in the recommended range (note: as discussed, you must know the true irradiance of your device), you will naturally end up in the range of ideal treatment duration. That's another critical reason that these dose and irradiance guidelines are so important to follow.

Treatment times typically range from 60 seconds to 30 minutes per treatment area, though this varies based on several factors. I believe that somewhere in the range of 3 to 40 minutes is likely optimal in most cases, but we don't have definitive evidence for ideal durations for every conceivable goal.

Remember that you do *not* simply want to optimize for the highest possible irradiance to deliver a dose in the shortest time. More, or faster, is not always better—and it certainly can be worse.

In summary, irradiance, duration, and ultimately the dose (J/cm²) should all fall within reasonable ranges. Again, duration itself appears to be a critical factor in treatment efficacy, independent of the total dose delivered. Extremely short treatments (under a minute) may not give tissues sufficient time to respond biologically, even if the correct total dose is achieved. Conversely, extremely long treatments (over an hour) may lead to diminishing returns or even counterproductive effects, regardless of low irradiance used.

Duration should be treated as its own factor influencing results, not merely a mathematical byproduct of whatever arbitrary dose and irradiance you choose.

Yet, practically speaking, for home PBM device users, the easiest way to arrive at your ideal treatment duration is still to focus on irradiance and dose, but doing so *by using the specific recom-*

mended safe and effective irradiance ranges in this book.

You don't really need to overthink the factor of treatment duration or worry about it as a separate variable, because if you're following the dose/irradiance guidelines here, it will automatically ensure you virtually always land in the ideal range of 3- to 40-minute treatment durations.

For practical home use, the process is straightforward:

- Verify your device's actual irradiance
- Confirm it's within the recommended safe and effective ranges
- Choose your target dose from the guidelines
- Calculate how many minutes you should apply the device to reach that dose

Follow these steps, and you'll automatically land in the ideal duration range.

SKIN CONTACT VS. NON-CONTACT

The method of applying a PBM device—whether through direct skin contact or with the device positioned at a distance—plays a significant role in how light penetrates tissues and the effectiveness of treatments. Each approach has its advantages and challenges, depending on the target tissues and treatment goals. However, there is a potentially large advantage to the skin-contact method of applying a PBM device, particularly for facilitating deeper penetration of the light.

When a device touches the skin directly, two key things happen:

1. **THE AIR GAP IS ELIMINATED.** Air between the device and the skin surface can cause light to scatter or reflect away before it enters the body. Skin contact removes that air interface and allows more of the light to pass directly into the tissue.

2. **TISSUE COMPRESSION IMPROVES PENETRATION.** Gentle pressure on the skin can physically shorten the distance that the light has to travel to reach deeper targets (like muscle beneath fat). It also temporarily pushes blood and water out of the area, reducing the amount of light-absorbing material in the upper layers and letting more light to pass through to deeper tissues.

These effects likely matter less when treating superficial targets, but they are extremely beneficial for reaching deeper tissues.

When light devices are used at a distance from the skin of several inches or more, several factors reduce their effectiveness:

- More light is reflected or scattered before it enters the skin.
- The beam spreads out as it travels, lowering the irradiance that hits the tissue.
- The angle of light entry becomes less optimal (perpendicular), reducing penetration capacity.

These factors can significantly reduce the amount of light actually reaching the target. Most of the energy might instead be reflected or remitted by the skin or absorbed in superficial layers compared to the result of the same device applied in direct contact with the skin.

Light Penetration of Non-Contact vs Contact

Non-Contact

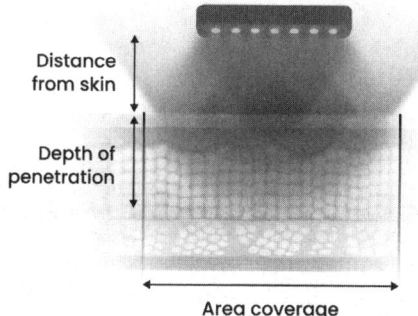

- Covers larger area
- More reflection losses
- Less deep penetration
- Better for superficial and systemic goals than deep tissues

Contact

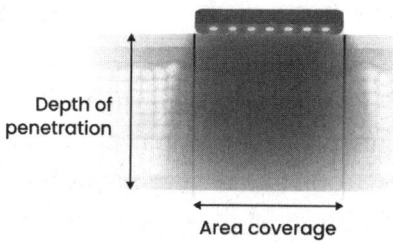

- Deeper light penetration
- Less reflection losses
- Often limited by coverage area and/or having good contact
- More optimal for deep tissues

So how much does skin contact actually help? While research is still limited and results are mixed, several studies have shown that skin contact can significantly increase light penetration to the deeper tissues.

Using dogs, researchers in Thailand demonstrated that NIR had similar penetration ability through the skin (3 mm) whether in contact or 5 cm (2 inches) away, and that light was also able to penetrate to reach muscle tissue 15 mm (1.5 cm) into the body using both the skin contact method and when the laser was moved 1 cm away from the skin surface, but no light was detectable at this tissue depth when the laser probe was moved 5 cm away from the skin's surface.[38]

Another study using dog cadavers found that on-contact application increased transmission by up to 67 percent compared to non-contact.[39]

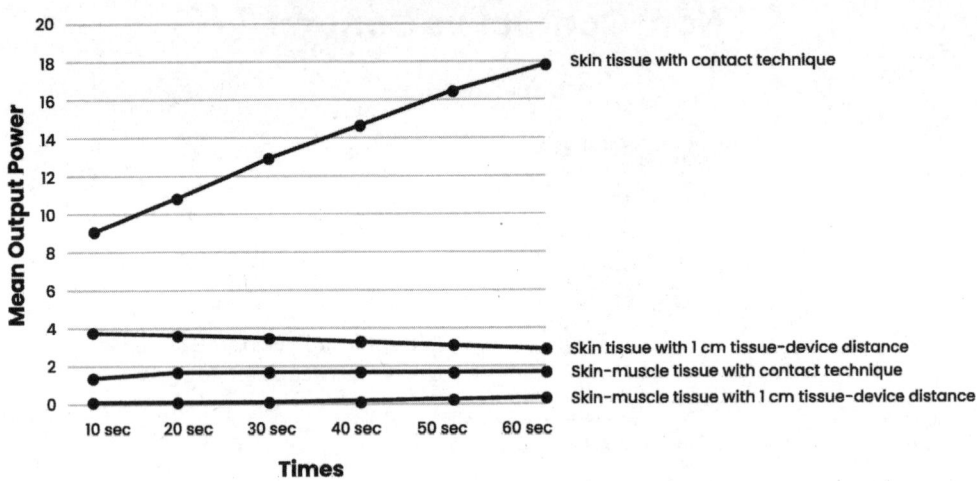

An Average of Mean Output Power During 60 Secs of Superpulsed and Multiple Wavelength Irradiation in Dog Tissue

An average of mean output powers (MOP) penetrating dog tissue during 60 secs of simultaneous superpulsed and multiple wavelength photobiomodulation therapy.

A third study by the same Thai researchers reported that skin contact delivered about four times more light to muscle tissue than non-contact.[40]

However, not all studies show large differences like this. For example, one study using rats showed only 5 to 12 percent differences in the detectable light intensity at a given depth of tissue between contact vs. non-contact (differences that could

likely be easily compensated for by slightly increasing the treatment time).[41]

A further nuance is that the physical structure of the device will influence whether skin contact enhances light penetration or not. For example, one study found that a laser device with a hollow tip actually had slightly *reduced* light penetration when applied with skin contact vs. non-contact.[41] On the other hand, a laser device with a convex lens had improved light penetration with skin contact vs. noncontact.

(This detail matters because many devices—particularly flexible pad-style devices—have recessed LED chips that don't make firm contact with the skin unless the device is tightly strapped down, and this could create a similar effect.)

As you can see, there are a wide variety of findings from research on this topic, and unfortunately, these data are often with dogs, or dog cadavers, or rats, and using lasers (rather than LED devices), so there are significant limitations in how much we can extrapolate this data to humans using LED devices.

Moreover, the data are relatively inconsistent—some show large changes in penetration from contact (vs. non-contact) and other studies show much more minor changes.

As far as expert opinion on the subject, here's what Dr. Hamblin had to say:

> My advice to somebody who has a big panel is treat it like a bed and lie on it, because the coupling from the LEDs into the skin is much better in contact, for sure, there's no much less diffuse reflection.

So clearly Dr. Hamblin believes light penetration will be superior with skin contact. (Note: If you're wondering about EMF exposure from being in close contact with the device, we'll cover that in another section shortly.)

On the other hand, here are Dr. Arany's thoughts on the subject when I asked him about it:

> The more studies we do, especially clinical research studies that we do, we have started to realize that is not very practical. . . . We find that it's much easier to be in noncontact and the loss that people are worried about in terms of reflection or whatever distance that you're accounting for is very minimal. You can easily account for that by increasing the amount or time, which seems to help a lot. I'm open to both, and I think the contact is more precise, but I'm leaning towards a noncontact. This becomes a practical thing when you're thinking of clinical care, because if you're in contact, you have to disinfect that surface pretty rigorously.

So we have a serious limitation with the current body of evidence on this topic, and as you can see, there are significant differences in opinion among PBM experts. Nevertheless, even with simple at-home tests that you can do in a few moments (like shining a flashlight through your hand/fingers with or without contact, you can see a large increase in light coming through with skin contact and pressure), so it is clear that using the device with skin contact certainly does enhance the penetration of light into the deeper tissues. I've done quite a bit of self-experimentation in dark closets with various PBM devices, and while my "testing" doesn't involve sophisticated technology and certainly couldn't be published in a peer-reviewed journal, it has made it very clear to me that skin contact greatly increases light penetration to deep tissues compared with non-contact with the same device. So despite mixed results in the literature, my bias is to believe that skin contact will, in most contexts, significantly enhance tissue penetration.

THE LIMITATIONS AND PRACTICAL DIFFICULTIES OF SKIN-CONTACT PBM

While skin contact with PBM devices offers real advantages for increasing light penetration, especially for deep tissues, this method also comes with several practical challenges and limitations. In principle, skin contact is ideal—but in practice, it's often more difficult than you might imagine.

Low-Irradiance Issues with Contact Devices

While theoretically, skin contact dramatically increases penetration depth, the reality is that most devices designed for skin contact—particularly flexible, neoprene-style pads—are very limited in their ability to deliver an effective dose to deep tissues by virtue of their very low irradiances. (There are exceptions, like most laser devices. There are also a handful of specialized LED devices that I'll mention in chapter 6, where we'll cover device selection for specific treatment goals.) If you have a very low irradiance device, you're simply not going to be able to treat deep tissues effectively, even with skin contact.

This raises an important question about trade-offs. What delivers more light to deep tissues: a 10 to 15 mW/cm² flexible pad in contact with the skin, or an 80 to 120 mW/cm² (higher-power) LED device that's not in contact with the skin? In other words, does the penetration advantage of skin contact compensate for the significant irradiance disadvantage of most contact devices? There are many scenarios where using skin contact with a low irradiance device simply won't allow you to effectively do PBM to deep tissues, even though you are using the skin contact method. But there are scenarios—let's say, as an example, treating an injured knee—where a 40 mW/cm² device in direct contact with the knee joint would likely deliver more light to deep tissues in the knee than an 80 mW/cm² panel used from 6 to 12 inches away. In this case, contact wins. So the answer really depends on the differences in the specifications of the device and what you're trying to accomplish. Factors like the exact differences in irradiance between the devices, the distance of the non-contact device from skin, the size of the device and the size of the body area you're trying to affect (which we'll address below), and other factors may all influence which approach delivers more therapeutic light.

Low-LED Density Issues with Contact Devices

Many devices designed for contact treatment (like most flexible neoprene pad-style devices) also often suffer from low LED density (i.e., lots of space between each two LED chips), creating "hot spots" and "cold spots"—areas that are receiving light, and an inch away from them, areas that are not receiving any light. Space between LED chips is much less of an issue when the non-contact method is used, because the light spreads out and allows uniform coverage by the time it reaches the skin. But if you take a device with lots of space between LEDs and press it against the skin, much of the skin surface in that area will be receiving little to no light, while the spots right under the LED will get most or all of the light.

So pressing a device with low LED density against the skin will technically get deeper penetration, but only right beneath the LED chips; much of the surface area under the pad may receive no light at all.

On the other hand, if you take the same device and move it a few inches away from the skin to get uniform light coverage, the irradiance may drop off so much that the PBM treatment is ineffective. This creates a fundamental engineering issue with many of these devices, which likely makes them largely ineffective for deep-tissue treatments using either the skin-contact or the non-contact method of application. If you have a very low irradiance device with large gaps between individual LEDs, it's likely to not be very effective for most treatment goals.

Device Heat-Transfer Problems

Another seldom-discussed and frequently overlooked problem is heat transfer from the device itself. As we've discussed, even low-irradiance pads (e.g., 15 to 20 mW/cm²) can generate significant heat when used in direct contact for 15 to 20 minutes. This happens not because of excessive light intensity being transformed into heat in the cells, but due to simple conduction of the device's own heat—especially when airflow is restricted and the skin can't cool itself. Direct skin contact can increase this heat transfer via conduction, and also can, with some devices like neoprene pads, limit skin ventilation. Some of my low irradiance pads (around 20 mW/cm²) actually cause far more skin heating than 80 to 90 mW/cm² lights used from several inches away. When I use my neoprene pad LED devices on my kids, they'll often complain it gets too hot after about 20 minutes or so. Again, this is just a result of heat conduction and lack of airflow.

Practical Surface-Coverage Challenges

Beyond these issues, there are challenges related to surface contact. The skin-contact approach originated with laser devices (often pen-shaped with fine points), which can easily be pressed against most body areas. But with larger-surface-area LED devices, maintaining consistent contact becomes problematic.

Imagine trying to place large flat tiles on a curved wall—you'll inevitably have gaps. Human anatomy generally isn't flat. Most body surfaces, from face to limbs, have curves or irregularities. While skin contact works well with small devices like torch-style units on small areas of the body, larger areas generally require flexible devices that can conform to body contours to maintain skin contact.

Even flexible pad-style devices often struggle to maintain uniform contact across curved surfaces like the spine or joints. You might achieve partial contact, but complete surface coverage is rare. And again, the most flexible devices (neoprene pads) often come with issues with both irradiance and LED density.

Treatment Time and Efficiency

Due to the difficulty of getting good skin contact with larger devices, the contact method often requires treating smaller areas sequentially using smaller devices, which significantly increases total treatment time compared to larger devices. While it's easy to justify contact treatment for specific, small target areas (like an injured ankle or elbow), treating larger surfaces (let's say your upper leg, or your upper arm muscles) with the same targeted device might require numerous 5-to-10-minute sessions to achieve complete coverage of that body area. On a practical level, this can be a significant time investment and inconvenience for many people (particularly if the device needs to be held in place with one hand), and many people just won't be willing to consistently treat large body surfaces with small contact devices, despite the potential advantages of the skin-contact approach.

Special Considerations for Skin Treatments

One of the primary uses of PBM is for superficial treatment, such as on a wound or to enhance skin health on the face. As such, it's important to recognize that for facial skin treatments, uniform light coverage may actually be more important than skin contact. That's because most masks designed to be in skin contact with the face struggle to maintain consistent contact across facial contours, and even if they do, most masks will still have the issue of "hot spots" and "cold spots" (i.e., too low of LED density) described previously.

Using a device designed to sit several inches away from the skin, which provides perfectly even coverage of the facial skin (with the appropriate irradiance), may be superior to trying to maximize skin contact. While it hasn't been tested directly, I would expect devices that give uniform coverage from several inches away from the skin to be more effective than low LED-density devices applied directly to the skin. The light from multiple LEDs also can converge before entering the skin, which can enhance the effect (something we'll discuss more in another section).

Contact vs. Non-Contact: Recap

In summary, skin contact during PBM is a great option for treating deep tissues, but it's not without some drawbacks and practical difficulties. Most devices on the market that are designed for skin contact suffer from inadequate irradiance, poor LED density, excessive device heat, low coverage area, or difficulty maintaining contact across complex surfaces. Ideally, we need devices that offer:

- Effective skin contact
- Adequate irradiance
- Optimal LED density
- Minimal heat transfer
- Ability to maintain contact over large surfaces

These are difficult engineering problems, and few devices have solved them well. For deep-tissue work in small areas of the body, direct skin contact with targeted devices is likely the best approach. Dr. Hamblin has even recommended lying directly on large panels to take advantage of partial skin contact across broad surfaces like the back.

Yet practical limitations exist with current technology. Most of the devices currently on the market that are designed for use with skin contact have extremely low irradiance that limits their efficacy for deep tissues. Also, many devices either struggle to maintain effective skin contact or require multiple time-consuming treatments with smaller, targeted devices to cover larger areas.

Overall, the evidence makes a compelling case that skin contact can significantly enhance light penetration in PBM treatments and is likely especially useful for deep tissue treatments of smaller body areas (e.g., ankle, knee, elbow, wrist, etc.) where you can use a targeted device directly on that area. However, it's not ideal in every context, and current device limitations (irradiance, coverage, LED density, flexibility) make it difficult or inconvenient in many circumstances.

Personally, when treating muscles, joints, tendons, or other deeper tissues in smaller areas, I strongly prefer doing PBM treatment using targeted devices directly applied to that area whenever possible.

LIGHT CONVERGENCE (LED SPACING, SPOT SIZE, BEAM ANGLE, AND WAVELENGTHS)

Spot size—the area of uniform light coverage—plays an important role in how light penetrates deeper tissues. Think of the difference between a narrow beam of light (like a laser pointer) versus a broader beam (like a floodlight).

With larger spot sizes, more light converges beneath the surface of the skin, creating beneficial overlap effects. This convergence helps maintain higher photon density at depth compared to smaller spot sizes, even when surface irradiance and other factors are equal. The broader coverage also reduces "edge losses"—where light scatters away at the boundaries of the treatment area—thus leading to more efficient energy delivery to deeper tissues.

This improved penetration through larger spot sizes occurs because light photons entering the tissue have more opportunities to interact and support one another's forward progression through the tissue, rather than being lost to scatter at the edges of a smaller beam. However, this effect depends on maintaining sufficient power density across the entire treatment area. (Think of arrays of LEDs that create more uniform coverage than single sources.)

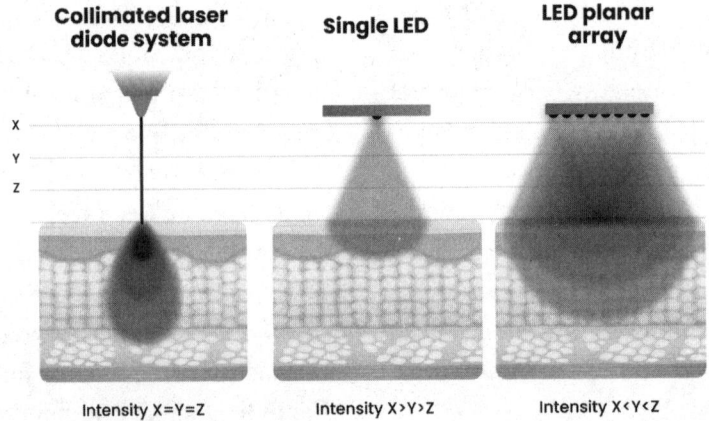

Intensity X=Y=Z   Intensity X>Y>Z   Intensity X<Y<Z

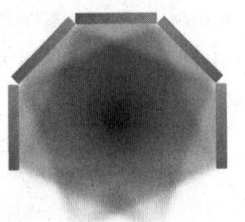

Concentrated photon density

Treatment with articulated arrays showing area of higher photon intensity where the individual beams intersect.

There's a limit to this benefit, though. One study found that increasing beam width from 1 mm to 10 mm nearly doubled penetration depth but expanding from 10 mm to 40 mm didn't produce further gains.[42] The advantage of increasing spot size appears to plateau once scattering in the tissue reaches a saturation point.

Although these findings are mostly from laser studies, similar—and potentially even greater—effects occur with LED arrays. Research by Tom Kerber has demonstrated that larger coverage areas dramatically enhance the amount of light delivered to a specific depth. As light scatters through tissue, photons from neighboring LEDs overlap, boosting light delivery to deeper regions.

Penetration of Light at 50mm and 75mm Depth

Light Intensity vs Illumination Field and Tissue Thickness (TK/PB Data)

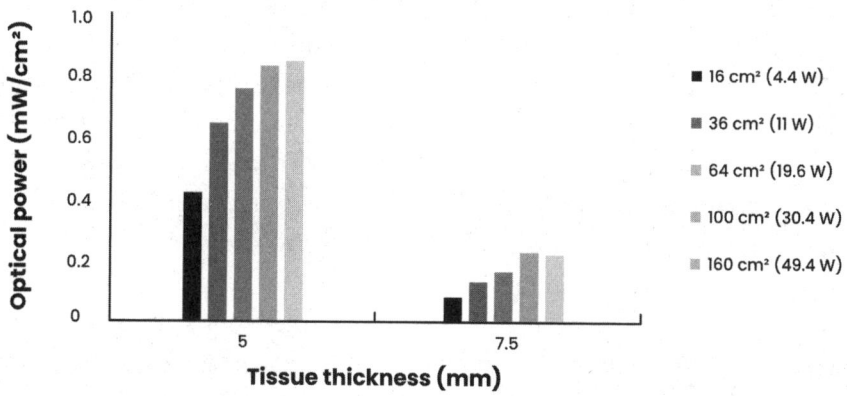

Importantly, this isn't just about depth of light delivery. A larger spot size means you can treat more tissue at once. It's the difference between hitting 0.5 square inches of tissue at a given moment and hitting 10 square inches in the same moment. The spot size not only enhances light penetration but also greatly enhances the efficacy of treatment, since you'd have to do multiple treatments of a given area to cover the same area of tissue with a device using a smaller spot size.

This is a key distinction between LED and laser devices. Lasers often have smaller beam sizes and treat highly specific areas, while LED arrays can cover broader zones. Though lasers may offer better penetration in a small, focused spot due to their beam properties, LEDs offer advantages in coverage, efficiency, and potential convergence effects.

A related concept is the effect of overlapping beams of light, which creates a light convergence effect that greatly improves the effective light intensity both above and especially below the surface of the skin.

When several beams (especially of the same or similar wavelengths) are directed at the same area, their intersecting photons create zones of increased light intensity. This is like multiple spotlights focused on the same stage actor: The point of convergence becomes much brighter than any single beam.

These overlapping beams can create higher effective irradiance beneath the skin than what's measured directly at the surface. And this convergence can happen both in air (before entering the body) and inside the tissue, reinforcing photon density and enhancing depth of penetration.

While a single beam may struggle to maintain sufficient power density at depth, like a flashlight beam becoming dim in fog, multiple overlapping converging beams create concentrated zones of light that help get more light to the deeper tissues.

Critically, this isn't about making each individual LED more powerful. The key advantage lies in their arrangement. By overlapping the right wavelengths at the right angles and spacing, manufacturers can achieve superior energy delivery to deeper tissue targets.[4]

As shown in the image below, different light sources, such as laser diodes and LEDs, produce distinct beam patterns that affect their penetration and intensity in tissues.[4]

Laser diodes create a coherent beam with minimal loss of intensity, thus enabling deep-tissue penetration. Scattering within the tissue concentrates the intensity just below the skin surface, enhancing therapeutic effects. In contrast, single LEDs emit noncoherent, divergent beams that lose intensity as they spread, resulting in poor penetration and extremely low photon intensity that's limited to superficial skin layers.

An array of LEDs, however, creates this light convergence effect, where overlapping beams increase photon intensity at the points of intersection. With the right engineering—high LED density, optimal spacing, and matched wavelengths—an LED array can significantly increase light delivery to the deep tissues.

So, to recap:

- Larger spot sizes or areas of light coverage lead to better penetration and efficiency.
- Light convergence from multiple LEDs enhances irradiance at depth.
- Curved or articulated panels may further concentrate photon intensity.
- Beam convergence may be more effective than simply increasing irradiance of the individual LEDs.
- Engineering—including LED spacing, density, and alignment—is critical to maximizing these benefits.

Now that you understand the principle of beam convergence, let's explore two major obstacles that can potentially sabotage this effect: poor LED spacing and mismatched wavelengths.

The Issue of LED Spacing in Contact Devices

The spacing between LED chips in PBM devices is a key factor that relates to light convergence, and this issue presents a significant limitation that's often overlooked by consumers and most PBM device manufacturers.

As we've discussed, tightly packed LEDs allow for overlapping light beams that reinforce one another, increasing both the depth of penetration and the irradiance at a given depth. But when LEDs are spaced far apart, those beneficial convergence effects largely disappear. The device stops functioning as a unified light field and instead becomes a collection of isolated light points—each one trying (and failing) to do all of the work alone.

This issue is especially prevalent in the pad-style devices that are designed to be used in direct contact with the surface of the skin. Most of these devices have gaps of one inch or more between LEDs—far too wide to allow for meaningful convergence effects when used in contact with the skin.

Types of Devices

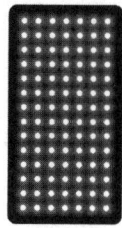

Panels

Good for large body areas and systemic benefits

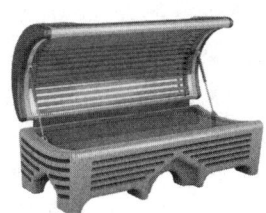

Pods

Best for systemic benefits and skin health

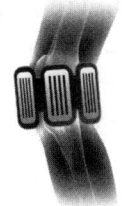

Flexible Targeted Devices

Best for deep tissue

When these pads are pressed against the body, there's no space for the light to spread and overlap before hitting the skin. Instead, each LED's beam acts alone. Any overlap that does occur within or beneath the tissue is severely limited—especially given that most of these devices are low in irradiance to begin with.

More critically, the common practice of spacing LEDs an inch or two apart in most of these pad-style devices creates significant inconsistency in light delivery. This creates a patchwork effect of treatment "hot spots" surrounded by undertreated or untreated areas ("cold spots") that aren't receiving light.

This problem is often masked by the physical appearance of the pad itself. Because the pad covers the entire treatment area, users naturally assume that the light coverage is uniform across that area. However, on the underside of the pad, the reality is quite different: The actual light delivery occurs at discrete points with significant gaps between them.

This is especially problematic for goals that demand uniformity, like facial anti-aging treatments. Most LED face masks on the market suffer from this issue. The low LED density and wide spacing simply don't provide the even distribution needed for consistent results.

The few pad-style devices that pack their LEDs in much tighter configurations offer superior treatment by minimizing these dead zones and providing more uniform coverage. Such devices are less common, however, and I believe that this is because of concerns about heat dissipation from the device, since the pad-style devices do not come with built-in fans, so pad-style devices typically rely more on low power and large spaces between LEDs to prevent the device from getting too hot. Unfortunately, the low LED density in most pad-style devices severely limits light convergence, and thus light penetration.

The Potential Problems of Multiple Wavelength Devices

There is a related and overlapping potential issue at play in many PBM devices (especially panels but also some pads)

that's subtler and harder to detect but may be just as big a factor in limiting results. Having a different wavelength in each LED chip may act in a way that's similar to using large gaps between LEDs: There may be light present, but it's of a different wavelength from one inch to the next.

It's difficult to paint with broad brushstrokes here, because this issue is complex, and this effect will differ depending on the specifics of the device design (LED spacing, beam angle, and distance from the skin). And to my knowledge, no study has adequately tested this, so what I'm about to describe should be considered largely speculative.

Let's say a device has separate LEDs for each wavelength—for example, 660 nm in one diode, 850 nm in another, and so on—and they're spaced about an inch apart. This setup creates a patchwork effect across the treatment area. One part of your skin might be getting mostly 660-nm red light, the next patch might get 810-nm NIR, another might get 480-nm blue, and so on. Some overlap happens due to beam spread, but it's minimal at best. Beneath the skin, where deeper convergence is needed for effective penetration, the overlap may be even more limited—especially since different wavelengths penetrate to different depths.

This creates two main problems:

- **REDUCED BEAM CONVERGENCE:** When LEDs emit different wavelengths, the overlapping convergence effect that enhances penetration is weakened or lost entirely. We lose the benefit of multiple beams of the same wavelength reinforcing one another at depth.

- **UNEVEN WAVELENGTH DISTRIBUTION:** Instead of every area of the tissue receiving all wavelengths, different areas receive different wavelengths in isolation. From close range or in contact mode, this means tissues are not getting uniform exposure across the full spectrum, which is particularly problematic if the therapeutic effect depends on synergy between wavelengths.

You can potentially move far enough away from the device to allow the beams to mix more evenly through diffusion, but this comes at a cost: irradiance typically drops off quickly with distance, and the angle at which photons strike the skin becomes less favorable for penetration. So, while distance may help blend the light, it reduces both irradiance and light penetration into the body.

Perhaps the best way to understand this is through LED density, or LEDs per 100 cm². This is not a measurement currently used by almost anyone in the industry, with the exception of Tom Kerber (who uses this metric to help differentiate his devices—which are designed with high degrees of light convergence—from others on the marketplace).

A device with six different wavelengths and 100 LEDs per 100 cm² may only have about 16 LEDs per 100 cm² of a given wavelength. In contrast, a single-wavelength device or one using multi-wavelength chips can concentrate more LEDs of a given wavelength into the same area—possibly offering 20 to 25 LEDs per 100 cm² of that wavelength—potentially leading to more light convergence at different levels of the tissue, and ultimately deeper, more effective penetration.

Most manufacturers of LED panels appear unaware of these potential effects. To my knowledge, SunPower LED and Thor Photomedicine are among the few manufacturers intentionally designing their devices with these concepts in mind to maximize light-convergence effects through optimal spacing of LEDs and wavelength choices.

This is one reason why, when using devices with multiple wavelengths, it may be preferable to opt for devices that use multi-wavelength LED chips, where each LED emits more than one wavelength, rather than devices where each LED only emits one wavelength. This helps ensure uniform delivery of all wavelengths to all areas of tissue and can allow for better beam convergence. While multi-wavelength chips may have slightly lower power efficiency per wavelength than dedicated single-wavelength chips, the benefits in convergence and uniform exposure probably outweigh that drawback. I want to be clear that much of this is still very speculative. Until controlled studies comparing these different approaches are conducted, these ideas should be considered a logical but speculative framework for device selection.

But ultimately, convergence of light (of the same/similar wavelengths) may be a critical factor that influences PBM treatment efficacy, particularly for getting light to the deeper tissues. And especially if you're using the device within close distances or with skin contact, it's likely that this factor influences one's results.

FLAT VS. BODY-CONFORMING DEVICES: TREATMENT ANGLE AND REFLECTION LOSSES

Think about shining a flashlight into a swimming pool. When you point it straight down, the light penetrates deep into the water. But angle it to the side, and far more of the light just bounces off the surface. There's a similar principle at play with light penetration into the body—perpendicular angles allow better penetration, while light at steeper angles is more likely to essentially reflect off the skin and superficial layers of tissue.

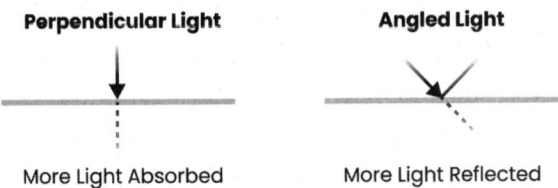

Light Absorption vs Reflection at Different Angles

Perpendicular Light — More Light Absorbed

Angled Light — More Light Reflected

This simple fact plays a key role in the types of devices that are likely to be best for various body areas. Most PBM devices currently on the market are either rigid flat panels or flexible devices that conform to your body. The key difference here is how well they maintain the more optimal angles of light relative to the body's surfaces.

When you place a flat panel on a curved area—like your shoulder, face, or thigh—only the part directly facing the panel gets light at that ideal perpendicular angle. On areas where your body curves away from the panel, the light hits at increasingly oblique angles.[43] This creates two problems:

1. **MORE REFLECTION LOSSES:** A lot of light essentially "bounces off" your initial skin layers instead of penetrating through them.

2. **LONGER PATH THROUGH TISSUE:** Light entering at an angle has to travel farther to reach the same depth, meaning more gets absorbed or scattered along the way.

A Curved Panel Allows for Better Penetration

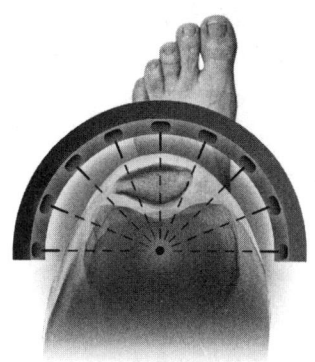 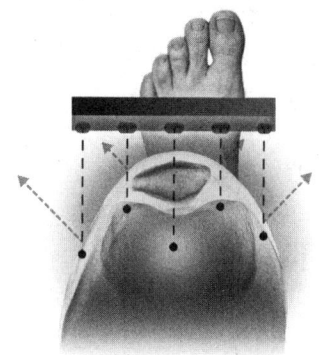

This is why conforming devices can give you better results in certain situations. They keep the light hitting your skin at more optimal angles across the entire treatment area. This becomes especially important when you're treating curved areas like joints or your face.

However, flat panels remain practical for treating larger and flatter body areas where perpendicular light delivery can be better maintained.

When choosing between flat and conforming devices, consider:

- The shape of the area you're treating (flat vs. curved surfaces)
- Target tissue depth
- Size of the treatment area
- Need for uniform coverage of an entire area

While researchers haven't thoroughly studied this issue specifically for PBM yet, basic physics—and simply observing how light interacts with your body—suggest that devices shaped to fit your body's curves will likely work better for many treatments. Until more research emerges, choosing body-conforming devices whenever possible is probably ideal, especially for curved areas and when targeting deeper tissues.

TISSUE OPTICAL PROPERTIES

The way light interacts with biological tissue significantly impacts PBM effectiveness. Several key factors determine how well light can reach its target:

Melanin

Melanin—the pigment that gives skin its color—is a primary chromophore in the epidermis and acts as the first major obstacle to light entering the body. Melanin strongly absorbs UV and blue light, moderately absorbs red light, and has much less impact on NIR light in the 800 to 1,000 nm range. In darker skin types, melanin is more concentrated, meaning more light is absorbed and scattered in the upper skin layers, which limits penetration. This creates two important considerations:

- Longer treatment times may be necessary to reach deeper tissues.
- Red wavelengths are more prone to being absorbed in the skin and can create excess heat. For this reason, darker skin types may benefit more from using NIR wavelengths, which both penetrate deeper and generate less surface heating.

Body Composition

Subcutaneous fat has a major influence on light penetration. Fat tissue has a high scattering coefficient, which means it tends to diffuse light in all directions. Even with optimal wavelengths and decent irradiance, each additional millimeter of fat significantly reduces light transmission. In people with thicker fat layers, light may be attenuated to very low levels before it ever reaches deeper tissues like muscle or joints. In some cases, too much body fat over an area may make direct treatment of deep tissues unachievable, and the only path to benefit from PBM is through systemic effects (see the section on how to maximize systemic benefits in chapter 6).

TISSUE-SPECIFIC PROPERTIES

Different tissues present unique optical challenges:

- **SKIN** forms the first barrier. The outer layer (epidermis) blocks light with melanin, while the inner dermis scatters it due to collagen and blood vessels.

- **FAT** allows more light through than other tissues due to its low blood content but scatters it significantly.
- **MUSCLE** is more challenging due to its dense structure and higher blood volume, both of which absorb and scatter light.

- **BONE** is the most difficult. Its mineral density causes extreme scattering and absorption, which is why targeting the brain requires higher power levels—the skull is a major barrier.
- **BLOOD VESSELS** act as light sinks. They absorb so much light that they can create "shadows" behind them, where less light is available for therapy.

This is why it's too simplistic to say something like "red light penetrates 3 cm into tissue." The reality depends entirely on what types of tissue the light encounters along the way. For example, light will travel much farther through 3 cm of mostly fat than through 3 cm that includes bone or dense muscle.

PRACTICAL IMPLICATIONS

Here's how to apply this knowledge when designing or adapting PBM treatments:

- Choose longer wavelengths (e.g., NIR) and higher irradiance when targeting deeper or more light-resistant tissues (like bone or muscle).
- Adjust treatment based on individual characteristics:
  - Darker skin may warrant extra care to avoid surface overheating, and opting for NIR over red light.
  - People with higher body fat may require longer sessions or stronger devices to compensate for light loss through fat.
- Select treatment areas where the target tissue is more easily accessible (e.g., closer to the skin surface).

Understanding these interactions enables optimization of treatment parameters while maintaining safety and efficacy.

LASER VS. LED

Modern PBM looks vastly different than it did in its beginnings. Originally, PBM-like therapies used simple incandescent bulbs in "light baths," where people would sit surrounded by broad-spectrum light. These early devices emitted a wide range of wavelengths—visible and infrared—but were not targeted to specific therapeutic wavelengths. As the science of PBM evolved, so did the tools. Today, PBM primarily uses two technologies: lasers (light amplification by stimulated emission of radiation) and LEDs (light-emitting diodes).

Laser technology was initially developed at the Hughes Research Laboratory by Theodore Maiman in May 1960. By the late 1960s, laser technology had been disseminated, and the historical evidence of light being utilized to improve health conditions prompted various research groups to examine how this new technology could be used. The greater control over wavelengths, location, and power meant that researchers could conduct more closely controlled experiments on more specific questions, and modern PBM (utilizing targeted, specific wavelengths of light) initially focused on laser as the primary application tool.

Interestingly, LED technology emerged around the same time as laser technology. The first LED light was invented on a small scale in 1961 by two scientists, Robert Biard and Gary Pittman, from Texas Instruments. This first LED was, coincidentally enough, an infrared light. Over the next few decades, LED technology continued to improve, larger LEDs that could be commercialized were developed, and, in the 1990s, LEDs began to be used in earnest as tools for PBM.

It is believed that NASA developed the first sufficiently narrow-banded LEDs with enough power density to be used for PBM. It is reported that NASA originally used red LED lights to improve plant growth in space and found that the researchers growing these plants who were exposed to the light experienced much higher rates of wound healing on their hands.[46-48] (This was one of the key insights that led to the modern field of PBM.)

Over the last several decades, both laser and LED light technology have been utilized as tools for PBM, but most of the original PBM therapies and research were done using lasers rather than LEDs. This is a critical point, because this fact has shaped the overall body of evidence on PBM, and it has led to the widespread belief that many of the benefits of PBM are dependent on the unique properties of light from lasers. A comprehensive review of the literature from Dr. Hamblin and Vladimir Heiskanen described it this way:[49]

To this day, more than 3500 scientific articles on photobiomodulation have been published. Approximately 85–90 percent of the original research has utilized lasers as light sources. Practically all of the photobiomodulation research before the twenty-first century was based on lasers.

This laser-centered history of PBM has been the reason for the assumption that the beneficial physiological effects of red and NIR light are somehow dependent on the "laser properties" of light, such as monochromaticity, coherence, collimation, and polarization. According to current knowledge, this is certainly debatable and probably not true. (We'll discuss the evidence for this later.)

While both lasers and LEDs deliver photons to tissues, they differ in how that light is generated and delivered:

- **WAVELENGTH SPECIFICITY:** Lasers emit highly monochromatic light (±1 to 2 nm bandwidth), while LEDs have broader spectra (±10 to 30 nm). Newer LED designs have narrowed this gap, achieving near-monochromatic output, especially in red and NIR ranges.
- **COHERENCE AND BEAM TYPE:** Lasers produce coherent, collimated light—the photons travel in sync and in parallel. This can allow for deeper penetration in some contexts. LEDs emit noncoherent, divergent light, which spreads quickly but is excellent for covering large areas.
- **POWER DENSITY:** Lasers typically deliver much higher irradiance (1 to 5 W/cm² or more), making them ideal for short, high-intensity treatments on small targets. LEDs, operating at 10 to 100 mW/cm², are more suitable for longer treatments across larger areas.
- **SAFETY AND ACCESSIBILITY:** Lasers require trained operators and strict safety protocols to avoid burns or eye injury. LEDs are much safer and more accessible for home or unsupervised clinical use.
- **COST AND USABILITY:** Lasers are more expensive, with focused applications. LEDs are cheaper, safer, and better suited for treating large areas and following general wellness protocols.

A long-standing argument is whether lasers can penetrate deeper than LEDs. Laser proponents point to their high-power beams as superior for reaching deep tissues. However, recent research and optical modeling challenge this view. Many studies show that once light enters tissue, even coherent laser light quickly becomes diffused due to scattering—losing the "beam-like" quality. Arrays of LEDs, especially when designed with proper spacing and convergence, can deliver significant doses of light deeply, especially when using high-density layouts.

Tom Kerber's research has shown that at equivalent levels of power, LED arrays can match or exceed laser light penetration in some cases, especially when considering beam convergence from multiple directions. He does note that ultra-powerful, super-pulsed lasers might still offer unique benefits, but that for most practical purposes, well-designed LED systems can be equally effective.

On the other side of the discussion, Dr. Theodore Henderson, a psychiatrist in Denver, Colorado, with a substantial research interest in the use of PBM to treat brain disorders, has carried out extensive measurements of the optical depth of penetration into sheep and human cadaver skulls by lasers and LED devices. His published works show that very little LED light can penetrate the skull, and that it takes a high-power laser device to deliver significant doses of light to brain tissues. He does, however, accept that there are valid treatment outcomes from LED-device studies on some brain disorders and leaves open the question as to the mechanisms by which the PBM treatment can operate (i.e., he's hinting that it could be more from systemic effects or perhaps other mechanisms).

But at least one study has shown that, depending on the area of the head, between about 1 to 12 percent of NIR light (830 nm) is able to penetrate into the brain (through soft tissue and bone) when delivered by an LED device.[50] Given that the brain is extremely rich in mitochondria and highly sensitive and responsive to light, this research indicates that it's actually perfectly reasonable to suspect that properly designed LED devices (with adequate irradiance) can deliver significant doses of light directly to the brain.

The question of greatest importance, and the one that has been most hotly debated by scientists and clinicians, is: What is the difference in actual efficacy of PBM treatments using lasers vs. those using LEDs? Many practitioners who have used laser devices in their clinics will swear that lasers are unique, have different effects than LEDs, and yield superior benefits.

Laser proponents suggest three theoretical advantages:

Coherence effect: Laser light creates tiny, regular patterns in tissue called "speckles." These speckles are about the same size as mitochondria, the cellular structures that produce energy. Proponents argue that this precise match in size allows laser light to stimulate these cellular powerhouses more effectively than the irregular light patterns from LEDs.

Deeper penetration: Some lasers can produce very powerful, extremely short pulses of light. The idea is that these intense pulses can push deeper into tissue than the steady, lower-power light from LEDs.

Better forward scattering: Laser light travels in an organized, parallel beam, while LED light spreads out in all directions. Laser proponents suggest that this organized beam structure helps the light maintain its path as it moves through tissue, potentially delivering more energy to deeper layers than the scattered LED light.

While these theories are intriguing, it's important to note that research is still ongoing to determine how significant these differences are in actual therapeutic outcomes, and some of these claims have been shown in several studies to be inaccurate. For example, studies have found that coherent light isn't necessary for PBM benefits.

Possibly the earliest report came from Pal Greguss Jr. in 1984, who concluded that "low-level laser irradiation, when having a biostimulating effect, is not laser specific."[51] Later, in 1993, some researchers were already pointing out that research shows noncoherent, non-laser light can stimulate the same or similar benefits.[52]

For most of the last few decades, we simply haven't had the body of evidence necessary to answer this question—the research comparing similar parameters of LEDs and lasers for specific outcomes simply hadn't been done. Now, we have some semblance of a body of evidence that has compared the two technologies in a scientifically rigorous way (though the overall size and quality of the evidence is still not great).

The weight of research evidence to date indicates that there are few convincing arguments for the use of true laser. Photostimulation occurs using both true laser light and noncoherent, non-collimated light from LEDs or other light sources. In their review of the literature, Heiskanen and Hamblin cited roughly 40 more recent studies that largely indicate that lasers and LEDs have similar efficacy in various contexts.[49] They describe it this way:

As can be noted from these tables, most of the comparisons have a very high risk of bias due to differing key parameters between the LED and laser groups. In almost every study the wavelengths, power outputs and spot sizes are different between the groups, which makes it impossible to make reliable comparisons between lasers and LEDs in PBM. Despite these notable shortcomings, most of these comparisons provisionally suggest that lasers could indeed be replaced by LEDs without significant worsening of the results.

If we examine the scientific literature that directly compares laser and LED-based approaches to PBM, we actually see they report similar outcomes for most use case. This is the entire reason why, in 2016, the National Library of Medicine added the term "photobiomodulation" to its database upon petition from researchers.[53] The prior term, "low-level laser therapy," was simply no longer accurate given that LEDs were being used with similar success.

LED PBM has been shown in hundreds of trials to improve many conditions, such as temporomandibular joint disorders, knee osteoarthritis, and as well as skin quality and reducing skin aging.[54–59] Recent studies have compared the efficacy of both laser- and LED-based PBM for many of these popular PBM-treated conditions. At a mechanistic level, one study compared 800- and 850-nm lasers to an 810-nm LED for effects on cytochrome c oxidase (CCO) redox activity and vascular hemodynamics in the forearm of adult volunteers.[60] While the time to achieve an effect varied between devices, they all led to similar effects within an 8-minute exposure time. This was despite the laser power density of the 800-nm laser (310 mW/ cm^2) being 2.3 times higher than that of the 810-nm LED (135 mW/ cm^2).

In a direct comparison of laser- and LED-based PBM for temporomandibular joint disorders, both laser and LED showed very similar improvements in temporomandibular joint related pain, with both groups showing a nearly 50 percent improvement in symptoms.[61] Unfortunately, the LED and laser emitted different wavelengths of light (660 nm with LED vs. 810 nm with laser), although the exposure time was different to help equalize the dose of light applied (5 minutes per pain point with LED vs. 30 seconds with laser).

Effects of LED vs. Laser on TMD Associated Pain

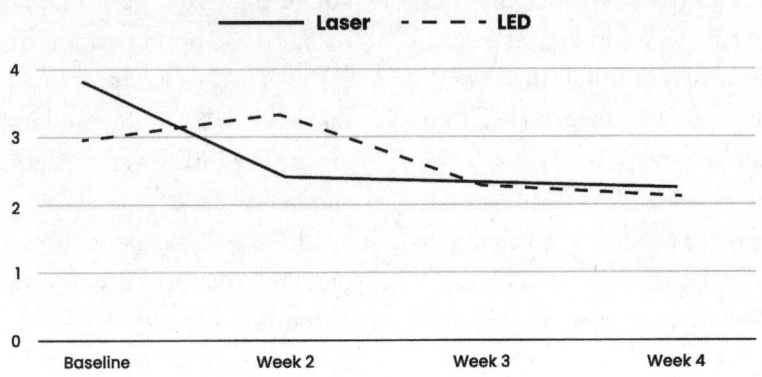

Pain Intensity Before and After LED or Laser Therapy

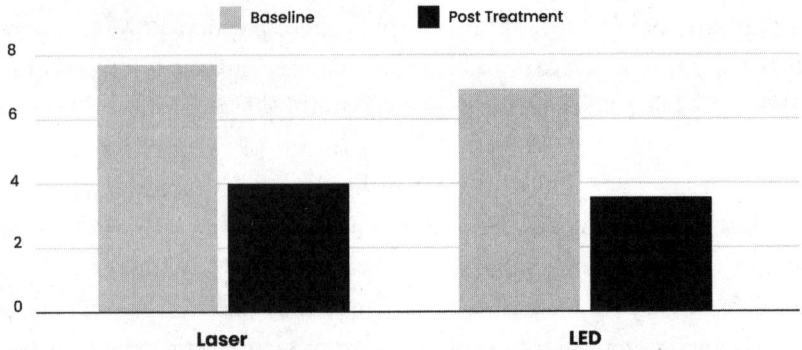

In another direct comparison study among individuals with knee osteoarthritis, both laser and LED reported similar improvements in arthritis-associated pain.[62] Once again, the wavelengths were not perfectly matched (890-nm LED vs. 860-nm laser), but the dosing parameters were similar due to different treatment times (30 minutes with LED surrounding the knee vs. 2 minutes of laser at each of five pain points).

Similarly, skin aging appears to be improved similarly by both laser and LED PBM. However, they appear to have different applications as it relates to dermatological uses.[58] LED-based PBM appears to be utilized more for general skin aging and skin quality, specifically with improving collagen, reducing wrinkles, and improving overall skin structure. Laser-based PBM may be more effective for addressing specific conditions in a faster time frame such as photodamaged skin or specific cases of acute wound healing. However, following up laser-based PBM therapy with LED-based PBM therapy appears to increase overall efficacy.[63, 64]

Even for brain applications—previously believed to require lasers—evidence is emerging that well-designed LED systems can produce beneficial effects, including for mood, cognition, and neurodegeneration.[65]

These are just a handful of studies that have compared LED- vs. LED-based PBM, and if you wish to do a deep dive into the full list of relevant studies, I encourage you to explore the review put together by Heiskanen and Hamblin in 2018. The larger literature base—flawed as it may be—shows that for most applications, laser and LED often yield similar results.

Lasers and LEDs are both effective forms of PBM. Lasers may offer advantages for precise targeting, rapid dosing, or reaching specific internal structures. But for general use, large surface areas, safety, cost, and accessibility, LEDs are often the better choice. LEDs have been validated across a wide range of conditions—from skin rejuvenation and pain relief to joint support and brain health.

As Heiskanen and Hamblin concluded,[49] *"Photobiomodulation is not dependent on lasers or coherence . . ."*

LED vs. Laser: Safety and Practical Differences

While both lasers and LEDs can be effective for PBM, several important considerations make LEDs the better option for most people looking to use an at-home device for PBM.

Perhaps the strongest reason to favor LED-based PBM is safety. Red and NIR LEDs are extremely safe to use, even without professional training. Lasers, on the other hand—particularly the high-powered ones used in clinics—come with much greater risks. Laser light can damage the eyes (including causing permanent retinal injury) and burn or blister the skin if misused. For this reason, laser-based PBM typically requires specialized training, and devices are often only legally available to licensed practitioners. LED devices don't carry these risks and are safe for everyday use, as long as general usage guidelines are followed (many of which are provided throughout this book).

Another compelling reason to choose LEDs over lasers is practicality. LEDs are far easier to use in daily life. You can set up a panel in your home or use a mask or wrap-style device and then go about your normal routine. Read, work, stretch—PBM can become part of your lifestyle. Lasers, by contrast, typically require you to hold a device still over small treatment areas, often for many separate points, or "optically scanning" the device (moving it around constantly), which can be time-consuming and difficult to manage without assistance.

Also, and very important for most people, LED products (with the exception of very expensive whole-body pods) tend to be substantially lower in cost than laser products. High-quality laser devices typically cost more than $10,000, and often more than $30,000 (and in many cases can only be purchased by a licensed practitioner). Quality LED devices (other than whole-body pods) generally cost less than a few thousand dollars, with many excellent devices in the neighborhood of $500.

Lastly, LED-based PBM can be integrated into myriad different devices that can be used to provide different therapeutic benefits. For example, you can achieve large surface-area coverage for various large body areas using LED PBM devices, whereas lasers generally have a very small surface area, and typically rely on manually doing point-by-point treatments over the same area. You can also have more targeted facial skin therapy and ensure that your face gets even light exposure by using contoured masks with built-in LED lights. You can also get devices that will hold red and NIR lights directly on your skin and increase the depth of light penetration to reach deeper into joints and musculature.

Overall, based on the existing evidence, laser and LED PBM appear to provide relatively similar outcomes (e.g., muscle-pain relief, anti-aging in skin, improvements in overall skin quality, help for osteoarthritis), outside of very specific-use cases (e.g., brain tissue or very targeted ablation-based therapy). But keep in mind that it's difficult to design studies to adequately compare lasers and LEDs, so the evidence is of limited quality and strength, and more research is needed to draw definitive conclusions.

Notwithstanding my preference for LEDs, I've seen interesting data on differences in how laser light penetrates to deep tissues vs. LED light, and I've heard enough anecdotes to believe that lasers may be uniquely effective in certain contexts—particularly for targeting very deep tissues in a precise way. It is likely that there are specific contexts where lasers will be shown to clearly outperform LED devices.

It could turn out that lasers have truly unique benefits above and beyond what can be achieved with LED PBM, or that (as most current evidence suggests) they are similarly effective in most contexts. If well-designed research emerges that shows clear superiority of lasers over LEDs in certain contexts, I'll certainly update this section to reflect that.

PULSING

Pulsing in PBM refers to the delivery of light energy in an on-off pattern rather than a continuous emission. While continuous wave delivery maintains consistent light output throughout treatment, pulsed delivery alternates between periods of light emission and of none, with the alternation at specific frequencies, typically ranging from 1 to 1,000 Hertz (Hz).

The development of pulsing has strong historical roots in the practical challenges of delivering high-powered light therapy. As researchers and clinicians began using increasingly powerful lasers to achieve deeper tissue penetration, heat management became a crucial concern. Pulsing emerged as an elegant solution, allowing for high peak powers while maintaining safe average power and preventing excessive tissue heating. This was a legitimate and evidence-based application that solved a real problem in PBM delivery.

As practitioners gained experience with pulsing devices, they began to observe various clinical effects and outcomes in their practices. These observations led to the development of hypotheses about why certain parameters (e.g., certain pulse frequencies) might offer specific benefits, and researchers began to explore potential mechanisms of action, and to hypothesize about the unique benefits of specific pulse frequencies. Some researchers hypothesized that certain pulse frequencies might interact with specific cellular rhythms or oscillatory processes in biological tissues.

As interest in frequency-specific effects grew, device manufacturers began to incorporate various pulse protocols into their designs, offering practitioners more options for treatment customization and starting to make claims about the unique physiological effects of specific pulse frequencies.

While many of these frequency-specific applications still require more research to validate their effectiveness, many studies do show superior efficacy for pulsing over continuous- wave treatments, while other studies have shown equal efficacy compared to continuous wave, and some studies even show continuous wave to be superior. Further, the pulse frequencies used in studies are often all over the map, from perhaps 10 to 3,000 Hz. The field continues to evolve, with ongoing research investigating potential mechanisms and applications for different pulsing protocols.

There are two key areas where pulsing has strong, evidence-backed benefits:

1. **HEAT MANAGEMENT IN HIGH-POWER DEVICES:** In devices with high irradiance, pulsing allows for delivery of higher peak power while avoiding

overheating the tissues. This enables deeper tissue penetration of high irradiance light while keeping skin temperatures safe. This is the most well-established, scientifically supported reason to use pulsing.

2. **BRAIN APPLICATIONS:** The second area where pulsing shows clear advantages is in brain treatment. Two mechanisms are supported by research:

   a) **METABOLIC EFFECTS:** Studies show that 10-Hz pulsed light enhances brain metabolism more than continuous wave or other frequencies, improving mitochondrial function, ATP production, and cerebral blood flow.[66] These effects have been linked to improved memory, focus, and reaction time—especially in models of traumatic brain injury.

   b) **BRAINWAVE ENTRAINMENT:** Pulsing light at certain frequencies can synchronize with natural brainwaves. For example, alpha waves (8 to 12 Hz) are linked to relaxation, beta (13 to 30 Hz) to focus, theta (4 to 7 Hz) to deep relaxation, and gamma (~40 Hz) to higher cognitive function. EEG studies show that light pulsed at these frequencies can shift brainwave patterns. In particular, 40-Hz pulsing has shown strong potential for helping with Alzheimer's disease.[67, 68] Overall,

there is clear evidence that specific frequencies of pulsed light can indeed alter brain function in unique ways.

The Nogier Frequencies

If you've spent any time looking into PBM, you've probably heard about Nogier frequencies. These are among the most widely circulated claims about specific pulse frequencies in light therapy. According to proponents, each precise frequency does something remarkably specific in your body—like 73 Hz for stimulating bone growth and cellular activation, or 4,672 Hz for controlling pain through specific nerve fibers. The frequencies in between supposedly target everything from scar tissue to specific embryological tissue types, each with its own detailed explanation.

But despite these frequencies being promoted for decades, there appears to be almost no peer-reviewed research supporting the specific effects they're supposed to have. Though these frequencies are heavily promoted by certain PBM device manufacturers, I was unable to find any actual peer-reviewed studies that have confirmed these frequency-specific responses, or studies supporting their proposed applications. To go further, there's no compelling scientific explanation (no body of evidence or known physiological mechanisms) for why these exact frequencies would affect the body in such specific ways.

The issues with these claims go deeper. Most of the "evidence" is anecdotal—basically, people reporting what they've observed without proper controls. Many claims come from theoretical models rather than actual experimental data. We also can't ignore how confirmation bias might influence clinical observations—when you expect to see a specific result, you're more likely to notice it. Without proper controls in these reported cases, it's impossible to draw reliable conclusions.

When you think about physiological plausibility, these claims become even more questionable. There's no clear biological reason why 73 Hz would affect bone differently than 70 Hz or 179 Hz (i.e., I can't find any research indicating that bone tissue oscillates at this specific frequency or responds to this specific frequency). Many of the claimed effects don't align with what we know about tissue specificity. The precision of these frequency claims just doesn't match up with how biological systems typically respond to light therapy, which tends to be much broader.

In a conversation I had with Dr. Hamblin on pulsing, he shares his thoughts on this topic:

Actually, you probably know people have been talking about Nogier frequencies for 100 years . . . and there's no hard evidence for them that I'm aware of—zero. A lot of people, alternative complementary type swear by them. If there was anything real

there, wouldn't there be hard peer-reviewed studies showing it?

I replied that "absence of evidence is not the same as evidence of absence" and that the issue here is less that we have lots of studies that have shown no effect, and more that there doesn't appear to be any studies on it at all. He then replied:

Probably because people think it's junk science, right? The general consensus. . . . Perhaps they don't even want to embarrass themselves by trying to study it.

Having said that, this is an area that could use more research, particularly given the abundance of claims that exist (from PBM device companies and/or practitioners). When I asked Dr. Hamblin about the possibility that other tissues of the body beyond the brain could respond in different ways to specific frequencies of light, he had this to say:

I don't know, really. Yes, one theory is that if photons of light can open ion channels, ion channels have a distinct half-life, right, which is measured usually in a few milliseconds. It varies, but you can find papers that report the half-life of ion channels and there are many ion channels and they have different half-lives. If the half-life is the order of tens of milliseconds, then that is equivalent to a pulse frequency of 100 Hertz. It's possible that the half-life of ion channels could sync with the frequency of the light. In other words, if the photons came in pulses, they hit an ion channel, they opened it, it would be more efficient if the next bunch of light could open it again. Whereas if the pulse was too short, it would still be open, it wouldn't do anything. To have the pulses of light coinciding with the ion channels opening and shutting is more efficient.

Overall, this is an area where claims abound that are very detached from the actual body of scientific evidence. But the fact that some research has clearly shown that pulsing can provide increased benefits over continuous wave light, we should be open to the possibility that we will eventually discover other examples where specific pulsing frequencies do indeed have unique physiological effects on various tissues of the body.

Practical Recommendations

Current evidence suggests that pulsing in PBM should be approached strategically rather than arbitrarily. Some key points:

- **USE PULSING WHEN IT MAKES SENSE—** like in high-powered devices, where it helps minimize tissue heating, or in brain treatments where specific frequencies (e.g., 10 Hz, 40 Hz) have genuinely been proven to have unique benefits.
- **OUTSIDE BRAIN TREATMENTS AND HEAT MANAGEMENT,** the evidence for pulsing, and certainly for specific

pulse frequencies, is inconsistent. Many studies show that it works equally well as continuous-wave light, some show it's better, and others show it's worse.

- **FOR MOST APPLICATIONS,** continuous-wave delivery likely represents the most efficient approach, and an equally effective approach.
- **IF YOU'RE USING A LOW-POWERED LED DEVICE,** pulsing often adds unnecessary complexity and reduces efficiency. Since the light is off for part of the time, it takes longer to deliver the same total dose. A 20-minute continuous treatment might now take 30 to 40 minutes to reach the same energy.
- **BEWARE OF MARKETING HYPE.** The marketing of devices with complex frequency protocols and claims about specific frequencies for particular conditions should be viewed with skepticism unless the claims are supported by robust evidence. While such protocols may not be harmful, they often add unnecessary complexity and cost to treatments without clear benefits. In many cases, these protocols seem to be based more on theoretical models or historical practices (or sometimes just marketing gimmicks) than on empirical evidence.

Looking forward, the field would probably benefit from a return to evidence-based principles rather than being influenced by claims about frequency-specific effects. Future research should focus on controlled trials of specific frequencies, mechanistic studies of frequency-dependent effects, and comparative effectiveness research.

This doesn't mean that pulsing is useless; just that we should treat it as an experimental variable that deserves further research in various contexts, not as a proven key to better results. As research continues, we may discover that certain pulsing frequencies do have unique benefits across different types of tissues (as is the case for the brain), but until such evidence emerges, we should focus on well-documented applications of pulsing and maintain skepticism toward unsupported claims about frequency-specific effects by those selling devices.

For now, pulsing should be used with a clear, evidence-based purpose—not simply because it sounds more advanced.

DISTANCE FROM THE DEVICE (AND USE OF PANELS)

Another important topic (related to and overlapping several factors we've already covered) is how far away you are from the PBM device.

Unfortunately, this isn't just an easy answer where we can say, "you always want to be X inches away from the device." This is a nuanced discussion because there are many variables, regarding both the treatment goal and the type of PBM device. Do you want to treat skin or deep tissue? What kind of device do you have—a flexible pad or a large, rigid panel, or another kind of device designed for a specific purpose, or designed to be used from a specific distance away from the body? Do you need uniform light coverage on the skin over a large area? Do you want a targeted treatment in a specific area or a whole-body systemic effect?

All of these questions lead us to differ-ent potential answers for how to best use the device. Let's break this complexity down into some practical rules and principles.

Skin vs. Deep-Tissue Treatment

As we've discussed, as light travels through the air, it scatters more and hits your skin at steeper angles, increasing reflection and reducing how much light actually enters your body. The farther away the device is, the more the irradiance is attenuated (with almost all devices), the more the light tends to diffuse outward, and the more that light will tend to reflect and remit (essentially "bounce off") from the surface of the skin.

That's why for deeper tissues, closer is generally better, with direct skin contact often being most ideal—unless the device has been specifically engineered to deliver deep penetration from a distance using beam convergence.

- **FOR DEEP-TISSUE TREATMENTS,** it's generally best to use the device in direct contact with the skin or very close to it. The closer it is, the more of the light will penetrate into the tissue.
- **FOR SUPERFICIAL OR SYSTEMIC (WHOLE-BODY) EFFECTS,** distance matters less. In fact, moving the device a bit away from the skin may improve uniformity of coverage, which is likely more important than depth of penetration in the context of skin rejuvenation.

Device Type

Some types of devices are designed to be used on or very close to the skin, while others are designed to be used from specific distances from the skin, such that the light becomes uniform.

- **FLEXIBLE PADS, MASKS, TORCHES, AND LASERS** are meant for direct skin contact or very close to it. Use them that way.
- **FACIAL SKIN DEVICES** often work best from a short distance—usually 1 to 6 inches—to ensure even coverage across the contours of the face. Many facial skin devices, such as DermaLux and several others, are designed to be used from several inches away so that the light covers all areas of the face in a uniform way.
- **SOME ADVANCED PBM DEVICES** (like SunPower LED's "Palm" devices) are specifically designed to be used from a precise distance away from the skin (about an inch away) to maximize penetration through beam convergence.
- **WHOLE-BODY PODS** typically place the LEDs 6 to 20 inches from the body to ensure even coverage across all body surfaces. These pods cost $30,000 to $130,000, but the idea is the same: uniform light coverage over a large surface area.

Panels

Large LED panels don't have a universally accepted "optimal distance." Some use them 6 inches away, others at 24 or 36 inches, and some place them directly on the skin. Many people advise simply adjusting the distance from the device to get different irradiances that are appropriate for different goals. (This is what I advised in the first version of this book, in 2018.) If you want to treat skin and cover a larger body area, you'd move farther from the device (perhaps 12 to 36 inches), and if you want deeper penetration, you'd move closer—about 6 inches from the device. In the early days, panels only had on/off switches and no ability to control the intensity of light, so the only way to lower the intensity was to move farther away from the device. Now, most panels have adjustable light intensity that allows one to control the irradiance without altering the physical distance your body is from the panel.

Now while almost everyone talks about using panels from around 6 to 24 inches away from the body (something we'll discuss more in the upcoming section on EMFs), consider that Dr. Hamblin himself uses panels directly applied to the skin. He explains:

It doesn't have to be on the skin; I put it on my skin because I think it's more efficient. The LEDs touch your skin, more of the light goes in rather than being diffusely reflected. The LED light is not focused, so if you stand in front of an LED panel, a surprising amount of the light is diffusely reflected off your skin. If you lie on the LED panel, much more of it goes in.

Several important factors complicate the distance question:

- **Coverage vs. efficiency:** As distance increases, light spreads out, covering more body area—a clear benefit for time efficiency. However, this also leads to steeper angles of light hitting the body surface, which means that the light is more likely to reflect off the skin rather than penetrate. (This effect depends on the device's beam angle—panels with narrow beam angles like 30 or 60 degrees—may show little change

when moved 6 or 12 inches away, making this device-specific.) The major benefit of increasing the distance from the panel is to get light coverage on a larger area of the body at once.

- **Measurement accuracy:** Discussions about optimal distance away from the device to modulate the irradiance assume we know the panel's true irradiance. Since manufacturers often misrepresent irradiance by 30 to 50 percent, accurate dosing becomes nearly impossible without independent verification.
- **The multi-area challenge:** Full-body panels expose different body areas to the same irradiance simultaneously. While 80 to 100 mW/cm² might be ideal for deep tissues, these levels could be excessive for facial skin. With targeted devices, you simply avoid sensitive areas. With full-body panels, you must either use intensity controls, select red-only wavelengths, physically shield sensitive areas, or accept that you're optimizing for skin and systemic benefits rather than deep-tissue penetration.
- **Modern solutions:** Years ago, adjusting distance was necessary to control irradiance, hence widespread recommendations to use panels from 12 or 24 inches away in certain contexts. But today's panels with intensity controls and wavelength selection offer more flexibility. You

can maintain a comfortable 6-inch distance while adjusting power to 30 to 50 percent or using red-only modes to achieve appropriate irradiances for different goals.

The bottom line is that there's no single ideal distance away from panels. Panels can be used from direct skin contact (like Dr. Hamblin) to several feet away. The main advantage of using the LED panel at a greater distance away from your body is if you want to cover a larger area of your body with light. Outside of that use case, closer is generally going to be better.

While we used to have to alter the distance from the device to control irradiance, now with modern panels, we can just adjust the irradiance in the device settings. Once you know your panel's actual output, you can position yourself at any comfortable distance and adjust power settings accordingly. As a general rule, if you're trying to affect deep tissues, you generally want the device closer to or in contact with your skin, whereas for superficial and systemic treatments, there is a lot of flexibility in terms of the distance from the device.

EMFS

One topic that commonly arises when discussing PBM devices is electromagnetic fields (EMFs). PBM devices, like many electrical appliances, emit magnetic and electric fields around the device, and many people are concerned about potential health hazards from these fields.

This is a complex topic with numerous EMF types (Wi-Fi, Bluetooth, magnetic fields, electric fields) and varying exposure intensities and durations. This will not be a comprehensive treatise on all EMF safety—there are areas of legitimate concern where evidence shows harm, and other areas where evidence demonstrates safety. The field remains controversial, with experts arguing for either relative safety or danger of various EMF expo-

sures. In general, I do think one should be cautious about exposure to certain types of EMFs, particularly those they may be exposed to for many hours daily. For those wanting to explore EMF safety more broadly, Nick Pineault's work is an excellent resource.

For our purposes, I'll address the specific concern about the types and dosages of EMFs from PBM devices. Fortunately, the EMF considerations for PBM devices are far less complex and controversial than many other EMF types.

PBM devices emit extremely low frequency (ELF) electromagnetic fields, like many common electrical appliances from computers to blenders to hair dryers. These fields occupy the lowest frequency portion of the electromagnetic spectrum, below 300 Hz, with most common sources operating at 50 to 60 Hz (household electrical power frequency).

ELFs are fundamentally different from higher-frequency radiation like X-rays, UV light, or radio waves. The electromagnetic spectrum ranges from lowest to highest frequencies, with the primary health risks increasing at higher frequencies where radiation becomes "ionizing"—meaning it carries enough energy to strip electrons from atoms and break chemical bonds. Gamma rays and X-rays can directly damage DNA, while UV light can cause sunburn and skin cancer with intense exposure.

ELF fields, however, aren't ionizing and don't damage DNA or break apart molecules. They behave more like slowly fluctuating magnetic bubbles around the device. The magnetic fields from these sources decrease rapidly with distance, which is why field strength drops off quickly as you move away from electrical devices.

When we talk about many other types of EMFs, we're dealing with electromagnetic radiation that propagates through space at much higher frequencies. ELFs create localized "near-field" magnetic fields similar to a permanent magnet, except they alternate at 50 to 60 Hz. Like a permanent magnet's field, these drop off rapidly with distance.

For context, static magnetic fields have been heavily studied for safety due to MRI machines, which use magnetic fields far more powerful than any PBM device (1.5 to 3 Tesla—over 30,000x stronger than PBM panels emit). Research has found no cancer risk from MRIs, including long-term studies of MRI technicians, animal studies with prolonged exposure, and cellular studies examining DNA damage mechanisms.

Because ELF EMFs are weak and drop off quickly with distance, most health authorities (WHO, IARC, and IRPA) don't consider them a major health concern at household levels. However, the science isn't entirely one-sided.

The International Agency for Research on Cancer (IARC) has classified ELF EMFs as "possibly carcinogenic to humans" (Group 2B)—the same category that includes lead and DDT.[69] That doesn't mean they are carcinogenic. It just means there's some evidence they could be (perhaps with extreme exposures), though not enough evidence to be sure.

Research has identified several potential mechanisms of biological interaction. Studies indicate that ELF EMFs may induce cellular stress responses, with some researchers noting that exposure "turns on" various intracellular mechanisms and modifies stress-related functions in nervous, hormonal, and immune systems.[70]

The Occupational Safety and Health Administration acknowledges that research has investigated potential "carcinogenic, reproductive, and neurological effects" as well as possible "cardiovascular, brain and behavior, hormonal and immune system changes."[71] Multiple peer-reviewed studies have examined possible connections between ELF EMF exposure and various health conditions, including cardiovascular effects,[72] neurological conditions,[73] effects on fertility,[74] impacts on the immune system,[75] potential influences on cellular stress responses,[76] and possible effects on hormonal systems.[77]

However, while these studies suggest correlations and potential mechanisms, there isn't definitive proof of causation between ELF EMFs and specific diseases.

More importantly, any intelligible discussion of the dangers of ELFs needs to be grounded in the context of dose. Almost everything can cause harm at a high enough dose, from water to exercise. Understanding EMF exposure requires applying the principle that "the dose makes the poison." Just as moderate sunlight exposure is beneficial while 8 hours of tropical sun exposure may cause severe sunburn and contribute to skin cancer, EMF exposure follows the same dose-dependent relationship. The critical variables are intensity (field strength) and duration (length and frequency of exposure).

PBM sessions typically last 10 to 30 minutes and emit modest magnetic fields of 20 to 150 mG within the first 1 to 6 inches away from the device. This exposure level is remarkably common in daily life. Common household devices produce similar exposures: hair dryers generate

10 to 90 mG at 6 inches, microwaves produce 10 to 50 mG at 1 foot, bedside lamps create 10 to 80 mG at one foot, and computer monitors emit 2 to 30 mG. Cell phones generate 10 to 40 mG when held against the ear during calls. Laptops create comparable field strengths when used on your lap, driving a car often subjects you to 20 to 50 mG during long drives, and people routinely experience similar levels from electrical outlets and bedside devices for 8 hours nightly while sleeping. LED panels at 20 to 150 mG fall well within this normal range of everyday household and personal device exposures that most people encounter multiple times daily without concern. So the first important piece of context here is that there isn't anything unique about EMF exposures from PBM devices compared to the many other common sources of EMFs in most people's daily lives.

But that doesn't tell us necessarily that all of these exposures are safe, only that they're common. So the next important context we need is to understand established safety guidelines. The distinction between brief therapeutic use and concerning exposure scenarios is dramatic. International safety organizations have established clear exposure limits based on extensive research. The International Commission on Non-Ionizing Radiation Protection (ICNIRP)—the WHO-recognized authority for EMF safety guidelines—sets the global standards that most countries adopt.[78]

For ELF magnetic fields at 50 to 60 Hz, ICNIRP guidelines establish:

General public limits:

ICNIRP 1998 guidelines: 1,000 mG continuous exposure limit

ICNIRP 2010 guidelines: 2,000 mG (though many countries still use the more conservative 1,000-mG limit)

Occupational exposure limits:

5,000 mG for trained workers during 8-hour workdays

To put PBM device exposure in perspective: Most LED panels emit 20 to 150 mG during use, which represents only 2 to 15 percent of the general public safety threshold for *continuous* exposure. Even at the upper range, PBM devices operate at exposure levels similar to common household appliances that people use regularly without concern.

The duration comparison is equally important. International safety limits are designed for *continuous, all-day exposure* scenarios. PBM treatments typically last 10 to 30 minutes, representing a tiny fraction of the exposure duration these safety standards are in reference to. While safety guidelines assume 24-hour daily exposure at these field strengths, PBM users experience these modest field levels for less than 1 percent of their day.

This means PBM sessions have substantial safety margins—both in intensity (7 to 50 times below safety limits, depending on device strength) and duration (representing less than 1 percent of the exposure time used to establish safety thresholds).

The cumulative exposure from a PBM session represents a small fraction of what international safety authorities consider safe for *continuous* exposure. In contrast, concerning scenarios involve industrial workers facing powerful magnetic fields for over 2,000 hours annually, or residents near major power lines with persistent exposure—situations combining both high intensity and chronic duration, fundamentally different from brief therapeutic sessions.

So Why Do People Worry About EMFs from PBM Panels?

If we look to the actual research, you can scarcely ever find even so much of a mention of EMFs as they relate to PBM, and it doesn't appear to have been studied to any significant degree in the context of PBM treatments.

If we look to see what PBM experts have to say about the issue of EMF exposure from using PBM devices, shockingly, they seem to rarely ever discuss it. I've been struck by the gap between public perception of concern over EMFs from PBM devices vs. the level of concern by PBM researchers. When I bring up the issue of EMFs from PBM devices to researchers in this field, most of them have no idea what I'm even referring to! They're often not even aware that consumers are worried about EMFs from PBM devices, and they generally don't express much concern about it. (Of course, it could be that some experts are concerned about it and I'm unaware of their views.)

When I asked Dr. Arany about it, he initially didn't realize there was a specific consumer concern about this issue. When I spoke with Dr. Hamblin about it, he was similarly unconcerned and remarked that ELF exposure safety thresholds are many orders of magnitude greater than the very low levels emitted by PBM panels. He went on to say:

My advice to somebody who has a big panel is treat it like a bed and lie on it, because the coupling from the LEDs into the skin is much better in contact, for sure, there's much less diffuse reflection. If you have a strong panel, it's not going to buckle, just put it on the bed and lay on top of it.

As evident from this exchange, Dr. Hamblin recommends using devices pressed directly against the skin, showing little concern about EMF exposure from panels even with your body pressed right up against them.

All of this begs the question: If it's not in the literature on PBM devices, and not generally talked about by PBM experts, where did the idea come from that EMFs from these devices pose some kind of critical health hazard and that panels should be used from 6 inches or more away from the device?

Based on my observations in the industry, I believe that this recommendation

(using the lights from several inches away to minimize exposure to magnetic fields) was never grounded in solid scientific evidence, but was mostly the result of psychological dynamics where:

- The general population started to become more EMF-aware and concerned with minimizing EMFs, making the assumption that such exposure could be harmful, and that it would be better off avoided. People started asking PBM device manufacturers about the EMFs from their devices.
- Manufacturers of PBM devices tried to overcome this common concern/objection many people were having to buying their devices and thus started to make public claims about "no EMFs" from their devices when used 6 inches away, and recommending customers to use the devices from 6 inches or more away from the devices for this reason.
- Other newer manufacturers basically conformed to this general trend of assumptions from the general public and the first manufacturers, who all seemed to be making a big deal over the concern with EMFs from these devices.

In my view, a psychological phenomenon was at play here, where, in the absence of any significant evidence suggesting any harm from this type and intensity of EMFs, people simply followed the assumptions of other people (the bandwagon effect), and businesses followed the assumptions (and marketing practices) of other businesses, and almost everyone was operating in a way that was largely detached from the actual scientific evidence.

While the precautionary principle of avoiding potential hazards is generally sound (i.e., we might say "why not just avoid the EMFs, because it's better to be safe than sorry"), its application here creates an important conflict. The reason why is that PBM efficacy is generally best with close proximity to the device (or skin contact), which is precisely where EMF exposure would be highest. So moving further away from the PBM device therefore potentially compromises PBM treatment efficacy—greater distance generally reduces light penetration to deep tissues and causes more light to reflect off the skin instead of penetrating and being absorbed by our cells.

In my opinion, the only way we should be willing to limit the effectiveness of our PBM sessions for the sake of minimizing our exposure to EMFs is if there is a significant body of quality evidence that strongly indicates harm to human health from this intensity and duration of exposure to magnetic fields. Currently, there isn't.

Now, to be charitable, there isn't a great deal of evidence on this topic in general, and absence of evidence is not the same as evidence of absence. I personally believe there's far more reason to be concerned with chronic multi-hour exposures to things like Wi-Fi and the radio frequencies from phones and computers, or even the magnetic/electrical fields from the lamp on my nightstand for 8 hours while I sleep each night, than I am with a sub 30-minute exposure to ELFs from LED devices.

It's also worth saying that if you have found yourself to be EMF-sensitive (if you have found that you react with symptoms to exposures to man-made EMFs of various types), that could certainly be justification for you to avoid exposures to EMFs from any device, whether a phone, computer, car, or PBM device. While this topic is controversial, it's plausible that someone in poor health generally would be less resilient to any exposure to any type of stress on their cells.

In a perfect world, PBM devices would have zero detectable ELFs. Alternatively, another perfect scenario would be that we could simply modify the way we use PBM devices to eliminate EMFs without affecting the PBM treatment. Unfortunately, that's not the scenario we're in, and the reality is that we face a trade-off with many PBM devices: minimize EMF exposure at the expense of treatment efficacy or optimize treatment parameters while accepting brief EMF exposure.

If I had any real concern that brief exposure to this intensity of ELFs was likely to be harmful to human health, of course, I would never advise it.

But my current interpretation of the evidence (which could, of course, eventually turn out to be flawed) is this: If you have to choose between optimizing for PBM efficacy versus minimizing EMF exposure, it's wise to prioritize PBM treatment effectiveness rather than being overly concerned about short-duration exposure to low-level ELFs. The current concern over 10-to-30-minute exposures to these fields seems greatly disproportional to what the scientific evidence says about their dangers.

Nevertheless, science evolves, and future research may show this type of ELF exposure is indeed harmful. In such a scenario, I'd modify my views accordingly. For now, I suggest focusing on optimizing your PBM treatment effectiveness.

PBM TREATMENT FREQUENCY

Dosing frequency refers to how often treatments should be administered to achieve optimal results while allowing sufficient time for the body to respond and adapt to the stimulus.

Just as with many biological interventions, the frequency of PBM treatments likely plays a crucial role in their effectiveness. A fundamental principle in biology is that beneficial adaptations occur during the recovery period between stimuli, not during the stimulus itself. This is well illustrated in exercise science: When we work out, we actually create minor damage to our muscles and stress our systems. The improvements in strength, endurance, and fitness happen during the recovery period between sessions. If we exercise too frequently without adequate recovery time, we can impair those adaptations and cause overtraining syndrome.

If we exercise only once every 15 days, whatever adaptations are stimulated are largely lost in the two weeks between bouts of exercise. It's just not happening frequently enough to do much of anything. On the other hand, if we do intense bouts of running or weight training three or four times a day, we have a different problem: The body simply doesn't have the downtime to rest, repair, and create adaptations, so we end up overtrained, fatigued, with sore and inflamed muscles, injuries, and stress fractures.

This same basic principle applies to many other things, like fasting, sauna therapy, cold plunging—and PBM. With PBM, each session triggers a cascade of biological responses—including changes in cellular energy production, gene expression, and inflammatory mediators. These changes need time to fully develop and stabilize. Many changes take place in the period *after* PBM treatment, not only during it. So just as with exercise, too frequent application of PBM can potentially interfere with these adaptive processes and lead to diminished returns or even negative effects. Fasting may be beneficial when done one day every week or few weeks, or more mild fasting done more frequently (e.g., 16-hour daily fasting windows), but extreme fasting will start to result in more harm than good.

When sessions are too frequent, the total dose (of multiple daily treatments combined) can become excessive, or the tissue may simply not get enough "downtime" in between treatments, potentially leading to a biphasic dose response (where more treatment actually produces fewer benefits or may even be harmful rather than beneficial). This is sometimes called the "too much of a good thing" effect, where oversaturation of the therapeutic stimulus can overwhelm the body's adaptive capacity.

Unfortunately, we don't have a significant body of evidence that compares different treatment frequencies for every conceivable treatment goal. Moreover, there is a huge variety of different frequencies of treatment used in studies, from single treatments, to once weekly treatments, to multiple treatments per day. I could potentially list out hundreds of studies here to give examples of different frequencies of treatment used in various studies, and the findings from each of them, but the differences in specifics—types of devices used, different irradiances, different dosages, methods of application, for different goals—introduce too many confounding variables for meaningful patterns to be extracted from the body of evidence. Some

studies might compare one treatment per week to two or three, while another study may find that daily treatment was too much, while another study did twice daily treatment with good results. You can even find studies where researchers have specifically advised having 48 to 72 hours between treatments for best results. Further complicating things is that in studies where a very large dose was administered, it is likely that they may find a lower frequency may be best (e.g., one treatment every 3 days), whereas with a more moderate dose, a higher frequency (like daily) may be perfectly appropriate. We also have to consider that different studies use different kinds of devices (from lasers applied to a handful of specific treatment points, or similar small devices applied to small areas of the body to full-body pods that irradiate the entire body from head to toe), and thus radically different total doses delivered—which is likely to hugely influence optimal treatment frequency.

Ultimately, all of these limitations and confounding variables mean that the current state of the evidence simply doesn't allow us to make definitive conclusions about the optimal frequency of PBM treatments that would apply universally to at-home use of various PBM devices.

When I asked Dr. Hamblin his thoughts on this issue, our conversation went like this:

ARI: Do you feel there's a concern with the biphasic dose response of doing the light therapy at too high a frequency? Doing it multiple times a day, for example?

DR. HAMBLIN: I think doing it multiple times a day is probably good.

ARI: You think two times a day in general is perfectly fine?

DR. HAMBLIN: That's perfectly fine.

ARI: Is that context-specific? Does that apply to pretty much everything, whether you're treating skin, anti-aging on your face, or treating your joints or muscles or things like that, or the brain?

DR. HAMBLIN: As far as I know, I'm going to stick my neck out and say this would apply to every site on the body. As far as I know, twice a day should be fine.

So we can conceptualize the range of expert opinion among PBM researchers as being from twice daily to once per 3 days. It's fair to say that almost everyone would agree that the optimal frequency is somewhere in that range.

Here are several factors that might influence optimal frequency (please note that some of this should be regarded as speculative):

1. **THE CONDITION BEING TREATED** (acute vs. chronic vs. general wellness). Acute injuries may respond well to multiple daily treatments. Some researchers use more frequent PBM treatments to invoke a biological response in chronic conditions. And in general wellness, less-frequent treatments (perhaps once a day or once every other day) may be more ideal.

2. **TISSUE DEPTH AND TYPE.** Deep tissues like the brain and muscles are especially light-sensitive and may be more prone to biphasic dose responses with too frequent treatments.

3. **INDIVIDUAL RESPONSE AND HEALING CAPACITY.** Frail or chronically ill people may be more prone to biphasic dose responses from more intense or frequent PBM treatments. Healthier individuals may be more tolerant of higher frequencies, analogous to what you'd expect to find in terms of tolerance to physical exertion.

4. **WAVELENGTH AND POWER DENSITY OF THE DEVICE.** A very intensive treatment with a high dose using a high irradiance device may stimulate a stronger response and may also require more downtime before another treatment takes place. In contrast, low-irradiance devices could potentially be applied multiple times per day without any concerns.

Again, this is somewhat speculative, but this could serve as a reasonable framework to guide your thinking and self-experimentation.

Perhaps most significantly, the World Association for Laser Therapy (WALT) dosing recommendations generally advise daily to every-other-day treatments in various specific treatment contexts.

Some researchers also note that higher frequency doesn't always mean better outcomes. For example, one study showed that once-daily PBM had stronger effects than three-times-daily PBM,[79] again reinforcing the importance of balance and incorporating adequate "rest" between PBM sessions.

It's also worth thinking in terms of local vs. total dose. Treating different body parts throughout the day is likely fine—as long as you're not overtreating one specific area multiple times daily. You could, for example, treat your shoulder in the morning and your knee and your low back in another session without issue. This would be three PBM sessions in one day, but only one session per body area. The concern over too-high frequency is more about multiple sessions on the same body area in one day.

It's also worth considering the dosing of light on the human body through an evolutionary lens. When we view PBM from the perspective of a random technological intervention, it is perhaps a complete question mark as to the ideal frequency of exposure. But if we look through an evolutionary lens—understanding that the original form of PBM was sunlight, and that our human ancestors spent most of their time outdoors being exposed to sunlight on a daily basis—it becomes logical

to presume that since our species evolved over millions of years with at least one daily outing in the sun, once-daily PBM (at least systemically, but not necessarily intensive treatment of a specific area) should be perfectly biologically appropriate. On the other hand, still operating within an evolutionary frame, we might consider more recent ancestry, and whether our personal ancestral line is of darker skin and have lived in sunnier regions of the world—or, for example, if our ancestral line comes from Northern Europe (perhaps England or Ireland) and tend to have very fair skin. It might be the case that, since full sun exposure in those regions is not a daily occurrence for much of the year, there is a lower tolerance for both sun exposure and PBM treatments in those with paler skin, and a schedule of dosing once every other day or every 3 days may be ideal. This is all speculation, because the studies to determine this kind of thing definitively have not been done, but it's a potentially useful perspective for personal experimentation and figuring out what works best for your biology.

The scientific evidence on PBM frequency is still limited, but this much seems clear:

- It needs to be frequent enough to derive a benefit (once a week or every 2 weeks is likely not sufficient to get meaningful benefit in most contexts).

- But more isn't always better; once you get beyond twice daily, it becomes questionable.
- Consistency matters.
- "Rest" periods (adequate time with no PBM) may be necessary between sessions to get the full benefits.

So what's the ideal frequency? Based on a combination of the available (limited) evidence and expert opinion, here is a simple framework to use:

- Acute conditions: one to two times per day
- Chronic conditions or general wellness: once per day, every other day, or every third day
- Full-body PBM (e.g., using a pod): potentially once per day, but given the high systemic load, two or four treatments per week may be more ideal

Overall, as a general rule, it's likely that somewhere between twice per day to once every three days is ideal in most contexts. Twice per day is likely preferable in the context of acute issues like injuries, which require more intensive healing, whereas once per day or every other day may be ideal in more general wellness contexts. (This may also differ depending on whether we're talking about targeted use of small devices on a specific body area, like the ankle or shoulder, or going into a full-body pod; we might expect that targeted use could be done more frequently, while whole-body pods may be a powerful systemic stimulus that should be used less frequently, perhaps every other day or every third day.)

The bottom line: Most people will likely do best with treatments once per day or every other day on a given body area, depending on the condition, device intensity, and personal factors. But there may be times when twice per day is desirable, or where one treatment every 3 days is more desirable. For me personally, I typically use it once daily or every other day in most contexts (on a given body area), but for acute injuries, I might use it twice per day. For example, I recently sprained my ankle playing tennis and over the last few days, I have been doing a PBM treatment on it in the morning and again in the evening. Now, keep in mind that all of this is referring to PBM treatments on the same body area. When you introduce treating multiple different body areas, the picture gets more complex. Over the course of a single day, I will almost always do at least one PBM treatment on one body area or another, and often multiple treatments daily on different body areas. For example, I may treat an injured ankle with a targeted device, use an LED mask on my face, use a laser cap to prevent hair loss while brushing my teeth, and use a large LED panel on my torso for systemic effects all in the same day. It's rare that a day goes by where I don't do at least one PBM treatment somewhere on my body.

TIMING: WHEN TO DO PBM TREATMENTS

One of the most common questions about PBM is: When's the best time to do it? The answer depends on your goals: whether you're looking to enhance energy, improve sleep, recover from workouts, or lose fat. But broadly speaking, we can break it down into categories based on the timing of the day and the specific outcome you're targeting.

Morning Treatments: Boosting Cellular Energy and Circadian Alignment

If PBM originally came from the sun, it makes sense that our biology is most adapted to getting red and NIR light during the daytime. And that's exactly what some research supports. Studies from Dr. Glen Jeffery's lab show that mitochondria are most responsive to light in the morning, when ATP production is naturally at its lowest.[80]

One study showed that PBM done between 9:30 a.m. and 12:30 p.m. during the winter significantly improved mood, alertness, and sleepiness—basically restoring energy and mood levels to what people felt during the summer.[81] No such effect was seen in the summer, suggesting that PBM may be especially helpful during times of the year when sun exposure is low.

Other studies show that enzymes like cytochrome c oxidase—key players in the body's use of light energy—follow circadian rhythms and are most sensitive to light earlier in the day.[82–84] These effects support the idea that morning PBM may enhance cellular energy and help regulate circadian gene expression.

Evening Sessions: Supporting Sleep

Surprisingly, red and NIR light may also have benefits in the evening. Unlike blue light, which suppresses melatonin, red and NIR light may actually support melatonin production and help with sleep.

Studies have found that red light exposure 90 minutes before bed can improve sleep quality,[85] and athletes have experienced better sleep after evening red light treatments.[86] Other research shows lower nighttime cortisol after PBM, another sign of improved relaxation.[87–89]

That said, some people find that using high-powered panels right before bed actually disturbs their sleep. Why? Because our biology likely doesn't expect bright, intense light after dark, even if it's red. Red light might not suppress melatonin, but the brightness alone could still signal wakefulness.

To minimize disruption, evening PBM should:

- Be done 1 to 2 hours before bed
- Be at low irradiance levels ($<50 \text{ mW/cm}^2$)
- Avoid direct eye exposure
- Possibly prioritize NIR over red, since it's less visible

Exercise Timing: Performance and Recovery

Before Exercise

PBM is well-studied in the context of exercise. Using PBM 10 to 30 minutes before a workout can boost performance, improve muscle power, increase oxygen efficiency, and reduce inflammation. These effects are strongest in that short window just before training, especially with NIR light, or red and NIR light combined.[90]

After Exercise

There's also a key post-workout window where PBM can amplify recovery and training adaptations. Studies show that applying PBM within 2 to 3 hours after exercise reduces muscle damage and soreness, speeds recovery, and improves energy replenishment.[91]

Even more interesting, PBM after training can amplify the adaptations from exercise themselves—like improving strength, endurance, and mitochondrial function.[92–98] This makes sense given that PBM enhances many of the same cellular pathways that exercise activates, like mitochondrial function and protein synthesis. By applying PBM during this post-exercise window, you may be able to maximize both the recovery process and the adaptive response to training.

The research points to that 2- to 3-hour post-workout "therapeutic window," with the benefits declining after 4 hours. It's possible that you might get even better results with follow-up treatments at 24 and 48 hours, especially when combined with proper nutrition timing.

Preconditioning Before Stress of Various Kinds (Exercise, Sun Exposure, Psychological Stress, Chemotherapy, and More)

There's strong evidence supporting the use of PBM as a preconditioning therapy— that is, applying light before a stress-inducing event to protect the body and enhance performance.

For example, studies show that using PBM before exercise can improve endurance and reduce the risk of injury. There's also evidence that it can work to precondition the skin before UV/sun exposure to reduce or prevent skin damage. Similarly, PBM has been successfully used ahead of chemotherapy or radiotherapy in cancer patients to prevent severe side effects like oral ulcers, which can be so painful that they force patients to be fed through a stomach tube. Applying PBM a day before these treatments can dramatically reduce both the severity and number of ulcers.

This approach is backed by high-level evidence and endorsed by global authorities in cancer care, such as MASCC/ISOO. Unfortunately, despite its proven efficacy, PBM is still rarely offered in mainstream cancer treatment. I asked Dr. Cronshaw about this:

DR. CRONSHAW: PBM preconditioning is incredibly effective—especially for reducing oral ulcers and skin damage from radiotherapy. Some large-scale studies even show reduced cancer recurrence and improved survival rates in PBM-treated patients. One study by Antunes showed a 20-percent reduction in recurrence and a 16-percent improvement in overall survival over 9 years.

ARI: So why isn't this more widely used?

DR. CRONSHAW: A survey of MASCC/ISOO members revealed that the biggest barriers are cost, time, lack of training, and fear that PBM might stimulate cancer. There are also country-specific bureaucratic hurdles.

ARI: Since PBM can promote cellular growth factors and repair, many people often ask me if it could potentially promote cancer or cancer growth. Is there any evidence that PBM might promote cancer?

MARK: After over 15 years of clinical studies, there's no evidence that PBM causes harm. In fact, PBM often improves treatment outcomes. While some lab studies have hinted at risks, these are highly artificial setups, and the consensus is that PBM is safe and effective. Of course, it should never be used as a stand-alone treatment on undiagnosed suspicious areas.

ARI: Can LED devices be used at home for self-treatment?

MARK: That's where the future is headed. Once proper protocols are established, PBM devices could become a standard part of home care prescribed by oncologists.

For those interested in cancer care and PBM: Dr. Cronshaw gave an online lecture on this subject for the laser company Biolase in December 2024. You can access it at the following link: https://www .biolaseacademy.com/webinar/photobio modulation-cancer-safety-concerns-and -proficiency-an-evidence-based-approach/.

A wide variety of in vitro, animal studies, and human studies have shown that PBM can serve to precondition cells or organs prior to exposure to a wide variety of stressors, including toxins, to help reduce their negative impact.

Timing for Brain Health and Learning

PBM applied to the brain shows promise for enhancing learning, memory, and mental performance. It likely works by increasing BDNF, boosting mitochondrial function, improving blood flow, and reducing inflammation—all of which support neuroplasticity.

Since learning and neuroplasticity are energy-intensive processes, PBM might create an optimal cellular environment for forming new neural connections. Therefore, it's very plausible that PBM could synergize with learning or the practicing of any brain-related skill, and thus that doing PBM before and/or after such activities could amplify the effects.

Using PBM about 15 to 20 minutes before intensive learning may be ideal, similar to how pre-workout PBM primes muscles for exercise. This timing allows for enhanced blood flow and energy production before tackling challenging mental tasks.[99] The benefits might extend through the learning period and into the consolidation phase, potentially supporting memory formation.

PBM seems particularly promising when paired with specific cognitive challenges like complex problem-solving, skill acquisition, language learning, and meditation practices. The benefits appear strongest when PBM precedes these activities.[100] For practical implementation, some people find morning treatments helpful for general cognitive enhancement, with additional sessions before important mental work.

That said, individual responses can vary significantly, and what works best likely differs from person to person. While these principles make logical sense given our understanding of PBM and brain function, we need much more research to develop evidence-based protocols. Consider this a framework for exploration rather than a definitive claim of proven benefits.

Fat Loss Timing: Supporting Mobilization and Oxidation

PBM may help enhance fat loss, particularly in stubborn areas, by improving blood flow to fat stores, reducing local inflammation, increasing mitochondrial activity, and potentially enhancing the release of stored fatty acids. Of course, you still need to burn these fatty acids off as energy. That's where exercise comes into play, as the body is already actively mobilizing and burning fat for energy. In my conversations with Dr. Hamblin, he has highlighted the particular effectiveness of using PBM *during* exercise for enhanced fat loss. This timing strategy may create a powerful synergistic effect, in which the combination of exercise-induced lipolysis and PBM's cellular effects could amplify fat mobilization and oxidation.

Logically, we'd suspect that it would best be paired with steady-state endurance exercise, particularly in Zone 2, the highest intensity of exercise where we're oxidizing almost entirely fat for energy. In contrast, we might expect it to synergize less well during weightlifting, high-intensity interval training, or other types of high-intensity training that rely more on carbohydrate metabolism.

For practical implementation, consider:

- Using flexible or wearable devices that don't restrict movement
- Focusing on specific stubborn fat areas during exercise

While the during-exercise application shows promise, a comprehensive approach might include several treatment windows.[101–103] The pre-exercise period can help prime tissues for enhanced performance and fat mobilization. During-exercise application, as discussed previously, may maximize fat release and oxidation when the body is actively burning fat for fuel. Post-exercise treatment might help maintain elevated metabolic activity while supporting recovery and cellular regeneration processes.

It's essential to remember that PBM is not a shortcut to fat loss but rather a potential optimization tool within a proper diet-and-exercise program. The therapy appears most effective when:

1. The body is in an overall caloric deficit
2. Regular exercise is part of the program
3. Treatment is focused on specific areas resistant to fat loss
4. Proper nutrition and recovery are prioritized
5. If you want to experiment with using it for fat loss, I recommend trying my "Stubborn Fat Protocol" presented earlier in the book in chapter 3.

CHAPTER SUMMARY

In this chapter, we've explored the key factors that influence the efficacy of PBM. We started with the basics—like choosing the right wavelength and achieving proper dosing in terms of energy delivered to a particular target tissue and for systemic effects. We looked at more technical aspects, such as how light convergence, LED spacing, LED density, and distance from the device affect light delivery and treatment outcomes. We examined how to optimize irradiance and wavelength depending on specific goals, and why treatment duration isn't just a leftover variable—it's a core part of the equation. We also broke down how the design of the device itself matters, especially when it comes to surface contact, anatomical fit, and how light enters the body based on angles and positioning.

Beyond the hardware, we also considered biological variables like tissue depth, optical properties, and body composition, which influence how light interacts with your body. We discussed the science and controversy around light penetration, pulsed vs. continuous-wave treatments, optimal treatment timing and frequency, and the concerns over EMFs.

Lastly, we covered how different treatment goals and body locations change how you should approach PBM, from deep-tissue treatments to full-body systemic effects, and why we generally want to leverage both local and systemic effects whenever possible.

Ultimately, understanding how all these

factors interact gives you the tools to get the most out of your PBM treatments. While research is still evolving, applying the best evidence we have now—and customizing it to your goals—can help you maximize the effectiveness of your PBM sessions.

To make things easier, below is a summary table of ideal dosing parameters and device types. Remember: While it's helpful as a quick reference for key dosing parameters, this table can't capture all the nuance we've covered throughout the chapter.

TISSUE TYPE	DOSE	IRRADIANCE	WAVELENGTHS	TYPE OF DEVICE AND METHOD APPLICATION
SUPERFICIAL TISSUES (skin, eyes, body fat and cellulite, hands, feet, mouth, thyroid)	3 to 20 J/cm²	10 to 50 mW/cm²	Prioritize red (630 nm and 660 nm)	Targeted device that contours to that area and is designed for that specific purpose (e.g., facial masks or pad-style devices), or, potentially, full-body panels used with lower irradiances (or farther distances away). Skin contact can be used, but even more important is a device that provides uniform coverage of the superficial tissue.
DEEP TISSUES (joints, brain, muscle/tendon, bone, fat, circulatory system, respiratory system, gut, glands, and internal organs)	20 to 60 J/cm²	50 to 120 mW/cm²	Prioritize NIR (810 nm, 830 nm, 850 nm, and 1,064 nm)	Targeted device designed to be applied directly to that specific area with appropriate irradiance and wavelengths (e.g., joint-specific devices) are ideal. Panels potentially can be used in some cases. Skin contact or high degrees of light convergence are optimal to facilitate deep penetration.

CHAPTER SIX

Guide to Red and Near-Infrared Photobiomodulation Devices

Choosing the right photobiomodulation (PBM) device has become increasingly complex as the market has evolved. This guide will help you understand the key principles for device selection, navigate common misconceptions, and make informed decisions based on scientific evidence rather than marketing claims.

Opinions about the best type of PBM device vary widely—from large panels to whole-body pods, to low-irradiance flexible pads, or other devices. It gets even more confusing when you start to consider different goals, like facial anti-aging, fat loss, hair growth, helping exercise recovery, enhancing performance, treating the brain, or deep-tissue muscle/tendon/bone/joint healing. Questions about lasers vs. LEDs, high vs. low irradiance, and pulsing vs. continuous-wave light only add to the complexity.

The market includes everything from home-use LED devices to professional-grade medical lasers used in clinical settings. Professional devices often include Class IV (>500 mW) or Class IIIB (5 to 500 mW) lasers that can deliver both red and NIR wavelengths, with some reaching incredible levels of power. These higher-powered laser devices typically require trained practitioners due to safety considerations, particularly regarding eye protection. Meanwhile, consumer devices tend to use LEDs (which are much lower-powered per square centimeter than lasers), but which deliver light over much larger surface areas.

When I wrote the first version of this book many years ago, the market had few high-quality options for devices, and my recommendations quickly became outdated as the industry expanded. At that time, there were only a few companies that existed selling PBM devices for at-home use and the options were very limited. Since then, the PBM market has exploded in growth, with dozens of new companies, and new devices are being brought to market every month.

Unfortunately, as a result of market dynamics, many manufacturers have been driven to change their devices in certain ways to gain a competitive advantage in the marketplace—perhaps relating to irradiance, wavelengths, pulsing, or size and power of their panels—and this has led to a growing gap between manufacturers' claims and the actual scientific data.

Further complicating this situation for the consumer is that different companies are making various kinds of claims for the superiority of their devices. One may claim their device to be superior based on its enormous size or wattage, another based on its use of many different wavelengths (some companies now have even started adding *blue* LEDs to try to claim that makes their panel superior). Others race to supply the highest possible irradiance, operating under the mistaken idea that higher irradiances are always better. And yet another claims that their *lower*-irradiance devices are more optimal, and that all other devices are in a dangerously high irradiance range. Still others make claims about proprietary technology, combinations of wavelengths, or pulsing frequencies, often with no basis in science. As a result, there is widespread confusion among consumers about what devices to buy for their goals, with many led to believe that simply buying the highest-wattage panel, or the largest panel, or the one with the most wavelengths is going to lead to the best results.

To make matters even more problematic, some device manufacturers use inaccurate meters to measure the irradiance of their devices and publish wildly inaccurate information about the irradiance of their devices (which their dosing guidelines are based on) on their websites. Before 2020, it was common for companies to use solar-power meters to measure the irradiance of these devices, and it has now been shown that these meters often give irradiance readings 30 to 50 percent higher than actual figures. (I made this mistake in the first edition of this book, by assuming that the meters were giving accurate data on irradiance, and I feel it's important to correct that mistake now.) Unfortunately, because some leading companies used these inflated figures from solar-power meters, many other companies followed suit and misrepresented their own devices' irradiance numbers in efforts not to be left behind.

While this was innocent and well-meaning many years ago—with people simply trying to measure and report irradiance data accurately—I know that virtually all of these companies are now aware of this measurement issue. Yet, many continue to misrepresent their specifications, no longer through ignorance but through deliberate choice. (I know this because of being involved in direct communication with many owners of companies and acquiring third-party lab reports on the true irradiances of their devices.) That's not the only form of misrepresentation, either: Many companies engage in various deceptive practices like measuring irradiance directly over the LED chip rather than average irradiance across the treatment area. (I have witnessed considerable dishonesty and unethical behavior among manufacturers of these devices, and I'd recommend avoiding manufacturers who engage in these practices until they demonstrate real transparency and integrity.)

As a result of all of this, we have one big mess of confusion. People don't really know what types of devices are best for a given goal, what makes them any better than another device, or how to dose with these devices because we often lack the true data on the light intensity of these devices.

One of my main goals for updating this book is to clear up this confusion, to bring greater transparency to the PBM device space, and to clean up many kinds of misrepresentation going on in the industry, so you can feel confident choosing the right devices for your goals. However, this is not an easy task. We don't have scientific consensus on many technical aspects of the devices, and there's no comprehensive body of research that definitively compares different types of devices against one another for specific purposes to give us objective data on which devices are best.

Given these limitations, we have to understand the *principles* of what makes a device effective for a particular purpose (which we've covered extensively in chapter 5 of this book), combine that knowledge with the limited selection of devices currently in existence (most of which are imperfect for one reason or another), and then use a bit of logical speculation to create a sort of blueprint of how to select the best device for your goals.

This is also somewhat difficult because the market for PBM devices now encompasses a huge range of different types of devices, with different specifications, with new generations and technological advancements entering the marketplace regularly.

To address the ongoing evolution of the PBM marketplace and avoid the problem of specific device recommendations quickly becoming outdated (which was a big issue with the original 2018 version of this book), this guide will focus on understanding the principles for selecting the right type of device for your goals. Rather than endorsing specific devices or brands, I'll explain the types of devices available, their best uses, and their limitations—with the ultimate goal of helping you select the right type of device for your specific goals. The idea is for this to be a resource for you to cut through the marketing hype, gimmicks, and inaccurate information that abound online about these devices and how they work. Additionally, I'll also give you real third-party data about the true typical irradiances from many of the panel devices from prominent manufacturers (so you can accurately dose these devices)—which is often not possible to do based on the inaccurate irradiance data that is on many manufacturers' websites. While I'll highlight some standout products from various brands in particular categories as examples, remember that these specific mentions may become outdated as new devices emerge.

For my specific product recommendations, I will maintain a constantly updated list of my top recommended devices across categories at www.redlightdeviceguide .com. This approach allows me to provide current, relevant recommendations as the market continues to evolve, while the principles and framework discussed in this book will remain valuable for evaluating any new devices that enter the market.

Most importantly, the goal of this section is to explain what types of devices are best for specific purposes and treatment goals, detail the pros and cons of each style of device, and identify which devices are supported by good evidence for specific treatment goals. By focusing on these core principles and maintaining updated specific recommendations online, this guide will remain valuable even as the market continues to evolve and new devices emerge.

WHAT'S YOUR GOAL?

Our deep dive into PBM devices begins with a simple question: What are you trying to accomplish?

As of this writing, there are more than 6,000 studies on PBM, for a huge range of specific treatment goals: wound healing, facial anti-aging effects on skin, athletic performance enhancement, brain enhancement, combating autoimmune disease, recovery from exercise, fat loss, improving joint health, fertility, oral health, pain relief, combating side effects of chemotherapy, overall systemic/metabolic health, and countless more.

Within this range of different potential uses, there is a huge array of different devices that could be used for various goals, with some being much better suited for a particular goal than others.

Given this landscape, we need to start by getting clear on what you are actually trying to do with PBM. Depending on what your goal is, we want to select the right type of device and the right specific device to best help you achieve that goal. This is a critical aspect of getting results with PBM: If you don't select the right device or use it properly, you're far less likely to derive meaningful benefit from PBM.

Generally speaking, we can break down all these PBM goals into three general categories:

1. Local effects on a specific tissue (e.g., facial skin anti-aging, wound healing, joint or tendon healing, treatment of internal organs, muscles after a workout, etc.). This can be further broken down by:
   a. Superficial tissues
   b. Deep tissues
   c. Photosensitive tissues
   d. Unique body parts where specialized devices are necessary
2. Systemic effects on the whole body (e.g., improving immune health, reducing chronic inflammation, improving metabolic health, stimulating stem cells, and general health/longevity)
3. A combination of local and systemic effects

Generally speaking, what's going to lead to the best results from PBM in most contexts is to leverage *both* local and systemic effects to the maximum, but there are many contexts in which you'd certainly want to prioritize one over the other.

Let's begin by discussing the most optimal ways to use PBM devices to reap systemic benefits. From there, we'll move into a section on more targeted goals and the best PBM device types for each of them.

MAXIMIZING SYSTEMIC EFFECTS

For general health and wellness, or for more generalized systemic illnesses not localized in any specific body part, the priority is harnessing the systemic benefits of PBM rather than targeting a specific tissue or body part.

As we've discussed in earlier sections, PBM offers a number of powerful systemic benefits:

- Reduces chronic inflammation and pro-inflammatory cytokines
- Promotes healing-focused immune response (M1-to-M2 macrophage shift)
- Improves mitochondrial efficiency and cellular energy production
- Enhances insulin sensitivity and glucose metabolism
- Mobilizes stem cells throughout the body for systemic repair
- Creates a more optimal healing environment in tissues
- Enables cellular healing and regeneration in both treated and untreated areas

By activating these pathways, PBM not only directly interacts with cells, but also triggers other complementary mechanisms that foster improved metabolic, mitochondrial, immune health, and cellular regeneration through systemic effects, making it a powerful tool for whole-body health, resilience, and maximizing healthspan and longevity.

Given this, I believe that the systemic effects of red and NIR light are basically analogous to an essential nutrient for the body: It provides a multi-pronged general wellness and anti-aging therapy that we should all be leveraging on a daily or near-daily basis.

With all this information in mind, let's discuss how to best harness the systemic benefits of PBM. Applying the principles we've covered should influence how we approach treatment protocols. While we don't yet have a comprehensive body of evidence providing explicit guidance (and thus these recommendations should be seen as somewhat speculative), the following strategies represent logical ways to maximize systemic benefits:

- **TREAT LARGER AREAS:** Targeting larger regions, the whole body, multiple areas, multiple different tissue types (and potentially some glands and organs), and areas of high blood flow (like major muscle groups) can stimulate systemic responses originating from different tissues and increase the total volume of blood exposed to the therapy. We want to treat the maximum number of cell types and volume of blood possible.

- **INCORPORATE BONE MARROW AND ADIPOSE-RICH AREAS:** Treating areas like the tibia (rich in bone marrow) or the abdomen (rich in adipose tissue) will likely enhance stem cell release into circulation, amplifying systemic repair capabilities.
  - › **COMBINE LOCAL AND STEM CELL-RICH AREA TREATMENTS:** When treating specific areas on your body (e.g., facial skin, muscles, joints, or brain), make sure to also incorporate PBM on stem cell–rich regions like the sternum, hip bones, ribs, spine, and tibia to mobilize stem cells into circulation for whole-body repair. Mobilizing stem cells with the more targeted treatment may create a synergistic effect.
  - › **UTILIZE NIR LIGHT WITH TARGETED DEVICES:** Use NIR light devices designed for deep penetration with skin contact and/or high irradiance, particularly in areas rich in bone marrow, to effectively stimulate stem cell release into the bloodstream.
  - › **ADOPT REGULAR MAINTENANCE TREATMENTS:** Frequent, consistent sessions support ongoing regenerative processes, maintaining an elevated baseline of circulating stem cells and other repair mechanisms. This could be daily or every other day.

- **DYNAMIC APPLICATION:** Rotate treatment areas across sessions to ensure that a variety of tissue types and blood vessels are exposed to PBM, maximizing systemic effects.
- **ENSURE ADEQUATE TREATMENT DURATION:** Longer sessions allow for more complete stem cell mobilization, increased exposure of circulating blood to therapeutic light, and greater systemic distribution of activated cells and signaling molecules, which all work together to help generate stronger systemic responses. Do this by treating multiple areas on the body rich in stem cells, like multiple bone and adipose tissue sites. You want to aim for 10-to-40-minute total durations rather than brief 2-to-5-minute sessions.

Combining all of this information, we can arrive at the conclusion that two general categories of devices are best suited to delivering systemic benefits:

1. Large LED panels (or whole-body pods) to maximize blood irradiation and stimulate as much total tissue as possible
2. Targeted devices with NIR and higher irradiances optimized for deeper penetration to deliver light into the bone marrow

Let's examine both of these types of devices and why they are likely to be effec-tive for maximizing the systemic benefits of PBM:

Panels and Whole-Body Pods for Systemic Benefits

This is where panels (especially large panels) probably have their biggest benefit: They are likely among the most effective methods to stimulate overall systemic benefits by delivering light to a very large surface area of the body.

A whole-body pod is arguably the most effective type of device for eliciting systemic benefits, as it provides near-complete body coverage. However, the difference in systemic benefits between using a pod and strategically placing multiple panels around the body may not be substantial. Given that whole-body pods are vastly more expensive (typically between $15,000 and $100,000)—often 10 to 100 times the cost of panels—they are likely to remain an option primarily for medical or wellness clinics and the very wealthy. There are several high-quality pods on the market, but as discussed previously, I have seen evidence of several manufacturers of pods massively misrepresenting the irradiance of their pods. So as always, but especially if you're going to spend tens of thousands of dollars, my advice would be to always opt for trustworthy brands that transparently provide third-party data on the irradiance of their devices.

It's also possible to arrange multiple panels in a way that approximates how whole-body pods deliver light to the body. If you have two to six large LED panels, you could fairly easily create a sort of "pod" setup that mimics the effects of a whole-body pod for a tiny fraction of the price. This setup can be achieved either standing (with panels in front and behind) or lying down (using an acrylic bed with panels above and below). For even better coverage, multiple panels can be positioned at angles to better conform to body curvature. For roughly $2,000 to $8,000, you can build a home setup that approaches pod-like parameters and coverage at a fraction of the cost. (Note that in this context of total-body treatment, you'd want to adjust the irradiance to approximately 20 to 50 mW/cm^2—particularly if you intend to expose your facial skin.) If you use parameters appropriate for skin health, this could be an excellent device that provides similar benefits to a whole-body pod, though definitely not nearly as nice to look at as a true full-body pod, so if you want to impress your biohacker friends, the real deal is probably the better choice over the DIY option.

Flexible neoprene pad-style "pods" may also deliver systemic benefits by virtue of simply irradiating so much of your body with light. The major flaw with these devices is that they are limited by their low irradiance, and by uneven coverage of the body surface due to LED spacing (low LED density). In pod-style devices using pads, skin contact with large portions of the body is going to be poor (the pad will be several inches away from the skin) because these pods don't wrap around our body surfaces the way that a belt or knee-wrap device would. That may seem like a small point, but these types of LEDs generally only have significant irradiance to induce PBM effects when pressed right up against the skin, and any gap of even an inch generally reduces the irradiance to very low levels. So much of the body—while technically being in the "pod"—may not be getting light with a high enough irradiance to induce significant PBM benefits.

But these flexible pods may still be a good option for some people, and I am confident that they, too, will elicit considerable systemic benefits based on the simple fact that they cover an enormous portion of the body surface (albeit with low irradiance and low LED density), and they likely have beneficial effects on skin health across all of the body. While this is speculative, there could also be a unique benefit to receiving PBM while lying down, as the relaxation might synergize with the treatment for added effects.

Overall, the greater the overall dose of light delivered to the body, the more tissues you can deliver light to, and the more of your overall blood that interacts with the light, the greater the systemic benefits are likely to be. For these reasons, true whole-body pods and large LED panels are likely to be the most ideal large devices for inducing systemic benefits.

Targeted Devices for Systemic Benefits

While this is still largely speculative as we don't yet have adequate research on it, it's logical that if you desire systemic benefits, you'd perform a treatment where a large portion of the body is being exposed to light from a large panel or pod, and you'd also use a more targeted device on specific areas of the body rich in stem cells to stimulate their release into circulation. (This is how I personally do almost all my PBM sessions.) Targeted devices with higher irradiances (50 to 150 mW/cm²) and ample power in the NIR wavelengths are ideal for penetrating deep tissues, including bone, to stimulate stem cells—one of the key mechanisms behind PBM's systemic benefits. These devices can effectively complement larger panels, maximizing the overall impact of PBM in terms of systemic benefits.

As of this writing, there are limited options for targeted devices with high irradiance and ample NIR power. Most pad-style devices on the market fall short in this regard due to their low irradiance, particularly in the NIR spectrum. Some standout devices currently on the market include the FlexBeam, SunPower LED's "Palm" products, Chroma Ironforge, and the Kineon Move Plus. Certain small panels may also work well for targeted applications when pressed directly against the skin. (Keep in mind that these recommendations might become outdated quickly—visit www.redlightdeviceguide.com for the latest updates.)

SunPower LED's "Palm" devices offer a higher irradiance (110 to 187 mW/cm²) and uniform coverage, though one downside with it is that it needs to be held in the hand and used manually (or with a makeshift strap to keep it on an area). This is one of my go-to devices for injuries and deep-tissue treatments.

FlexBeam from Recharge Health offers a nice irradiance of 110 mW/cm² (based on their website) and conforms to some extent to body surfaces. I have one of these devices, and it's solid, but the one major flaw I see is that the coverage could be improved.

Chroma's Ironforge is an extremely high irradiance device (>400 mW/cm²). Some people report excellent results with it, but I have some concern that it may be too high of an irradiance. (Using it at a greater distance from the skin may help mitigate this issue.) Remember, going much above 100 mW/cm² can result in excessive heating of tissues, and while the manufacturer avoids that effect through encouraging users to move the device around almost constantly, one also needs to consider that exposure time is a factor in the efficacy of PBM—that is, that it may be more ideal to use a more moderate irradiance for a longer period of time than a very high irradiance for a very short period of time, even if the end dosage in J/cm² or total joules is the same in both cases.

The Kineon Move Plus is a sophisticated device designed for joints that also includes lasers, though its overall irradiance and coverage are on the lower side for this category of device. But it's definitely a good device for targeted issues in small areas and on joints. Each one of the three light-emitting pods can be used in isolation for precisely targeting small areas.

Again, consider these as examples rather than definitive recommendations. Device options and innovations evolve rapidly, so check for updated device recommendations at www.redlightdeviceguide.com.

For systemic benefits, targeted devices are best applied to bone marrow–rich regions close to the surface (i.e., without a lot of fat or muscle between the skin and the bone). These include the sternum, ribs, upper spine, tibia, and hip bones. With the right device, significant light penetration to these areas can stimulate the systemic release of circulating stem cells.

Any of the above devices (or similar products from other brands available by the time you're reading this) could potentially be used in a targeted way to facilitate stem cell release to enhance the systemic effects of PBM.

Devices Likely to Be Relatively Ineffective for Systemic Benefits

Many devices on the market are unlikely to deliver significant or comprehensive systemic benefits from PBM. These include most low-irradiance devices (though large devices covering a substantial body surface may still provide some systemic effects) and small devices with limited coverage areas.

Pad-style devices, except for very large ones, often lack effectiveness due to low irradiance, uneven coverage from sparse LED spacing, and insufficient NIR power. Similarly, small devices designed for specific areas, such as mouth or brain applications, and other devices that fail to offer adequate body coverage or penetration depth—though they may be ideal for a specific kind of targeted treatment—are unlikely to be highly effective for achieving systemic benefits. In general, devices that deliver low overall doses of light (in total joules), with lower irradiances, to smaller surface areas of the body, are likely to be less effective in triggering the systemic benefits of PBM.

Personalizing PBM for Systemic Benefits: The Sunlight Factor

The relationship between natural sunlight exposure and artificial PBM therapy is an important but often overlooked factor when assessing the need for dedicated PBM devices. Sunlight is nature's original PBM source, delivering therapeutic red and NIR wavelengths along with a full spectrum of other beneficial light. Before implementing PBM therapy, it's important to consider your sunlight-exposure patterns.

On a sunny day in the tropics, you can expect to receive 80 to 140 mW/cm^2 of sunlight, of which 5 to 35 mW/cm^2 is NIR depending on the time of day.[1] These values obviously depend on where you live, but even in Europe during the summer you can expect to receive 20 mW/cm² of NIR from the sun around midday.[1]

Tropics: Summer Solstice

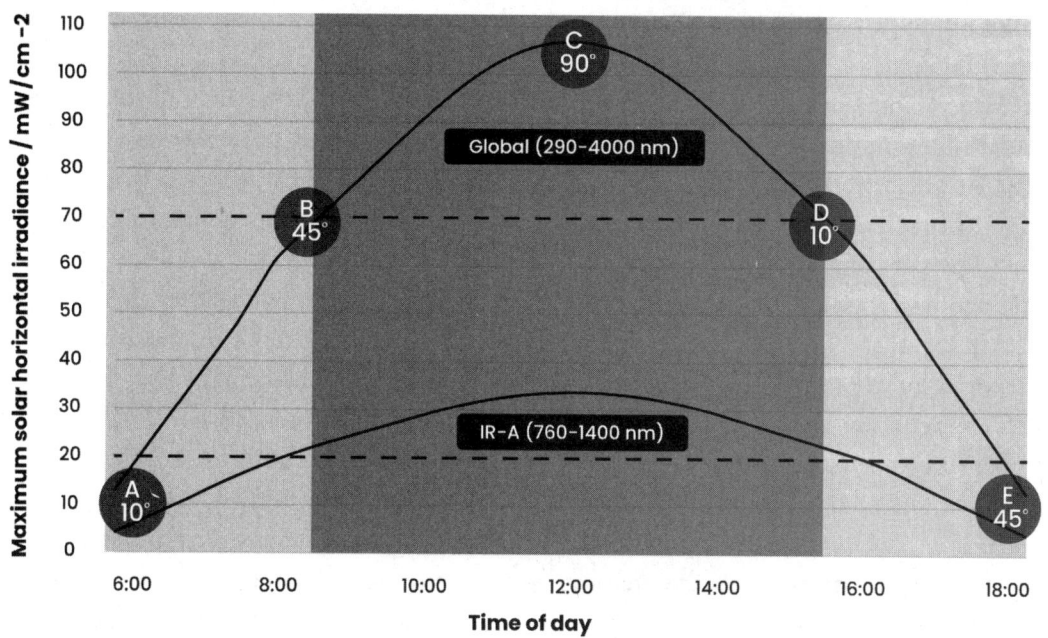

Barolet et al. J Photochem Photobiol B. 2016; 155: 78-85.

THE SUNLIGHT-SUFFICIENT INDIVIDUAL: For individuals who spend substantial time outdoors with significant skin exposure—such as those who exercise outside daily or practice regular sunbathing—many of the systemic benefits associated with red and NIR light therapy devices may already be covered. Sunlight stimulates mitochondrial function, improves circulation through nitric oxide release, and activates systemic signaling pathways. The broad spectrum of natural sunlight may even provide benefits beyond what artificial devices can achieve, given

that our bodies evolved to respond to sunlight's full-spectrum stimulation. Of course, efforts should be taken to minimize the risk of burning, and while sunblock may reduce some red/NIR penetration, it's still preferable to sunburn for maintaining regular outdoor exposure.

For these individuals getting regular and ample sun exposure on their full body, they may not need to do whole-body PBM devices for *systemic* benefits (though this is my own speculation, since it has not been tested scientifically). But targeted applications for specific concerns (e.g., joint issues or skin health), and use of targeted devices to enhance stem cell release, will still likely be beneficial. It's also worth noting that red/NIR light are anti-aging at the level of the skin, while the sun is linked with pro-aging effects (largely due to UV light), so those getting more sun exposure may also benefit from more red/NIR light on the skin.

THE MODERN INDOOR DWELLER: In contrast, most modern individuals spend more than 90 percent of their time indoors under artificial lighting, often with minimal skin exposure due to clothing, climate, or cultural norms. This lifestyle creates a "light deficiency" that results in a number of problematic systemic effects.[2] For these individuals, artificial PBM therapy can fill this biological gap, potentially improving energy, recovery, inflammation management, and overall health. Regular use of red and NIR light therapy devices could provide the systemic benefits their sunlight-deprived biology needs.

SEASONAL CONSIDERATIONS: A practical approach might involve adjusting PBM use seasonally. During summer, when natural sunlight exposure is feasible, PBM use could be reduced or focused on specific targeted treatments. Conversely, in winter or during extended periods of bad weather, PBM devices can help maintain the systemic benefits typically derived from sunlight exposure.

To determine your personal need for systemic PBM therapy, consider these factors:

- **DAILY SUN EXPOSURE:** Track how much time you spend in direct sunlight with a large portion of your skin exposed (e.g., in a swimsuit or shirtless). If it's less than 30 minutes daily, systemic PBM therapy is likely to be very beneficial.
- **SEASONAL PATTERNS:** Consider how your sun exposure varies throughout the year. Many people might need minimal PBM in summer but significant PBM in winter.
- **GEOGRAPHIC LOCATION:** Those living in higher latitudes or consistently cloudy climates might benefit more from PBM therapy, even if they spend time outdoors.
- **LIFESTYLE CONSTRAINTS:** If your work or lifestyle makes regular sun exposure impractical, PBM devices should help bridge this biological gap.

While all of this is speculative in the sense that it hasn't been formally tested by scientific research, it makes logical sense that our bodies evolved to receive PBM naturally through sunlight on a regular (daily or near-daily) basis, and it's best to see red and NIR PBM in this context. So if you're already getting ample sun exposure on a daily or near-daily basis, it's probably the case (though again, I must emphasize that this is my own speculation) that you're already getting a large portion of the systemic benefits of red and NIR PBM. You may still want to do some extra PBM with devices at targeted times of day (perhaps in the morning) or in a targeted way on bone marrow sites (to facilitate stem cell release) for example, but as far as systemic benefits go, it's likely that the sun is already giving you a good portion of those benefits. Based on this line of logic, your goal with PBM devices should be more about targeted use for specific purposes—for example, facial skin anti-aging, wound healing, muscle recovery, exercise performance, brain treatment, and treatment of deep tissues in a targeted way.

On the other hand, if your sun exposure is, like most modern humans, fairly low, you would likely benefit tremendously from regular use of PBM devices for the systemic/general wellness benefits—essentially to help replace some of what you're missing because of lack of sun exposure.

Ultimately, the goal is to optimize light exposure using available resources, whether through natural sunlight, PBM devices, or a combination of both.

Whereas I think it's likely that adequate sun exposure will have similar or equivalent systemic benefits to red and NIR PBM applied via something like a panel, I think it's also likely that we can amplify at least some of these systemic benefits through more targeted ways of using PBM devices (e.g., on bones, organs, or the thymus gland) to maximize systemic benefits, and perhaps most notably, the activation of stem cells by applying targeted devices on stem cell-rich sites in the body.

Now that we've covered using PBM devices for systemic benefits (and tailoring this use according to your sun exposure), let's cover more targeted uses of PBM devices.

TARGETED DEVICES FOR SPECIFIC BENEFITS ON SPECIFIC BODY AREAS

Let's dive into specific goals you might have and the types of devices I recommend for each. First, please keep in mind that many devices have yet to be formally tested for specific goals, and we lack head-to-head comparisons between different devices. Furthermore, the current range of devices on the market is limited, but PBM science and device development are rapidly evolving, so I anticipate significant advances in the coming years to better address specific goals.

Given these factors, what follows is largely based on logical speculation about which devices are likely to be most effective for specific purposes. We've covered the rationale and framework for dosing and choosing devices for specific goals in the dosing section, but here's a brief overview of how this applies to selecting specific devices for specific goals.

(As a reminder, the following devices are examples, not explicit recommendations. The market is constantly evolving, and these examples may already be out-dated by the time you're reading this. For my up-to-date recommendations on the top devices in each category, visit www.redlightdeviceguide.com.)

When targeting local effects on specific tissues or areas of the body, factors like wavelength, power density (irradiance), device design, and treatment parameters become crucial. Tailoring protocols to match tissue depth and sensitivity ensures both safe and effective results. These considerations will help guide your decision-making process when selecting devices to meet your specific goals.

FOR SUPERFICIAL TISSUES (0 TO 1 CM DEPTH), the focus should primarily be on red wavelengths (630 to 670 nm), which work effectively for surface-level therapeutic effects. NIR wavelengths can also be included. The ideal devices are those that conform to the body's natural contours, allowing for consistent light delivery across curved surfaces like the face, legs, arms, and joints. These anatomically designed devices should deliver lower irradiances, typically in the range of 10 to 50 mW/cm². This gentler approach is particularly effective for skin rejuvenation, surface wound healing, and addressing superficial vascular conditions.

- **BEST WAVELENGTHS:** Red light (630 to 670 nm); NIR (800 to 850 nm) may also help and be synergistic with red light.

- **IDEAL DEVICES:** Anatomically contoured designs that conform to body curvatures for consistent light delivery across curved surfaces like the face, joints, legs, and arms
- **IRRADIANCE:** 10–50 mW/cm²
- **APPLICATIONS:** Skin rejuvenation, surface wound healing, and superficial vascular issues
- **TREATMENT TIME:** 2 to 20 minutes to allow sufficient light absorption without overexposure

FOR DEEP TISSUES (1 TO 5 CM DEPTH), the emphasis shifts to NIR wavelengths (800 to 850 nm, 1,064 nm), as these penetrate more effectively through deeper layers. Devices for this purpose should be specifically engineered for deep penetration using higher irradiances (50 to 150 mW/cm²), skin contact, or high degrees of light convergence. Skin-contact devices may use compression to temporarily reduce tissue thickness, enhancing light penetration. Alternatively, devices designed for use just above the skin may employ high degrees of light convergence to achieve similar results. Lasers can also be useful for this purpose, as their collimated light enhances penetration, and very high irradiances can be used with pulsing to mitigate heat.

- **BEST WAVELENGTHS:** NIR (800 to 850 nm, 1,064 nm)
- **IDEAL DEVICES:** Engineered for deep penetration with higher irradiance

(50 to 150 mW/cm²) and LED light convergence or focused beams (lasers). Devices may apply gentle pressure with skin contact for better tissue penetration. For ultra-deep tissues (greater than 5 cm), it's possible that only high-powered lasers will deliver significant quantities of light.

- **APPLICATIONS:** Muscle, tendon, joint, or deep organ or other deep tissues
- **TREATMENT TIME:** 5 to 20 minutes for adequate energy delivery to deeper layers

FOR PHOTOSENSITIVE TISSUES, which include areas not naturally designed for significant light exposure—such as internal organs, endocrine glands, genitalia, mucous membranes, and possibly even the eyes—a more cautious approach is required. Even facial skin could be considered a sensitive tissue that is prone to being harmed by excessive irradiances and dosages (which may be a concern with high-powered panels that also subject the facial skin to high irradiances). These tissues are also more prone to biphasic dose responses, requiring moderate irradiances and precise control over treatment parameters, particularly irradiance, exposure duration, and total energy delivery. The focus should be on gentle, controlled application for longer periods of time with low-irradiance devices specifically designed for these sensitive areas.

FOR UNIQUE BODY AREAS, specialized devices are often necessary to ensure effective light delivery tailored to the anatomy and therapeutic needs of each region, such as the brain, facial skin, oral cavity, nasal passage, genitalia (e.g., intravaginal devices), scalp, and joints.

Let's now examine the most common goals of PBM and the best types of devices for each goal.

For Facial Skin Anti-Aging

PBM offers a powerful way to support facial skin health and rejuvenation. For effective results, devices should conform to facial contours, deliver moderate light intensity (10 to 50 mW/cm²), and avoid excessive heating. Treatments usually target the entire face, with extra focus on areas prone to aging, like around the eyes and mouth. While red wavelengths should likely be prioritized, research has also shown benefits from NIR, and given their differing penetration depths, it's likely that they are synergistic.

When choosing a device, consider face masks or hood-style devices that provide even light coverage and are designed to be used a few inches from the skin. Masks on the market vary widely in quality, with issues like uneven light distribution or light intensity that's either too low or too high. The best options prioritize uniform LED placement to avoid "hot spots" and "cold spots" and use primarily red wavelengths (630 nm and 660 nm), with some NIR for added benefits. Whenever possible, opt for devices that have been tested in scientific studies and shown to deliver real results. This ensures you're using a product that's both effective and safe.

Some of the devices I recommend in this category currently are:

- The Dior face mask (though it's very pricey compared to competitors), but it has been tested in peer-reviewed research and shown to have benefits
- JOVS 4-D (uses lasers and multiple wavelengths)
- Lumara (high LED density, ideal irradiance, and uniform coverage)
- Celluma
- Dermalux

Using light panels for anti-aging skin effects is feasible but requires thoughtful adjustments, since most panels have irradiances higher than ideal for facial skin. To use panels effectively:

- **POSITIONING AND DURATION:** Place two panels at 45-degree angles to the face or use a single panel for 5 to 10 minutes per side. Adjust the power level to 20 to 30 percent of the panel's full intensity or position it 18 to 36 inches away to achieve a suitable irradiance. For panels with narrow beam angles and unpredictable irradiance drop-off, a closer distance of 5 to 10 inches may work better, provided intensity is adjusted down to 10 to 20 percent.

- **STARTING SAFELY:** Many manufacturers misrepresent irradiance figures, making it challenging to determine actual intensity without an accurate spectrometer or third-party lab data. I recommend only buying panels from manufacturers that share third-party lab data. If you already have a panel and you don't have access to that data, to stay safe, begin with lower intensity— around 20 to 40 percent of maximum power, typically equating to 10 to 35 mW/cm² for most panels. If your panel lacks intensity adjustment, position it 18 to 36 inches away for an estimated suitable range for facial anti-aging effects.

- **CHALLENGES AND LIMITATIONS:** Panels lack the peer-reviewed evidence that supports specialized facial masks for anti-aging, and factors like light angles and distance can affect penetration and efficacy. This may lead to less predictable results compared to face-specific devices.

CAUTION: *Avoid* using high-irradiance panels close to your face at full intensity, especially within 12 inches. Doing so risks doing more harm than good in terms of facial skin health. Always prioritize moderate, safe doses over high-intensity exposure for facial skin (i.e., follow the irradiance guidelines in the dosing guide).

Given these considerations, face-specific

devices are strongly recommended for facial anti-aging unless you have verified the exact irradiance of your panel at a given distance. Without reliable irradiance data, relying on a panel introduces unnecessary guesswork and potential risks.

Another device people often use on the face is a PBM wand. Perhaps I'm missing something, but in general, I don't find these devices compelling, as they come with several significant drawbacks. The most obvious downside is their extremely small coverage area. Using a wand requires holding it in place for several minutes on a specific spot, which makes consistent use unlikely for most people. To treat even a small area of the face, such as around the eyes, you'd need to hold the device on one to five spots per side, spending several minutes on each. This tedious process diminishes practicality and ultimately means that you're less likely to use it regularly (which is, of course, key to getting results). Unless someone has a very specific concern with a small area of their face *and* explicitly wants to *avoid* broader treatment with something like a face mask or the curved facial panels mentioned previously—which is a rare scenario— a wand doesn't seem like the best option. That said, if there's a targeted issue, such as fine lines or wrinkles near the eyes, a wand might serve as a supplementary device to facial masks. Being charitable, I'd say the one advantage a wand may offer is that you can get good skin contact and press it into the skin in a particular area,

which may allow for better light delivery to deeper layers of skin. Beyond that, it's hard for me to think of why someone would opt for a wand over a facial mask or a dome-style device that treats the whole face at once.

For Superficial Wound Healing

Surface wounds benefit from red wavelengths to stimulate cellular repair and regeneration processes. Deeper wounds benefit from NIR wavelengths to enhance tissue repair at multiple levels.

For wound healing, devices in the range of 10 to 50 mW/cm² applied directly over or in contact with the wound site, and emphasizing red wavelengths, are likely ideal. Given that the skin barrier is not present (or is compromised) and thus would not reflect and absorb light as it would in the absence of a wound, it stands to reason that lower irradiances may be optimal and higher irradiances (50 to 150 mW/cm²) may be more likely to induce a biphasic dose response (as the wounded tissues lacking skin covering may be sensitive to higher irradiances).

For this purpose, I'd favor flexible pad-style devices, ideally with high LED density. One of my current favorites is the Quad belt from Mito Red.

Other devices could certainly still work here, including panels used at a distance or with the intensity adjusted down so the irradiance is more in the range of 20 to 50 mW/cm², or some of the devices for targeted use like the Kineon Move Plus, the LumaFlex, or the FlexBeam. But again, especially with open wounds where the skin is damaged, I would generally favor a more cautious and lower-irradiance approach.

For treatment of diabetic ulcers, there are a number of flexible pad-style devices on the market that conform to specific body areas like the foot and lower leg, and while most of them suffer from low LED density and low irradiance, many users still report tremendous benefits.

(Also note that systemic effects also likely play a key role in wound healing of any tissue in the body, so you should pair any targeted PBM on a particular wound/injury with the previously covered ways to maximize the systemic benefits of PBM.)

For Brain Health, Cognitive Performance, Traumatic Brain Injury Recovery, and Mood Support

PBM has demonstrated significant potential for brain health and neurological function. When applied transcranially, NIR light can penetrate the skull and reach brain tissue, where it enhances mitochondrial function, reduces inflammation, increases blood flow, protects against neuronal death, and promotes neuroplasticity.

This application requires specialized (and generally higher-irradiance) devices capable of delivering NIR light (primarily 810 to 940 nm and/or 1,060 to 1,070 nm) through the skull. The most effective approaches often use arrays of emitters positioned to target specific brain regions in

direct contact with, or positioned very close to the skin of the head (commonly the forehead due to the lack of hair, but they may also be positioned between the hair shafts and pressed against the scalp).

For brain health, there are currently several device options, but I'm also aware of several more currently under development that may be available by the time you read this, including one from Thor Photomedicine. Below are some brief thoughts on some of the existing devices. Again, my constantly updated top recommended devices will be at www.redlight deviceguide.com.

My top choice for a light for brain health is currently the VieLight, because it has by far the most robust scientific literature clearly showing it supplies benefits for a number of brain-related conditions.

But there are several other devices on the market that may also turn out to be excellent devices. SunPower LED makes a large and powerful device for targeting the brain, and another company called Neuronic (the product is called Neuradiant) makes a helmet using 1,070 nm—both companies are currently involved in conducting clinical trials on their devices.

For Joint Health and Bone Healing/ Density, Targeted Deep Tissue Injury Healing, Post-Surgery Recovery, and Other Deep-Tissue Goals

For deep tissues like muscles, tendons, ligaments, joints, and bones; for deep internal bruising from injuries; and for after surgeries, it's likely best to use higher-irradiance devices that have ample power in the NIR wavelengths, ideally with skin contact or close to the body to help maximize light penetration to the deep tissues. PBM offers significant benefits for musculoskeletal conditions. In joint health and arthritis treatment, it reduces inflammation, increases synovial fluid production, and promotes cartilage repair, leading to better mobility and less pain. For bone healing, studies show that PBM speeds up fracture recovery by enhancing osteoblast activity and bone density, making it valuable for delayed unions, osteoporosis, and post-surgical recovery.

The therapy also boosts tissue regeneration through increased collagen synthesis and blood flow, helping heal tendons and ligaments while reducing scarring. For pain management, it provides both immediate and sustained relief by reducing inflammation and modulating pain pathways.

Treatment approach varies with joint depth and tissue thickness. Surface joints like fingers and wrists may benefit from red and/or NIR light, or combinations, while deeper joints like knees and hips likely need more power in the NIR wavelengths. Devices should ideally conform to the body surfaces being treated and either allow skin contact/compression or optimize for beam convergence to enhance light penetration. Treatment works best when targeting the area from multiple an-

gles, with some flexible devices able to do this simultaneously.

Here are some devices currently available that work for this purpose:

- SunPower LED's "Palm" devices offer excellent irradiance (110 to 187 mW/cm^2) for deep tissues, and uniform coverage, though they must be held in the hand and used manually (or used with some kind of makeshift strap to keep it on an area). It's not flexible, but you can do two to three positions (e.g., to cover a knee joint from multiple angles), with a few minutes in each position.
- FlexBeam offers a solid maximal irradiance (110 mW/cm^2) for deep-tissue treatments right over the LEDs, and conforms to some extent to body surfaces, but lacks somewhat in terms of light coverage with that irradiance.
- Ironforge—an extremely high irradiance device of more than 400 mW/cm^2. Some people report excellent results with this device, but I have some concern with how powerful it is. (They rightly advise moving the device around to avoid overheating the tissue, but I wonder if this may lead to treatment duration not being optimal.) This may be worth experimenting with for very deep tissues, but I advise caution due to the extremely high irradiance, and the potential to overheat tissues.

- The Kineon Move Plus—
  a sophisticated device designed
  for joints that also includes lasers,
  though its overall irradiance and
  coverage are on the lower side. But I
  think it's likely a good device for
  targeted issues in small areas and on
  joints.
- Lasers also make excellent devices
  for targeted treatment of deep
  tissues, but they tend to be vastly
  more expensive than LED products
  and require training to use safely
  (i.e., it's best to see a practitioner
  trained in the use of lasers if you
  wish to go that route), and one
  should also keep in mind that lasers
  are often narrow beams, so there is
  an enormous difference in coverage
  area that may or may not matter
  depending on the size of the area
  you're trying to treat. For extremely
  deep tissues, it may be the case that
  only high-powered lasers can
  effectively do PBM.

In the case of very targeted areas where
you might want to get skin contact on a
very specific small area of the body, torch-
style devices and lasers may be ideal. The
downside of these approaches is that it can
be very time-consuming and inconvenient
to treat larger body surfaces, because it
may require five to twenty applications
(each of several minutes) to cover, for example, the quadriceps or calf, and the device has to be physically held in place for
the entire period each time. It's enough of
an inconvenience for most people that they
just won't do this kind of thing regularly.

Lasers are likely the best option in cases
where one is trying to treat very small
areas of very deep tissue, but they're expensive and require professional training
to use safely (i.e., I don't recommend you
get one of these devices unless you are a
trained professional). It's currently still
unclear if, given equal treatment parameters, lasers are more effective than LED
devices, but there is certainly ample research supporting the benefits of lasers.

Again, note that systemic effects also
likely play a key role in the healing of any
tissue in the body, so you should pair any
targeted PBM on a particular area, such as
the injured or arthritic joints or other
physical injuries/damaged tissues, with the
previously covered ways to maximize the
systemic benefits of PBM.

For Exercise Performance and Recovery (Muscle Treatment)

Both pre-exercise preparation and post-
exercise recovery are wonderful times to
use PBM and some of my personal favor-
ite times to use it.

Pre-exercise PBM enhances workout
performance through multiple mechanisms. Red and NIR light primes muscles
by boosting mitochondrial function and
blood flow, leading to improved strength,
power output, and endurance during
training. Treatment typically targets large
muscle groups with NIR wavelengths to

maximize these effects and reduce injury risk through increased tissue flexibility.

After workouts, PBM accelerates recovery and amplifies training adaptations. It reduces inflammation and muscle damage while enhancing repair processes through increased growth-factor activity and stem cell responses. This leads to better gains in strength, endurance, and muscle growth. The therapy also supports connective tissue health by boosting collagen production, helping prevent overuse injuries like tendonitis.

Treatment involves 5- to 20-minute sessions targeting major muscle groups and joints. Timing is crucial: Pre-exercise treatment should occur within a small window before activity, while post-exercise applications are most effective within a few hours. Devices should provide adequate coverage and have high enough penetration to reach deeper tissues. Many athletes use both pre- and post-workout treatments for optimal results, though the focus shifts from performance enhancement to recovery and adaptation.

For smaller areas of muscle (e.g., biceps, triceps, shoulders), devices like the FlexBeam, the SunPower Palm, and the Kineon Move Plus could all still potentially be options here, but I would favor products with larger areas of coverage to be able to efficiently target large muscle groups, because otherwise it can be very time-consuming to treat them.

For larger areas of muscle (e.g., back muscles, chest, leg muscles), you could use panels (from close distance or potentially with skin contact), or targeted devices for multiple treatments (those listed above) in different spots, or a large flexible body-wrap style of device. I'd favor one with high LED density, adequate irradiance, multiple wavelengths per LED chip (rather than separate wavelengths in each chip), and adequate power in the NIR range. The main wrap I'm currently aware of that meets these criteria is the Mito Red Quad Belt (but this may change by the time you're reading this). This kind of device has considerably lower irradiance than the targeted devices above, but it has a much larger area of coverage with a high enough LED density and NIR wavelengths that it will still likely offer significant penetration.

The LumaFlex is another device with a moderate irradiance that offers some ability to conform to body surfaces and to get some skin contact, and it offers a larger surface area than many other devices, though with a lower LED density, so some degree of "hot spots" and "cold spots" will likely be present. It has 45 LED chips, but with roughly 1 inch of spacing between them. That's a lot of spacing for a device designed for skin contact.

Targeted devices like the FlexBeam or Sunpower's Palm are likely also good options here, though it would be time-consuming to treat large muscle groups with them because you'd likely have to do five to ten treatments in different spots to cover the back or the legs, for example. A large wrap like the one mentioned previously can treat much larger areas at any given time, albeit with a significantly lower irradiance. (Again, we don't have a perfect device that conforms to areas like the arms or legs and can treat large muscle areas with higher irradiances and skin contact all at once, so we have to deal with some trade-offs.)

Panels can also be great options for treating large muscle areas like the back or legs. You could potentially press yourself right up against the LED panel (if you're not concerned about EMFs and the device isn't heating up so much that it makes your tissues too warm), or you could use smaller or more moderate-sized panels from close distance or with skin contact on areas like the legs. Again, I'd favor panels with multiple wavelengths per LED chip rather than single wavelengths, and adequate power in the NIR range. If you have a higher-irradiance panel (e.g., 80 to 100 mW/cm²), you could experiment with using it with skin contact

and lowering the irradiance by simply turning down the intensity of the light if the device is warming your tissues excessively. This may actually be one of the best available options for efficiently treating large muscle areas, though the size and rigidity of panels can be cumbersome and difficult to use for some areas.

Eye Health

Recent research highlights the remarkable potential of PBM in supporting eye health and treating retinal conditions. The therapy works by enhancing mitochondrial function in retinal photoreceptors, which naturally decline in function with age. Notably, red light therapy has shown promise for challenging conditions like dry age–related macular degeneration (AMD), with studies indicating it can protect retinal health by reducing light-induced stress, improving contrast sensitivity, decreasing cell death, lowering inflammation, and enhancing visual acuity.

PBM has also shown promise for other

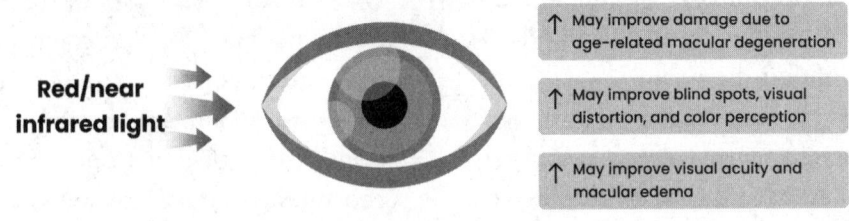

Improve Eye Health

Red/near infrared light

↑ May improve damage due to age–related macular degeneration

↑ May improve blind spots, visual distortion, and color perception

↑ May improve visual acuity and macular edema

*WARNING: Your eyes are a sensitive area. Use shorter sessions, increase distance from the light, and opt for lower irradiances.

conditions, including diabetic retinopathy. Devices like the Valeda Light Delivery System, available only in professional settings like eye clinics, have undergone successful clinical trials for dry age-related macular degeneration and have received regulatory approval.

For general eye health, low-irradiance red light from devices like flexible pads, face masks, and book-reading lights may be safe and potentially beneficial, though evidence is still emerging. At least one study has used "torch" style PBM devices on the eyes, with benefits. However, caution is advised when using moderate or high-irradiance devices near the eyes, as this tissue is potentially photosensitive. Treatments for specific eye conditions should ideally be performed by trained specialists using devices specifically designed for ocular health. I would strongly suggest caution using direct exposure of high irradiance panels or any other high irradiance PBM device—the full irradiance of many panels is likely higher than ideal both for eye health and facial skin health. (Note: Powerful lasers can permanently damage the eyes, so never experiment with lasers in your eyes.)

It's possible that some benefits to eye health may occur indirectly when using face masks designed for skin rejuvenation, as low-level red-light exposure to the eyes could provide some therapeutic effects. While this remains speculative and less targeted, it suggests a safe, low-risk option for supporting overall eye health. Other than that, if one does wish to experiment with PBM on eyes, I strongly advise sticking only to very low irradiances in the range of 10 to 25 mW/cm^2 unless otherwise guided by an eye health professional. It should be noted that red light at these irradiances is very intense for the eyes (although not harmful), while NIR light (800 to 940 nm) does not have this drawback.

For Oral Health

I'm a big fan of using the mouthpiece-style devices with red light for general oral health. They can improve gum health and tissue healing in the mouth, and perhaps also activate local stem cells to support cellular regeneration. Having said that, I've purchased many different oral devices, and there are enormous differences in the LED density and irradiance among them. One that is actually more affordable than many high-priced products and has vastly superior irradiance and LED density to many other devices I've bought over the years is the Starlite Smile oral device (which can be found on Amazon). I use it personally, after having tried several more expensive options that I found to be of lower quality. (Note: There are also devices with blue light, which has been used for tooth-whitening and antibacterial effects.) Again, I may have found better devices and have altered my recommendations by the time you read this, so check my website for the latest information.

For Genitalia/Fertility

Research indicates that PBM may support reproductive health in both men and women through improved cellular function and blood flow, though more clinical studies are needed. For women, PBM shows potential for promoting healthy vaginal tissue, reducing inflammation, and supporting hormonal balance. As discussed in chapter 3, clinical research demonstrates effectiveness in treating genitourinary syndrome of menopause and stress urinary incontinence. For men, studies suggest that PBM can enhance testicular function and testosterone production through improved Leydig cell activity and reduced oxidative stress. The therapy may also support penile health by promoting vasodilation and tissue regeneration. It's likely that these tissues are photosensitive, so lower-irradiance devices and lower dosing is likely the best approach.

Joylux makes a device for transvaginal PBM called vFit, which has received very positive feedback. To my knowledge, this is the only device on the market in this category that is supported by peer-reviewed research. The study (discussed in chapter 3) found clinically meaningful improvements in bladder symptoms, pelvic floor muscle strength, and quality of life in women with stress urinary incontinence.

There are also devices on the market designed for the penis and testicles, and even devices for women to use on the perineal area after childbirth (one from Mommy Matters called Neo Heat). I'm not aware of any research on any device intended for male genitalia, but if you have issues in that region, it's certainly worth experimenting with one of devices designed for that purpose.

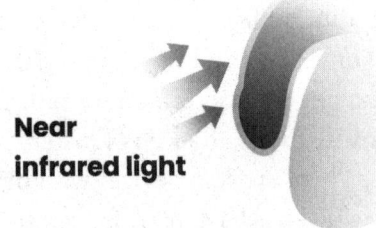

Near infrared light

850nm near-infrared light is applied to the perineal area (Nitric Oxide)

Nitric Oxide helps improve blood flow and erectile function.

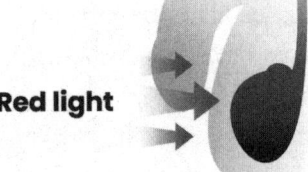

Red light

630nm red light is applied to the testicles (Leydig Cells)

Red light promotes the health of Leydig cells in the testicles, which are involved in male hormone production.

Hair Growth and Scalp Health

One of the other major categories of targeted PBM devices is to help combat hair loss. PBM can stimulate dormant hair follicles and enhance the growth phase of existing follicles. This application typically uses a combination of red wavelengths (630 to 670 nm) to energize the surface follicle cells, and less commonly, also NIR (800 to 850 nm) to penetrate deeper into the dermis and enhance blood flow to the follicles.

The scalp's curved surface requires specialized devices that can maintain good contact while delivering consistent energy across the treatment area. There is substantial evidence of efficacy of PBM for this purpose, and numerous quality products on the market (which give the proper dosing parameters aligned with the research). While it has not been well-researched, Dr. Hamblin believes it is possible that laser diode caps could be more effective than LEDs for this specific goal, and there are several laser caps on the market from reputable companies like Capillus, Kiierr, as well as other companies.

Intranasal Devices: Sinuses and Immunity

Intranasal PBM is an emerging approach that targets the nasal cavity, offering benefits for sinus health, for immune function, and potentially for brain health. The nasal cavity serves as both a gateway to the respiratory system and, theoretically, a path for light to reach the brain.

For sinus and respiratory health, intranasal PBM works by improving blood flow and reducing inflammation in the nasal tissues. The light penetrates the thin mucosal lining, enhancing cellular energy production and promoting better mucus drainage. This can help with conditions like sinusitis and allergic rhinitis, potentially reducing congestion and supporting respiratory health.

Some researchers suggest that intranasal PBM might benefit brain function through the thin bone separating the nasal cavity from the brain. For example, VieLight makes an intranasal device designed to stimulate the brain. NIR light, in particular, could potentially stimulate brain regions like the prefrontal cortex, enhance cerebral blood flow, support mitochondrial function in neurons, and reduce neuroinflammation. However, this remains debatable and controversial: Most current intranasal devices have insufficient irradiance to deliver meaningful light doses to brain tissue. Some argue that the brain benefits seen from intranasal devices are likely due to systemic effects rather than light directly reaching the brain.

Intranasal PBM may also support immune function, since the nasal cavity is a crucial first line of defense against pathogens. PBM can stimulate local immune cells and modulate cytokine production while improving lymphatic drainage, potentially helping protect against respiratory infections.

Several brands offer low-power devices for nasal health, but as of this writing, I'm not aware of any evidence that would cause me to favor any particular product.

Blood-Vessel, Circulatory, Lymphatic, and Nerve Health (Circulation Issues, Peripheral Neuropathy, Nerve Regeneration, and More)

PBM can be used to help other types of tissues and organ systems beneath the skin, like blood vessels, lymphatic vessels, and nerves.

For lymphatic health, it can enhance fluid movement and reduce swelling, making it helpful for conditions like post-surgical swelling and lymphedema. PBM can stimulate the formation of new lymphatic vessels (lymphangiogenesis) and enhance the contractility of existing ones. This boost in lymphatic flow helps clear excess fluid, waste products, and inflammatory mediators from tissues. Clinical studies have shown that PBM, when combined with standard lymphatic drainage techniques, effectively reduces lymphedema, making it particularly beneficial for post-surgical swelling, breast cancer–related lymphedema, and chronic inflammatory conditions. Treatment typically targets major lymph nodes and drainage pathways, with sessions lasting 10 to 25 minutes per area.

For nerve-related issues like peripheral neuropathy, PBM may help reduce pain and support nerve function. Treatment approaches vary depending on the condition—from targeting specific nerve paths in diabetic foot neuropathy to treating larger areas for chemotherapy-related symptoms. Circulatory support is another potential benefit, particularly for people with compromised blood flow in their extremities.

When treating peripheral neuropathy or supporting nerve regeneration, PBM can help restore nerve function and reduce pain. The treatment might focus on specific nerve paths, like in diabetic neuropathy of the feet, or target larger areas in conditions like chemotherapy-induced peripheral neuropathy. Beyond neuropathy, PBM can support general circulatory health in diabetic patients, particularly in the extremities, where circulation is often compromised.

For this purpose, I favor flexible pad-style devices with lower or more moderate irradiances used for 20 to 40 minutes and applied directly on the skin in the affected area. However, studies have been done on diabetic peripheral neuropathy using targeted laser devices as well, with beneficial results,[10] so it's likely that other types of LED devices (perhaps those mentioned in the deep-tissue sections above) are effective, and mini-panels applied directly to the affected area may also be effective.

Fat Loss and Body Contouring

Research has shown that PBM can help increase fat loss when combined with exercise and proper nutrition. The best use in this context is likely to support the loss of "stubborn fat" while you're already in a calorie deficit. In other words, please be aware that red and NIR light can't magically cause fat loss unless you are in a calorie deficit. Think of this in the same way as with muscle building, strength, and athletic recovery: In the presence of a solid workout routine and good nutrition, PBM on the muscles can speed up recovery from workouts as well as amplify growth and adaptations to exercise. In other words, it synergizes with exercise to amplify the effect. But if you were to just apply red and NIR light to your muscles without doing any workouts, there wouldn't be any notable gains in strength or muscle mass. With fat loss, it's the same idea: PBM shouldn't be thought of as a way to lose fat when applied by itself, but rather as a supplementary strategy that synergizes and amplifies the effects of diet and exercise on losing fat.

Many of the devices on the market for this purpose are clinical laser devices, which are both expensive and intended to be used by trained clinicians. While none of the LED devices on the market, to my knowledge, have been tested in formal scientific research for their effectiveness in fat loss applications, I recommend the use of a portable device with a fairly large area of coverage, moderate irradiance, and some use of NIR light that can be used during workouts. My current go-to choice is the Quad belt by Mito Red, and I would be inclined to wear it *during* exercise sessions (right over the target area) in a period of time which you are in a calorie deficit to facilitate fat loss.

I would also consider some of the other devices used for deep penetration with adequate coverage and portability, like the LumaFlex and the FlexBeam. (Again, by the time you read this, the products on the market may have evolved and I may have different recommendations, so make sure to check www.red lightdeviceguide.com for my updated recommendations.)

MORE THOUGHTS ON PBM DEVICE CATEGORIES

Heat Lamps

Heat lamps pose several significant challenges for effective PBM therapy when compared to targeted LED and laser devices. The main issues with attempting to use incandescent heat lamps for PBM are low irradiance in the PBM wavelengths, uneven light coverage, and tissue heating.

As discussed in chapter 5, research by Dr. Arany has demonstrated that tissue heating above 42°C begins inactivating re-active oxygen species (ROS) scavengers, and heating above 45°C can cause overt cellular damage.[3]

While there is certainly a place for hyperthermia (tissue heating) as a modality to get certain benefits, PBM's cellular benefits occur through mechanisms that can be disrupted when excessive heating occurs. If our goal is to stimulate tissue regeneration, we want to avoid excessive tissue heating, which can cause damage to the cells.

Heat lamps, which emit broad-spectrum radiation with significant infrared-B and infrared-C components, inevitably cause a great deal of tissue heating when used at intensities that would deliver therapeutic levels of red and NIR light.

It should be noted that the application of far-infrared (FIR) wavelengths (>3,000 nm) delivered by infrared saunas or infrared heat lamps can have many physiological benefits that may, in some cases, bear some similarities to those produced by NIR PBM. Moreover, the wearing of garments or fabrics containing FIR-emitting minerals (such as alumina, titania, or jade) can have beneficial effects on pain, inflammation, and muscle performance, despite there being no external power source capable of producing any heat. In this case, the explanation is that these FIR-emitting materials, worn next to the skin, can convert normal body heat into FIR radiation, which penetrates deeply into the body. It

is hypothesized that the FIR radiation can excite nanostructured water clusters and thus open heat-activated ion channels to produce cellular changes analogous to those produced by stimulating cytochrome c oxidase in mitochondria. Simple heating of tissues and the improved blood circulation that results from tissue heating can also speed up healing of damaged tissues and provide symptomatic relief.

The research supporting PBM's efficacy has predominantly used controlled applications of LED and laser light (rather than heat lamps), which generally does not cause excessive tissue heating. Heat lamps' broad-spectrum output and significant thermal components make it extremely difficult to do precise dosing while accounting for the PBM wavelengths (630 to 680 nm red, 810 to 850 nm NIR), or to control irradiance within therapeutic windows, or to avoid triggering counterproductive heat stress responses, or to maintain consistent treatment parameters across body areas. While not necessarily dangerous when used cautiously, the thermal effects of heat lamps are fundamentally problematic in the context of PBM because at close distances (where the irradiance for PBM in the 600 to 900 nm wavelengths may be adequate), tissue heating is likely to be excessive, and to avoid overheating the tissues, you are forced to move farther away from the device, which pushes you out of optimal PBM treatment parameters.

This creates a problematic trade-off: You

must either position the lamp close enough to achieve therapeutic power density for PBM effects but risk thermal damage or maintain a safer distance that avoids heating but results in inadequate photonic energy delivery for optimal PBM benefits.

Let's get more specific in discussing the actual distances and irradiances. The LED panel company Joovv paid for third-party lab data to test the irradiance of heat lamps in the 600 to 900 nm range and interviewed Dr. Hamblin on this topic. Here is that exchange:

DR. HAMBLIN: You would need to spend much, much longer in front of a heat lamp to receive a clinically relevant dose of near-infrared light. The difference between an infrared heat lamp and the Joovv [LED panel] is that the heat lamp puts out mid-infrared and far-infrared wavelengths in addition to near-infrared. These IR wavelengths are absorbed by the body and generate heat. As a result, a person cannot get too near a heat lamp or it will feel uncomfortably warm.

Isolines of Irradiance Between 600–900 Nanometers

4 Infrared Heat Lamps at Distance of 18"*

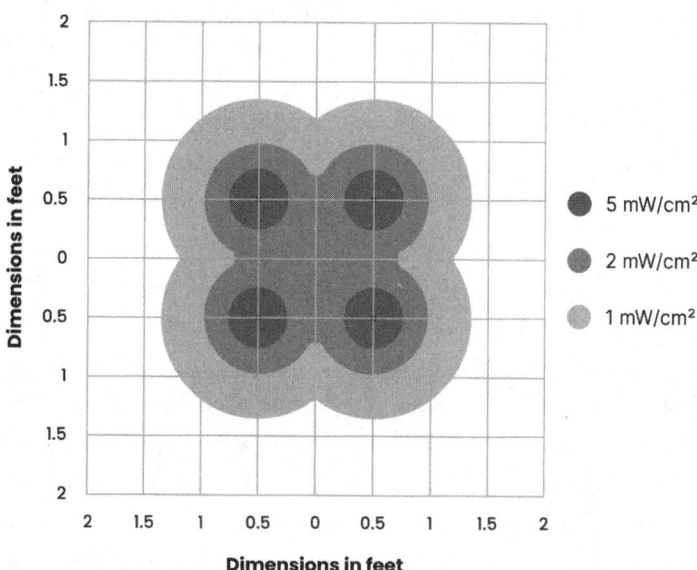

Unbiased 3rd party testing provided by Independent Testing Laboratories (ITL).
*Independent testing based on a distance of 18", per manufacturer's recommendations.

Note that this image has been altered from the original to better illustrate what's happening, but the overall data is very close to accurate. Depending on the position of the heat lamps, there may also be some light convergence that can increase these irradiance figures slightly.

JOOVV: We recently used a third-party diagnostic company, Independent Testing Laboratories, to test a series of 250-watt heat lamps. The total light output measured 27 watts within the 600 to 900 nm range and the average irradiance over the surface of the device was 2 mW/cm² at 18 inches away. By comparison, at 6 inches away from the Joovv Solo, the average irradiance over the surface area of the device was 30.4 mW/cm². Far more than the heat lamp.

DR. HAMBLIN: A distance of 18 inches from heat lamps is recommended, and with the highly divergent nature of the heat-lamp beam, the power density at that distance will be very low, in the region of the 2 mW/cm² that you measured.

Joovv published an image showing the data from the lab, indicating that even with four heat lamps, the maximal irradiance in the 600 to 900 nm range would only be 5 mW/cm², and that was directly across from the heat lamps, whereas the irradiance drops even lower as you go farther outside that zone of coverage.

Another subtle issue may be important. One argument that people make in favor of incandescent bulbs is that they more closely mimic the spectrum from the sun. On paper, the spectrum of incandescent bulbs mimics the spectrum of sunlight to an extent, certainly much more so than isolated wavelengths from lasers or LEDs do. However, with sunlight, the rays must first pass through the earth's atmosphere (which contains significant water in the form of clouds and humidity) before it arrives at our bodies. This is important because that water actually filters out part of the infrared spectrum.

When we use heat lamps on our bodies, that part of the infrared spectrum is not filtered out, which leads to an *unnatural* exposure to part of the infrared spectrum.

So the heat-lamp-style devices actually aren't as "natural" as many people believe, since they include some wavelengths we *don't* get from the sun, and which may actually be harmful to our skin. When your body is exposed to these wavelengths, the light is still absorbed in water—but it's the water in your cells instead of in the earth's atmosphere. (Also, logically, it's possible that the human body isn't well adapted to receiving these wavelengths.) Studies have shown that excessive heating of the skin likely does have aging effects,[1] and I do think it's a bad idea to use heat-lamp-style devices from a distance that causes significant heating of the skin. Of course, this is all still somewhat speculative as we don't have good evidence, and it could turn out that heat lamps used from a distance with low heating may be beneficial for skin health (I have seen some anecdotes of people claiming this).

A company based in Europe called HydroSun figured this out many years ago and created devices using a water filter to remove this part of the infrared spectrum, to allow for PBM benefits from

Energy Spectrum of Sunlight

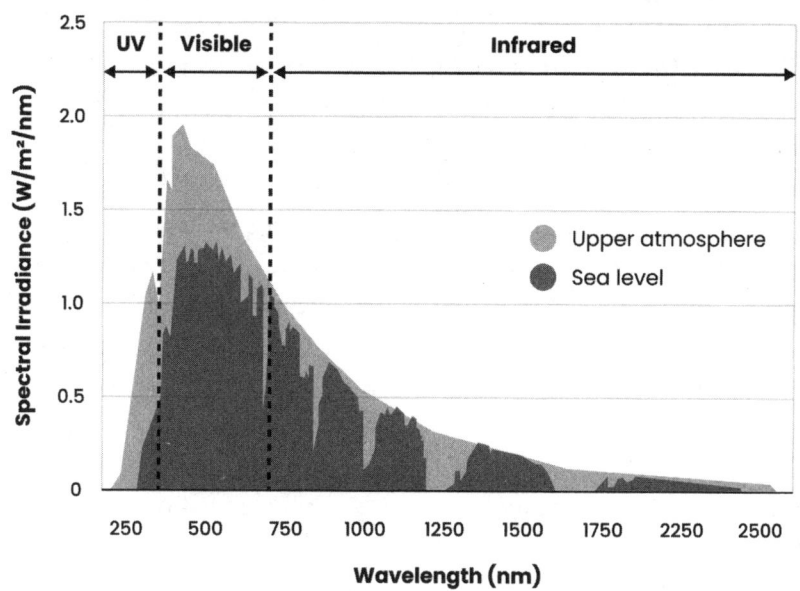

Wavelengths of Infrared Heat Lamps

R125 blown-bulb infrared heat lamps

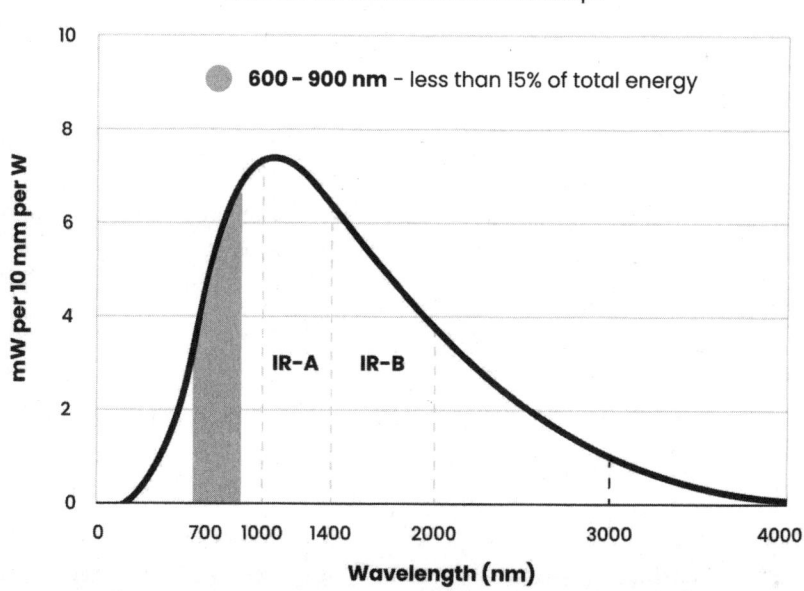

this type of device without nearly as much heating of the tissues.

As you can see in the previous image, the wavelengths around the border of infrared A and B (~1,350 to 1,400 nm) are filtered out by the Earth's atmosphere. But this part of the spectrum is *present* in very significant amounts from heat lamps. For this reason, I believe one should be cautious in using heat lamps on the body with no water filter.

I think it's worth comparing heat lamps to sunlight. With sunlight, we're getting a much higher irradiance of red and NIR light (roughly 20 to 35 mW/cm²), it's over a much broader area of the body, and we don't have the issue of getting unnatural wavelengths of infrared (which may be harmful to the skin).

For all of these reasons, I do not believe that heat lamps are well suited for PBM. Having said that, it is certainly possible that when used at a distance, heat lamps may provide some benefits of PBM without causing tissue overheating. An option that's likely to be both much safer and vastly more effective for PBM would be using these devices from closer distances with a water filter (as with the Hydrosun device). In general, however, I would strongly recommend LED or laser devices over heat lamps for PBM.

PANELS, PADS, AND OTHER DEVICES: PROS AND CONS

Let's discuss in depth some pros and cons of some of the major categories of devices.

Flexible Pads

These devices excel in treating contoured areas and specific body regions where maintaining consistent contact is crucial. Their ability to wrap around limbs and joints makes them ideal for targeted treatments of curved body areas like limbs and joints, but can be used on most areas of the body due to their flexibility.

Whereas they typically offer much lower power output than rigid panels, their direct-contact application can provide more effective treatment in some cases, particularly for superficial issues in curved body surfaces. The main trade-off is that they typically have low irradiance and low LED density, which may make them relatively ineffective for deep-tissue treatments. But their ease of use, portability, and ability to conform to curved body surfaces often make this a worthwhile compromise.

- **CONSTRUCTION:** Flexible pad designs using low- to medium-power LEDs arranged in arrays, typically in neoprene or similar flexible materials
- **POWER CHARACTERISTICS:** Lower irradiance (typically 5 to 30 mW/cm²) but designed for direct skin contact,

greatly reducing power loss from distance

- **APPLICATION METHOD:** Wraps directly around treatment areas, conforming to body contours and maintaining consistent contact
- **COVERAGE:** Targeted coverage of specific body regions like legs, arms, back, and joints. Design focuses on following anatomical contours.
- **SIZE OPTIONS:** Usually available in various sizes optimized for different body parts (e.g., knee pads, back pads, arm wraps, belts, and large whole-body pads and even pods)
- **ATTACHMENT:** Often include Velcro straps or other securing mechanisms for hands-free treatment
- **TREATMENT PROTOCOLS:** Longer treatment times (typically 15 to 45 minutes) due to lower power density, but potentially improved efficacy through direct skin contact

There are some key issues to be aware of when it comes to flexible pad devices. As with panels, there is a rampant issue of companies misrepresenting the irradiance of their devices. I commonly see manufacturers of these pad-style devices claiming that their devices emit 50, 75, or even 100 mW/cm^2. When actually tested by proper equipment, the real numbers are often 5 to 20 mW/cm^2. This creates an enormous problem for accurate dosing. People are wearing a device for 20 minutes thinking they are getting, for example, 10 J/cm^2 on that area, when in reality they may have only gotten 2 J/cm^2. Knowing the true irradiance numbers is key for accurate dosing, and when it comes to pad-style devices, one may need to wear them for two to three times longer than is recommended to actually end up at the dose one is aiming for (particularly if trying to affect deeper tissues). Fortunately, with low-irradiance devices, it's extremely safe to do this, and unlikely to cause harm.

Moreover, it also means that many of these devices—even though they may be ostensibly designed for deep-tissue treatments of a targeted area—are simply not high enough in irradiance to actually effectively treat the deep tissues in reasonable time frames, or at all. Another subtle and hard-to-identify issue is embedded here. That irradiance number (5 to 20 mW/cm^2) may be what is detectable *directly over the LED,* within an inch away from it. The problem is that with most of these devices there are large spaces between the individual LEDs, so the "20 mW/cm^2" irradiance is only directly on the LED chip, but if you move 0.5 inches away from that, it's at 0 mW/cm^2. There are "hot spots" and "cold spots"—that is, uneven coverage. This also means that there is likely going to be little in the way of beam convergence to offer deeper penetration.

Together, what all of these issues—low irradiance and low LED density—mean is that most of these pad-style devices aren't going to do much for deeper tissues like muscles and joints, even though they are often advertised specifically for that purpose. Most of the perceived effects may be derived from treating the more superficial tissues, perhaps bringing circulation to the area, and potentially inducing systemic benefits like modulating inflammation and stem cells. In some cases, the products are so low in irradiance and LED density that any benefits noticed may be placebo effects.

As of this writing, I'm only aware of a few pad-style devices on the market that are not subject to these major flaws—devices that have relatively higher irradiances (closer to 20 mW/ cm^2 rather than to 5 to 10 mW/ cm^2) and have high LED density.

Pad-style whole-body "pods," similar to smaller pad devices, face significant challenges in delivering effective PBM. They share the issues of low irradiance and sparse LED spacing, but with an added drawback: These pods conform to the body's contours far less effectively than wraps or belts do. This creates gaps where the LEDs are positioned perhaps 1 to 4 inches from the skin in certain body areas, causing the already low irradiance (15 to 20 mW/cm^2) to drop to as little as 1 to 5 mW/cm^2. Such a reduction severely limits the potential for deep-tissue benefits, as most light will be absorbed in superficial tissues and may be even too low for benefits to those areas. These limitations mean that while some skin-health benefits—such as improved wound healing, diabetic ulcer

treatment, and addressing circulatory issues—are possible, the primary advantage of these devices is likely their systemic effects, akin to full-body panels. However, due to the lower irradiance and less uniform coverage, the pods may deliver fewer total joules to the body compared to large LED panels, which likely provide greater systemic benefits.

Despite these limitations, many studies have in fact used pad-style devices and shown clear benefits from them. They are likely to be most beneficial for skin health, and also for things like diabetic ulcers, skin wounds, diabetic neuropathy, lymphatic issues, and circulatory issues—anything in more superficial tissues. Again, it's also possible that some of the benefits seen in research are due more to systemic benefits of irradiating the bloodstream rather than to direct local effects.

In summary, I think that most of these pad-style devices don't have a high enough irradiance or LED density to be truly effective for deep-tissue treatments (which many of them purport to do) but they can likely be highly effective for more superficial issues and systemic benefits.

Whole-Body Light Pods

Whole-body pods offer the most efficient full-body coverage in a single session. They're generally ideal for professional settings or serious home users who want regular full-body treatments. Generally speaking, these pods offer lower irradiances (under 50 mW/cm^2)—as you generally don't want high irradiance when treating the entire body at once. Given their full-body coverage with low to moderate irradiances, they are likely more ideal for maximizing systemic benefits of PBM, and likely also for improving the health of skin and other more superficial tissues throughout the body (e.g., blood vessels, lymphatic vessels). Notably, there are several studies using whole-body pods showing profound benefits.

While they require significant investment and dedicated space, they offer the most time-efficient approach to full-body treatment and probably the most powerful systemic benefits of any type of device. The main considerations are space requirements and initial cost, but for commercial facilities offering regular treatments, and serious home users (for whom neither money nor space in their homes are limitations), they are excellent options.

As discussed in chapter 5, several manufacturers of pods have been shown to be misrepresenting the irradiance of their pods (to a dramatic degree), so I'd strongly advise going through a reputable company and one that is transparent in sharing third-party lab data before spending tens of thousands of dollars on one of these devices.

- **SCALE AND DESIGN:** Largest PBM devices, similar to tanning beds in size and setup
- **POWER CHARACTERISTICS:** High total power output, but with lower irradiances

- **COVERAGE:** Provides full-body treatment in a single session, and the largest doses in total joules delivered to the body
- **TREATMENT EFFICIENCY:** Most time-efficient for full-body treatment, typically 10 to 30 minutes per session
- **TECHNICAL FEATURES:** Different brands now offer a wide assortment of wavelengths, sequences of treatment, and other novel features
- **INVESTMENT LEVEL:** Typically $17,000 to $120,000

Semi-Flexible/Targeted Devices for Deep Tissues

These devices bridge the gap between rigid panels and flexible pads, potentially offering higher irradiances while conforming to body contours. They're particularly effective for deep-tissue treatment around complex joint structures and areas requiring significant penetration depth. Their ability to maintain both higher irradiances and good tissue contact makes them ideal for deep-tissue PBM. They are generally imperfect, however, in bridging the gap between irradiance, body surface area coverage, and conformance to body curvatures; most devices in this category have issues with either lack of significant coverage, being too rigid, having too-low irradiance, or having too-low LED density. But I do like several devices in this category for many applications, and several strike an excellent balance between irradiance and skin contact (or very close to it), to allow for effective deep-tissue PBM.

- **CONSTRUCTION:** Typically a multi-layered design (usually using plastic and other flexible materials) with heat-dissipation systems
- **POWER OUTPUT:** Higher irradiance (25 to 150 mW/cm²) than standard pad-style devices
- **APPLICATION FOCUS:** Specifically designed for deep-tissue penetration around complex joint structures
- **TECHNICAL FEATURES:** Often includes both red and NIR wavelengths and sometimes pulsing modes for heat management
- **TREATMENT AREAS:** Ideal for shoulders, hips, spine, knees, ankles, muscles on limbs, and other complex anatomical regions

Handheld Torches and Wands

Portable devices excel in precision applications and small-area treatments, offering the distinct advantage of achieving good skin contact directly over the target tissue. For deep-tissue issues in small body areas like tennis elbow, trigger-point pain, or joint discomfort, these torch-style devices may be the best option. The maneuverability of facial wands allows for precise control and light pressure application, making them well suited for detailed work, especially on facial areas.

While some users report benefits from "photopuncture" (using torch devices on acupuncture points), research here is limited and the mechanisms are regarded as controversial in the Western scientific community.

The main drawback of these devices is that they require active involvement. Holding them in place for several minutes can lead to user fatigue during longer sessions, and many people may not take the time to use them regularly. They're also impractical for larger body areas, since point-by-point treatment is time-intensive. However, for individuals or practitioners focused on precision targeting of small areas, these devices are an excellent tool. And if you don't mind holding it in place for several minutes (perhaps while watching TV or listening to podcasts), these devices can work for you. (Note that many of these same pros and cons apply to many laser devices.)

- **DESIGN CHARACTERISTICS:** Portable devices with concentrated LEDs, usually in a pen-like or flashlight shape
- **ATTACHMENTS:** Sometimes feature interchangeable heads for different treatment approaches—broad heads for larger areas, focused tips for trigger points
- **APPLICATION BENEFITS:** Excellent for targeting specific points or small areas with precision, and users can adjust pressure and angle for optimal treatment

- **POWER DELIVERY:** Typically lower total power output but higher intensity at point of contact due to concentrated design
- **POPULAR USES:** Frequently used for facial treatments, joint pain, trigger points, and small-area targeting

Panels

Large LED panels deserve a special section for deeper discussion, because they have become the most commonly used and recommended PBM devices.

First, let's briefly describe what LED panels are:

- **CONSTRUCTION:** Rigid, flat panels constructed with high-powered LED arrays mounted on metal frames. Panel sizes range from portable roughly hand-sized units up to large full-body-sized panels. (Many of them are modular, so you can put multiple panels together to make them longer, wider, etc.)
- **POWER CHARACTERISTICS:** Irradiance typically ranging from 40 to 150 mW/cm² at 6 inches away from the panel. Need for heat management systems (fans) due to the higher power electronics.
- **DISTANCE USAGE:** Typically designed to be used 6 to 18 inches from the body, but can also potentially be used from closer distances (including skin contact) or farther distances.

- **COVERAGE:** Potentially provides broad uniform light coverage of large body areas. Larger panels can treat multiple body regions simultaneously.
- **WAVELENGTH DELIVERY:** Most quality panels combine both 630 to 670 nm red light and 830 to 850 nm NIR wavelengths (but sometimes include other wavelengths, like blue, amber, or 1,064 nm).
- **FEATURES:** Newer generations of panels often include built-in timing systems, pulsing options, and the ability to adjust light intensity (irradiance) and wavelengths

I actually have a long history with panels—before any companies even existed selling panels for PBM—I was getting them custom-built (for myself and my clients) by a company that made "grow lights" (that mainly provided lights for people trying to grow marijuana at home). For years, the company didn't even know why I was asking them to build these strange red and NIR light LED panels. I had been experimenting with them for years at that point, and this was all many years before the existence of any companies selling red and NIR light panels.

As these LED panels came onto the scene and became available to the general public, they hadn't been subjected to rigorous scientific study. (In fact, there is still a paucity of research on them as of 2025.) I was excited by the possibilities of the technology, and assumed that basically all the existing research on PBM (from various other kinds of devices) would also apply to LED panels—I believed that they represented the future of PBM and would be powerful universal tools, like Swiss Army knives, that could be used for almost every conceivable treatment context, from anti-aging effects on the skin, to treating muscles and joints, to brain health (which is how I was attempting to use them for years in my own self-experimentation). I felt they would be as effective as or superior to most targeted devices that were on the market (mainly the low-irradiance, low-LED density, flexible pad-style devices).

Fast-forward many years, and after vastly more self-experimentation with various kinds of devices, and through many conversations with PBM experts, I now understand subtler and more technical aspects of PBM device design and application, which has led me to the conclusion that many treatment contexts are better served by using more targeted devices designed for specific purposes, as discussed throughout this section and in chapter 5.

Having said that, I do still believe LED panels can be great wellness tools, particularly for getting the systemic benefits of PBM and treating large body areas. In fact, it's possible that panels deliver the systemic benefits of PBM more effectively than just about any type of PBM device (with perhaps the exception of the generally very expensive whole-body pods).

Let's dig a bit deeper and I'll explain what I believe they are well suited for, and not well suited for, based on my own perspective and the opinions of many other experts I have spoken with over the years.

Panels vs. Specialized Devices—The Case for Specialized Devices over Panels in Targeted Treatment

To begin to understand why LED panels are not necessarily the ideal option for various treatment goals, let's start by considering some of the basics of dosing for different tissues.

If one wants to treat the face for anti-aging effects in the facial skin, it's best to have an irradiance in the range of 10 to 50 mW/cm² and for the device to conform to the facial curvatures to deliver even light coverage to all sides/curves of the face.

On the other hand, if one wants deep penetration of light into deep tissues like muscles, tendons, and joints, it's ideal to have much higher irradiances (more like 75 to 150 mW/cm²), and ideally a device that is in contact with (or very close to) the skin while hitting the target area (e.g., a knee joint) from multiple sides/angles.

So just knowing this layer alone, we can see that using a large "whole-body" panel from head to toe (from 6 or 12 inches away) isn't going to do either of these two optimally.

If we choose to use it at a higher irradiance (something like 70 to 100 mW/cm²) from 6 inches away, for example, to try to get more light to the deeper tissues, the irradiance is likely too high for facial skin at that range and may result in an excessive irradiance or excessive dose (or both) for the face. But since it's a whole-body panel, many people *do* expose the face.

On the other hand, if you use it on a low irradiance (20 to 40 mW/cm^2)—perhaps by dialing back the intensity or by moving the device farther away—it may be ideal for skin health, but less light will penetrate to the deeper tissues. Moreover, even for the skin, because all the light is coming from one angle (the flat surface of the LED panel) and there is no conformance to the body's curvatures, areas like the face and other curved parts of the body like joints will receive fairly uneven light coverage. Adding to that issue, moving farther from the device means that the light will spread out more and start to hit the body surfaces at steeper angles such that less of the light will penetrate to the deeper tissues.

Another potential option is to use the panel with direct skin contact, but this, too, comes with certain potential drawbacks:

1. Because it's a large rigid panel with a flat surface and no flexibility to conform to body surfaces, you'll be very limited with how much skin contact you can actually get with most body areas (particularly with a very large panel).
2. Many panels produce a lot of heat in the device itself, which can heat the tissues (separately from the issue of the actual light being transformed into heat).
3. Many panels have significant spacing between LEDs (low LED density) and have different wavelengths in each LED chip—both of which make it less ideal for skin-contact treatments. You'll get the "hot spot" and "cold spot" effect of some areas receiving lots of light and areas next to them receiving little to no light.

These are not insurmountable issues, and almost all panels can be used in ways that have benefits, but we can see from these simple examples that large panels are generally a somewhat "blunt instrument" that aren't well-suited for many PBM treatment goals, and with which optimizing for one benefit may be problematic in other ways.

While LED panels can be used in some cases for more-targeted treatment goals, I believe that for most treatment goals other than general systemic benefits, specific targeted devices designed for particular body parts or conditions are likely to be more effective than LED panels.

Let's go over several examples of treatment goals, and I'll explain why panels are not likely to be as effective as targeted devices designed for that goal:

FACIAL TREATMENT

Dedicated facial masks provide optimal irradiance for facial skin, anatomically appropriate coverage, and specific wavelengths for skin health. They conform to facial contours and maintain consistent distance and energy delivery—something that's impossible with flat panels. While it's likely possible to use LED panels for facial skin anti-aging, it hasn't been formally tested in the research, and it would require knowing with some precision the actual irradiance of the panel you're using at a given distance, not to mention hitting the face from multiple angles—for example, 5 to 10 minutes on one side of the face (perhaps at a 45-degree angle) and then again on the other side, or perhaps using two panels at these angles simultaneously. Even then, the question remains as to whether this would be as effective as using one of the mask-style devices that is already in the optimal parameters and has shown in actual research to be effective for this purpose.

SCALP AND HAIR TREATMENT

Hair-restoration helmets offer uniform scalp coverage by conforming to the curvatures of the head and appropriate power density for follicle stimulation. They often use lasers (which may be more effective in stimulating hair follicles) and offer consistent treatment parameters across the scalp's surface. They're designed to penetrate through hair and maintain optimal contact with the scalp. A panel would have several basic problems in replicating this. It would be hard to replicate the ideal irradiance (you'd need to know the true irradiance of your panel at a given distance away and main-

tain that distance for the treatment). Panels will almost certainly be largely ineffective in getting light to penetrate through the hair into the scalp, as opposed to the helmets, in which the light can be pressed right up against the skin where much more of it is likely to get between the hair shafts. (Consider why your scalp doesn't get sunburn even after hours in the sun: the hair blocks too much of the light.) Perhaps most important, the helmet-style devices conform to the curves of the human head and deliver the light in a vastly more uniform way than could ever be achieved with a panel.

JOINT TREATMENT

Flexible, high-powered, wrap-around devices can deliver concentrated energy to multiple aspects/sides of a joint simultaneously, with appropriate power density for deep-tissue penetration. Unlike a flat and rigid panel, they can often conform to complex joint geometries and deliver light to a whole curved joint area (like a knee, ankle, or elbow) very efficiently. An LED panel can only treat one plane/angle at a time, and cannot maintain consistent power delivery (or angle of photons delivered) across curved surfaces.

As a result, treating a single joint requires multiple separate treatments from different angles (e.g., 5 minutes from the front, 5 minutes from the right side, 5 minutes from the left side, and 5 minutes from the back). This is possible to do in many cases, but it increases total treatment time, is inconvenient (especially if you have to stand in front of the panel), and potentially reduces consistency. Practically speaking, with large panels fixed on the wall or to a stand, it may also simply be physically awkward to position your inner elbow or inner knee or shoulder (for example) against the light from the ideal angles (as opposed to a small device that's very easy to reposition on a joint).

It may also be difficult to get skin contact where you need it, and many panels have too low LED density to be used effectively for this purpose. So while it is certainly possible to use panels for some types of joint treatment, I would strongly favor a more targeted and flexible device that can be used with skin contact or very close to the joint.

BRAIN TREATMENT

One area where I would not use panels is on the brain. There is no research testing this use of panels, and doing so is essentially a question of how much light penetrates into the brain and in which areas. The brain is strongly light-sensitive, and therefore it may be particularly easy to overdo the dose and create a biphasic dose response (which is counterproductive). At the same time, the brain's location inside the skull makes it difficult to deliver light to it. So without adequate research on a particular device used in a particular way, we don't know whether such a device is totally ineffective in delivering a significant amount of light to the brain, or far

too powerful and thus likely to have negative effect. It's just an unknown; to my knowledge, no research has been done on brain treatment using panels.

It's also difficult to do (on anyone with hair) except at the forehead, because without good skin contact, it may be hard to deliver light through the skull to the brain. Transcranial devices are specifically engineered for optimal skull penetration, precise targeting of brain regions, and appropriate power delivery for neural tissue—parameters that cannot be reliably achieved with general-purpose panels. I recommend a cautious approach if trying to affect the brain, and I would strongly suggest using a device that has been tested in formal research and shown to benefit brain function.

There are other potential examples, but the basic idea here is that panels are a great general tool for PBM in certain contexts like where they technically treat the "whole body" for systemic effects but tend not to be optimal for any specific treatment goal (i.e., skin benefits or deep-tissue benefits in joints and muscles). More targeted devices designed for specific purposes are likely to outperform panels in these situations.

When evaluating LED panel devices, it's important to approach marketing claims with a critical eye. Be wary of "all-in-one solution" marketing suggesting that a single device can be equally effective for all applications, from superficial skin treatments to deep-tissue therapy, and of claims that one device can completely replace specialized treatment tools. Power specifications also warrant careful scrutiny; as I've mentioned elsewhere, manufacturers frequently present inaccurate numbers about the irradiances of their devices, which makes accurate dosing very difficult.

Lack of Evidence for Efficacy

Surprisingly, there are still relatively few studies using large LED panels. And the studies that do currently exist aren't especially impressive.

In that sense, there is a gap between the popularity and the marketing of LED panels vs. the actual evidence supporting their use. Most of the studies on PBM have not used panels or treated the whole body but generally study more targeted use of devices on specific body parts.

It's worth noting that this is largely an issue of "absence of evidence" rather than "evidence of absence." In other words, this is more an issue of a lack of studies testing LED panels in various contexts than it is an issue of having dozens of well-controlled studies that have shown LED panels to be ineffective. Of the existing studies of panels, some are quite poorly designed; for example, one study of college athletes using LED panels used a total treatment time of 5 minutes (2.5 minutes on the front of the body and 2.5 minutes on the back). This is a very low dosage where it's not surprising that no benefits were shown. It would be like assessing the effects of doing only 25 minutes of exercise

per week. It's just a tiny dose. In this case, 10 to 30 minutes of total treatment time with the panels would be a far more effective dose. Most of the research on "whole-body" PBM has used pods, particularly the NovoThor device, and several studies have shown benefits for things like exercise recovery, long COVID–related brain fog, improved heart rate variability, and improvements in symptoms and blood markers associated with fibromyalgia.

On the other hand, we could say "light is light." In other words, different PBM devices delivering red and NIR light to the body in similar parameters should provide similar benefits. Stated differently, it's likely that large LED panels that are used in a way that mimics whole-body pods should yield a good portion of the systemic benefits as have been demonstrated with the studies on whole-body pods.

TRUE IRRADIANCE FIGURES FOR LED PANELS FROM THIRD-PARTY LAB DATA

As I've emphasized, a key reason for updating this book—apart from incorporating the latest research and devices since its initial publication in 2018—is to resolve the significant issue of inaccurate irradiance data on LED panels. This problem stemmed from widespread reliance on photosynthetically active radiation meters to measure devices' light output. It's now known that photosynthetically active radiation meters can overestimate irradiance by as much as 50 percent. This caused inaccurate irradiance data and exaggerated claims across the internet, in thousands of blogs, videos, and product descriptions (and in the original version of my book).

To improve the accuracy of available information, I linked up with a third-party light laboratory specializing in precise measurements of output for light-emitting devices. I then contacted all the major PBM device manufacturers, inviting them to submit their panels for independent testing.

Fortunately, many companies participated. (Some prominent companies declined, presumably because they did not wish to reveal the true performance of their devices.) The following data was obtained through rigorous testing conducted by LightLab International in Allentown, Pennsylvania. Using precision instruments under controlled conditions, LightLab provided accurate and reliable measurements. I am in possession of the actual lab reports, so I have verified all of the following numbers. I want to give special thanks to the companies that generously paid to have their panels tested by LightLab International and worked with me to bring this third-party lab data to all of you.

I hope that this data will offer clarity to consumers and help to set a new standard of transparency in the PBM device market. Here are the results from the brands that participated in this initiative:

BRAND AND DEVICE NAME	TOTAL RADIANT FLUX (WATTS)	IRRADIANCE (MW/CM²)	
		6 INCHES	12 INCHES
Hooga Health HGPRO4500	558	93	90
Mito Light Mitohacker 3.0	242	86	76
KOZE Health X Series	184	88	71
Hooga Health HGPRO1500	182	92	70
Bestqool Y-200	88	54	34
PlatinumLED Biomax 900	182	81	73
Red Therapy Co. RedRush Pulse	81	80	80
Rouge Light Therapy Rouge Pro Generation 3	155	76	71
Mito Red Light MitoPRO 1500	146	73	56
Red Therapy Co. RedRush 840 Pulse MAX	161	78	78
GembaRed Reboot	106	43	34
Luminous Labs Luminousred model 2+2	136	44	36
EMR-TEK Inc. Inferno	180	138	67

It's worth noting that most of these tests were conducted between roughly 2022 and 2024, and thus may not reflect the current offerings from these companies, as some companies may have released new generations of their panels since these tests were done. New generations of devices may have significantly different irradiances. Nevertheless, this can give you a good idea of the real irradiance range for most panels on the market, which can be used for accurate dosing.

There are a few more important points I want to make about panels:

1. Many companies claim irradiance figures above 150 mW/cm^2 for their panels. As you can see, almost no devices test in that range. For many companies, the real irradiance figures are often around half of what they publicly claim. So the first rule is simple: Do not trust irradiance claims on a manufacturer's website unless they provide third-party lab data to back them up. If a company refuses to share such data or advertises figures that differ significantly from verified measurements, it's a red flag, and I suggest not doing business with that company.

2. While higher irradiance isn't always better for every treatment goal, it does offer an important advantage: flexibility. A higher-irradiance panel can be adjusted to lower settings for treatments requiring lower irradiances (like facial anti-aging) or used at full intensity for deeper penetration into muscles and joints. In contrast, a low-irradiance panel limits your options, as it may not deliver enough intensity for deeper tissues even at maximum output. Essentially, a higher-irradiance panel provides versatility, allowing you to tailor treatments across a broader range of goals.

3. Many claims of superiority for one device over another are marketing rather than science, based on inaccurate data or minuscule differences in irradiance that have little practical impact. For instance, a panel offering 85 mW/cm^2 vs. one at 75 mW/cm^2 may only require an extra 30 to 60 seconds of treatment time to deliver the same dose. On the other hand, there are cases in which irradiance differences between panels are highly significant. For example, brands like Hooga, EMR-TEK, and Mito Light may offer panels with more than double the irradiance of some other brands. These differences likely would meaningfully affect treatment outcomes, particularly in terms of the advantage of higher irradiances (closer to 100 mW/cm^2) in delivering light to deeper tissues. But again, many of the brands offer very similar specs, so don't get too caught up in the marketing claims of various manufacturers, most of which are detached from the scientific evidence.

4. The given data is certainly not meant to be a comprehensive comparison of various panels. There are other factors that go into determining how effective a panel is likely to be. For example, how far apart the LEDs are spaced (particularly for contact treatments), and whether they use multiple wavelengths or only one wavelength per LED chip. It's also important to consider the number of wavelengths and portion of total light in those wavelengths. Some devices focus more on red wavelengths, while others emphasize NIR or offer a 50–50 balance. Certain panels even include blue LEDs, though these are less relevant (and potentially counterproductive) for some PBM purposes. Panels that allow users to customize settings—such as switching between red and NIR wavelengths or adjusting light intensity—are preferable for their added flexibility.

My hope is that with the publishing of this third-party data on the true irradiance of panels, and with your help of buying only from manufacturers that openly share the third party–verified irradiances of their devices, we can bring an end to the era of deceptive and low-integrity practices that have run rampant in the industry for years. This is crucial for people to be able to safely and effectively dose these devices for various treatment goals.

Optimal Use of Panels

Given this understanding, large LED panels might be best understood and utilized:

- For broad systemic benefits alongside targeted therapeutic interventions
- As part of a comprehensive wellness routine focused on general health maintenance
- For general skin health of the entire body (more moderate irradiances in the range 20 to 50 mW/cm^2 are likely best for this purpose)
- For delivering light to a large surface area of the body and effectively irradiating the bloodstream, when systemic benefits are the primary goal
- For maintaining general tissue health and function
- For treating deep tissues in very large areas like the back or legs (can be used from close proximity or in direct skin contact)

This suggests a paradigm shift in how we think about and use large LED panels—not as universal treatment devices for every conceivable goal, but as valuable tools for supporting systemic health and complementing more targeted therapeutic approaches, and perhaps also for treating large muscle groups. This understanding can help guide more effective treatment protocols and better outcomes by matching the right tool to the right purpose. Simultaneously, approaching things this way removes much of the potential for inaccurate dosing that comes with panels.

Remember, in most treatment contexts, it's wise to leverage both the local effects on a particular body area (ideally with a device specifically designed for that purpose) *and* to also leverage systemic effects, which will almost invariably contribute to a better treatment outcome for anything you might be doing PBM for. And panels are still likely to be one of the best types of devices (along with whole-body pods) for enhancing systemic benefits.

TEMPLATE FOR DEVICE SELECTION

While it's difficult to summarize all of this information succinctly, here is my best attempt to capture most of the key practical recommendations about device selection for specific treatment goals:

TARGET GOAL	BEST DEVICE TYPE(S)
Skin health	Facial masks Curved face-specific panel devices designed to be used from a distance Large LED panels (used at lower irradiances) Flexible pad-style devices Whole-body pods
Other superficial tissues (Skin wounds, etc.)	Flexible pad-style devices Potentially LED panels (set at lower irradiances)
Muscles, bones, joints, and other deep tissues	Semi-flexible higher-irradiance targeted devices Panels (from close distance or with skin contact for large body areas) Torch-style devices with skin contact (for small areas) Flexible pad-style devices with higher irradiances and LED densities than most pad-style devices
Body fat	Flexible pad-style devices (again, choose pads with relatively higher LED densities and irradiance), and semi-flexible devices
Genitalia	Genitalia-specific devices
Oral, nasal	Oral/nasal-specific devices
Hair	Laser and LED caps
Eyes	Eye-specific devices Other low-irradiance devices (used cautiously with medical guidance) Torch-style devices (making sure irradiance is not too high)
Brain	Brain-specific devices
Whole-body, systemic benefits	Large LED panels Full-body pods Higher irradiance semi-flexible targeted devices to increase stem cells in circulation

FINAL THOUGHTS

As we reach the end of this journey through the world of PBM, I hope you now feel equipped with the knowledge and confidence to harness this remarkable healing modality for your own health and wellness goals.

Throughout this guide, we've explored the fascinating science behind PBM—how specific wavelengths of red and NIR light can stimulate cellular energy production, reduce inflammation, accelerate healing, and support your body's natural regenerative processes. We've delved deep into the technical and scientific aspects that determine whether PBM will be effective for a particular goal, examining the critical factors of wavelength, irradiance, dose, and treatment protocols. We've covered the extensive research showing PBM's benefits for everything from skin health and wound healing to muscle recovery, pain relief, brain function, and beyond.

Perhaps most importantly, we've cut through the marketing hype and confusion in the device marketplace to give you the practical tools you need to make informed decisions. You now understand the principles of proper dosing, how to select the right device for your specific goals, and how to use PBM safely and effectively.

PBM represents one of the most promising and accessible therapeutic technologies available today. Unlike many medical interventions, it's remarkably safe, non-invasive, and free from significant side effects when used properly. It works with your body's natural healing mechanisms rather than against them, supporting cellular function at the most fundamental level.

The beauty of PBM lies not just in its broad therapeutic potential, but in its simplicity. With the right device and proper protocols, you can access these benefits from the comfort of your own home, integrating this powerful therapy into your daily routine.

As you begin or continue your PBM journey, remember that consistency is key. Like exercise or good nutrition, the benefits of PBM compound over time with regular use. Start with the protocols outlined in this guide, listen to your body, and adjust as needed based on your individual response.

The field of PBM continues to evolve rapidly, with new research emerging regularly that deepens our understanding of how light affects human biology. While we've covered the current state of knowledge comprehensively, new research will undoubtedly continue to reveal new applications and refine existing protocols.

PBM unquestionably works, but success requires the right mindset and realistic expectations. This isn't a magic pill that will instantly transform your appearance, melt away pounds overnight, regrow hair in days, or reverse decades of joint damage in weeks. I encourage you to approach red light therapy like starting a new exercise routine—with both enthusiasm and patience. Just as you might feel energized after your first workout but need months to build real strength and endurance, some PBM benefits may be noticeable quickly while others develop gradually over weeks or months of consistent use. Trust the process, stay consistent with your protocols, and give your body time to respond. Whether you're seeking peak performance, faster recovery, healthier skin, pain relief, or enhanced longevity, PBM offers a scientifically validated tool that amplifies your body's innate healing capacity.

You now possess the knowledge to see through the hype and gimmicks, select quality devices, dose properly, and integrate this powerful therapy into your life safely and effectively.

Here's to your health, healing, and the bright future ahead as you harness the power of red and near-infrared light.

Shine on.

References

Introduction: The Essential Role of Light in Human Health

1. Câmara AB, de Souza ID, Dalmolin RJS. Sunlight incidence, vitamin D deficiency, and Alzheimer's disease. *J Med Food*. 2018;21:841–8.
2. Wang J, Yang D, Yu Y, Shao G, Wang Q. Vitamin D and sunlight exposure in newly-diagnosed Parkinson's disease. *Nutrients*. 2016;8:142.
3. Tremlett H, Zhu F, Ascherio A, Munger KL. Sun exposure over the life course and associations with multiple sclerosis. *Neurology*. 2018;90:e1191–9.
4. New Research sheds more Light on Parkinson's Disease [Internet]. 2016 [accessed 2025 Jan 27]. Available from: http://sunlight institute.org/new-research-sheds-more-light-on-parkinsons-disease/
5. Egan KM, Sosman JA, Blot WJ. Sunlight and reduced risk of cancer: is the real story vitamin D? *J Natl Cancer Inst*. 2005;97:161–3.
6. Holick MF. Vitamin D, sunlight and cancer connection. *Anticancer Agents Med Chem*. 2013;13:70–82.
7. Holick MF. Cancer, sunlight and vitamin D. *J Clin Transl Endocrinol*. 2014;1:179–86.
8. van der Rhee HJ, de Vries E, Coebergh JWW. Does sunlight prevent cancer? A systematic review. *Eur J Cancer*. 2006;42:2222–32.
9. Fleury N, Geldenhuys S, Gorman S. Sun Exposure and Its Effects on Human Health: Mechanisms through Which Sun Exposure Could Reduce the Risk of Developing Obesity and Cardiometabolic Dysfunction. *Int J Environ Res Public Health* [Internet]. 2016;13. Available from: http://dx.doi.org/10.3390/ijerph13100999
10. Gorman S, Lucas RM, Allen-Hall A, Fleury N, Feelisch M. Ultraviolet radiation, vitamin D and the development of obesity, metabolic syndrome and type-2 diabetes. *Photochem Photobiol Sci*. 2017;16:362–73.
11. Frellick M. Avoiding Sun as Dangerous as Smoking [Internet]. Medscape. 2016 [cited 2025 Jan 27]. Available from: https://www.medscape.com/viewarticle/860805
12. Lindqvist PG, Epstein E, Landin-Olsson M, Ingvar C, Nielsen K, Stenbeck M, et al. Avoidance of sun exposure is a risk factor for all-cause mortality: results from the Melanoma in Southern Sweden cohort. *J Intern Med*. 2014;276:77–86.
13. Keshet-Sitton A, Or-Chen K, Huber E, Haim A. Illuminating a risk for breast cancer: A preliminary ecological study on the association between streetlight and breast cancer. *Integr Cancer Ther*. 2017;16:451–63.
14. Al-Naggar RA, Anil S. Artificial light at night and cancer: Global study. *Asian Pac J Cancer Prev*. 2016;17:4661–4.

15. De Nike L. Study links exposure to light at night to depression, learning issues [Internet]. The Hub. 2012 [accessed 2025 Jan 27]. Available from: https://hub.jhu.edu/2012/11/14/light-exposure-depression/

16. Rybnikova NA, Haim A, Portnov BA. Does artificial light-at-night exposure contribute to the worldwide obesity pandemic? *Int J Obes* (Lond). 2016;40:815–23.

17. McFadden E, Jones ME, Schoemaker MJ, Ashworth A, Swerdlow AJ. The relationship between obesity and exposure to light at night: cross-sectional analyses of over 100,000 women in the Breakthrough Generations Study. *Am J Epidemiol*. 2014;180:245–50.

18. Fonken LK, Nelson RJ. The effects of light at night on circadian clocks and metabolism. *Endocr Rev*. 2014;35:648–70.

19. University of Houston. Artificial light from digital devices lessens sleep quality. Science Daily [Internet]. 2017 Jul 28 [accessed 2025 Jan 27]; Available from: https://www.sciencedaily.com/releases/2017/07/170728121414.htm

20. Baker J, Putnam N, Kozlowski RE, Anderson M, Bird Z, Chmielewski J, Meske J, Steinshouer N, Kozlowski MR. Effects of chronic, daily exposures to low intensity blue light on human retinal pigment epithelial cells: Implications for the use of personal electronic devices. *Journal of Photochemistry and Photobiology*. 2022. 1;10:100118.

21. Serrage H, Heiskanen V, Palin WM, Cooper PR, Milward MR, Hadis M, Hamblin MR. Under the spotlight: mechanisms of photobiomodulation concentrating on blue and green light. *Photochemical & Photobiological Sciences*. 2019;18(8):1877–909.

22. Opländer C, Deck A, Volkmar CM, Kirsch M, Liebmann J, Born M, Van Abeelen F, Van Faassen EE, Kröncke KD, Windolf J, Suschek CV. Mechanism and biological relevance of blue-light (420–453 nm)-induced enzymatic nitric oxide generation from photolabile nitric oxide derivates in human skin in vitro and in vivo. *Free Radical Biology and Medicine*. 2013 65:1363–77.

Chapter One: A History of Red and Near-Infrared Light Therapy

1. Mathewson I. Did human hairlessness allow natural photobiomodulation 2 million years ago and enable photobiomodulation therapy today? This can explain the rapid expansion of our genus's brain. *Med Hypotheses*. 2015;84:421–8.

2. Bloch H. Solartheology, heliotherapy, phototherapy, and biologic effects: a historical overview. *J Natl Med Assoc*. 1990;82:517–8, 520–1.

3. Goyal M, Sasmal D, Nagori BP. Ayurveda the ancient science of healing: An insight. Drug Discovery Research in Pharmacognosy. *InTech*; 2012.

4. Gaddesden J. Rosa medicinae [Internet]. 1313 [accessed 2025 Jan 31]. Available from: https://archives.collections.ed.ac.uk/repositories/2/archival_objects/159481

5. Gusain P, Paliwal R, Joga R, Gupta N, Singh V. Ancient Light Therapies: A Boon to Medical Science. Science and Culture [Internet]. 2016;82. Available from: https://www.researchgate.net/publication/326367879_ANCIENT_LIGHT_THERAPIES_A_BOON_TO_MEDICAL_SCIENCE

6. Chesney RW. Theobald Palm and his remarkable observation: how the sunshine vitamin came to be recognized. *Nutrients*. 2012;4:42–51.

7. Holick MF. The one-hundred-year anniversary of the discovery of the sunshine vitamin D3: Historical, personal experience and evidence-based perspectives. *Nutrients*. 2023;15:593.

8. Findlay L. The etiology of rickets: A clinical and experimental study. *Br Med J*. 1908;2:13–17.

9. Zupanic-Slavec Z, Toplak C. Water, air and light—Arnold Rikli (1823–1906). *Gesnerus*. 1998;55:58–69.

10. Grzybowski A, Pietrzak K. From patient to discoverer—Niels Ryberg Finsen (1860–1904)—the founder of phototherapy in dermatology. *Clin Dermatol*. 2012;30:451–5.

11. Kellogg JH. *Light Therapeutics: A Practical Manual of Phototherapy for the Student and*

the Practitioner, with Special Reference to the Incandescent Electric-light Bath. Legare Street Press; 2021.

12. Kellogg JH. *The Battle Creek Sanitarium System*. Legare Street Press; 2021.

13. Bernhard, O. Light treatment in surgery. *Nature*. 1927;119:701–701.

14. Hobday RA. Sunlight therapy and solar architecture. *Med Hist*. 1997;41:455–72.

15. Rollier A. Heliotherapy with special consideration of surgical tuberculosis. *J R Nav Med Serv*. 1927;13:322–3.

16. Woloshyn TA. Soaking up the rays: Light therapy and visual culture in Britain, c. 1890–1940. *MUP*; 2017.

17. Russel EH, Russell WK. Ultra–Violet Radiation and Actinotherapy. *JAMA*. 1927;89:1715.

18. Einstein A. "On the quantum theory of radiation." In: D. Ter Haar *The Old Quantum Theory*. London:Elsevier; 1967. p. 167–83.

19. Maiman TH. Stimulated optical radiation in Ruby. *Nature*. 1960;187:493–4.

20. Mester A, Mester A. The history of photobiomodulation: Endre Mester (1903–1984). *Photomed Laser Surg*. 2017;35:393–4.

21. Mester E, Mester AF, Mester A. The biomedical effects of laser application. *Lasers Surg Med*. 1985;5:31–9.

22. Karu T. Primary and secondary mechanisms of action of visible to near-IR radiation on cells. *J Photochem Photobiol B*. 1999;49:1–17.

23. Palucka T. 50 years ago: How Holonyak won the race to invent visible LEDs. *MRS Bull*. 2012;37:963–6.

24. Whelan HT. The Use of NASA Light-Emitting Diode Near-Infrared Technology for Biostimulation. Second International Conference on Near-Field Optical Analysis: *Photodynamic Therapy and Photobiology Effects*. 2002.

25. Heiskanen V, Hamblin MR. Photobiomodulation: lasers vs. light emitting diodes? *Photochem Photobiol Sci*. 2018;17:1003–17.

26. Anders JJ, Arany PR, Baxter GD, Lanzafame RJ. Light-emitting diode therapy and low-level light therapy are photobiomodulation therapy. *Photobiomodul Photomed Laser Surg*. 2019;37:63–5.

27. Anders JJ, Lanzafame RJ, Arany PR. Low-level light/laser therapy versus photobiomodulation therapy. *Photomed Laser Surg*. 2015;33:183–4.

Chapter Two: How Photobiomodulation Works: The Mechanisms and Pathways of Red and NIR Light Therapy

1. Hamblin MR, Ferraresi C, Huang Y-Y, Freitas de Freitas L, Carroll JD. *Low-level Light Therapy*. Bellingham, WA: SPIE Press; 2018.

2. Cardoso FDS, Barrett DW, Wade Z, Gomes da Silva S, Gonzalez-Lima F. Photobiomodulation of cytochrome c oxidase by chronic transcranial laser in young and aged brains. *Front Neurosci*. 2022;16:818005.

3. Hamblin MR. The role of nitric oxide in low level light therapy. In: Hamblin MR, Waynant RW, Anders J, editors. *Mechanisms for Low-Light Therapy III* [Internet]. SPIE; 2008. Available from: http://dx.doi.org/10.1117/12.764918

4. Quirk BJ, Whelan HT. What lies at the heart of photobiomodulation: Light, cytochrome C oxidase, and nitric oxide-review of the evidence. *Photobiomodul Photomed Laser Surg*. 2020;38:527–30.

5. Farivar S, Malekshahabi T, Shiari R. Biological effects of low level laser therapy. *J Lasers Med Sci*. 2014;5:58–62.

6. Anderson AJ, Jackson TD, Stroud DA, Stojanovski D. Mitochondria-hubs for regulating cellular biochemistry: emerging concepts and networks. *Open Biol*. 2019;9:190126.

7. Caterina MJ, Schumacher MA, Tominaga M, Rosen TA, Levine JD, Julius D. The capsaicin receptor: a heat-activated ion channel in the pain pathway. *Nature*. 1997;389:816–24.

8. Sharma SK, Sardana S, Hamblin MR. Role of opsins and light or heat activated transient receptor potential ion channels in the mechanisms of photobiomodulation and infrared therapy. *Journal of Photochemistry and Photobiology*. 2023;13:100160.

9. Caterina MJ, Rosen TA, Tominaga M, Brake AJ, Julius D. A capsaicin-receptor homologue

with a high threshold for noxious heat. *Nature.* 1999;398:436–41.

10. Juárez-Contreras R, Méndez-Reséndiz KA, Rosenbaum T, González-Ramírez R, Morales-Lázaro SL. TRPV1 channel: A noxious signal transducer that affects mitochondrial function. *Int J Mol Sci.* 2020;21:8882.

11. Zhang Z, Zhang Z, Liu P, Xue X, Zhang C, Peng L, et al. The role of photobiomodulation to modulate ion channels in the nervous system: A systematic review. *Cell Mol Neurobiol.* 2024;44:79.

12. de Oliveira ME, Da Silva JT, Brioschi ML, Chacur M. Effects of photobiomodulation therapy on neuropathic pain in rats: evaluation of nociceptive mediators and infrared thermography. *Lasers Med Sci.* 2021;36:1461–7.

13. Ma H, Du Y, Xie D, Wei ZZ, Pan Y, Zhang Y. Recent advances in light energy biotherapeutic strategies with photobiomodulation on central nervous system disorders. *Brain Res.* 2024;1822:148615.

14. Wang W, Sun T. Impact of TRPV1 on pathogenesis and therapy of neurodegenerative diseases. *Molecules* [Internet]. 2023;29. Available from: http://dx.doi.org/10.3390/molecules29010181

15. Arany PR, Nayak RS, Hallikerimath S, Limaye AM, Kale AD, Kondaiah P. Activation of latent TGF-beta1 by low-power laser in vitro correlates with increased TGF-beta1 levels in laser-enhanced oral wound healing. *Wound Repair Regen.* 2007;15:866–74.

16. Arany PR. Photobiomodulation-activated latent transforming growth factor-β1: A critical clinical therapeutic pathway and an endogenous optogenetic tool for discovery. *Photobiomodul Photomed Laser Surg.* 2022;40:136–47.

17. Clark DA, Coker R. Transforming growth factor-beta (TGF-beta). *Int J Biochem Cell Biol.* 1998;30:293–8.

18. Whitten A. The Nitty-Gritty Science Of Photobiomodulation with Dr. Praveen Arany [Internet]. *The Energy Blueprint—Cutting-Edge Science For Overcoming Fatigue and Increasing Your Energy.* The Energy Blueprint; 2024 [cited 2024 Nov 30]. Available from: https://theenergyblueprint.com/dr-praveen-arany-part-1/

19. MacFarlane EG, Haupt J, Dietz HC, Shore EM. TGF-β family signaling in connective tissue and skeletal diseases. *Cold Spring Harb Perspect Biol* [Internet]. 2017;9. Available from: http://dx.doi.org/10.1101/cshperspect.a022269

20. Pan X, Chen Z, Huang R, Yao Y, Ma G. Transforming growth factor β1 induces the expression of collagen type I by DNA methylation in cardiac fibroblasts. *PLoS One.* 2013;8:e60335.

21. Rathbone CR, Yamanouchi K, Chen XK, Nevoret-Bell CJ, Rhoads RP, Allen RE. Effects of transforming growth factor-beta (TGF-β1) on satellite cell activation and survival during oxidative stress. *J Muscle Res Cell Motil.* 2011;32:99–109.

22. Beanes SR, Dang C, Soo C, Ting K. Skin repair and scar formation: the central role of TGF-beta. *Expert Rev Mol Med.* 2003;5:1–22.

23. Janssens K, ten Dijke P, Janssens S, Van Hul W. Transforming growth factor-beta1 to the bone. *Endocr Rev.* 2005;26:743–74.

24. Travis MA, Sheppard D. TGF-β activation and function in immunity. *Annu Rev Immunol.* 2014;32:51–82.

25. Xu X, Zheng L, Yuan Q, Zhen G, Crane JL, Zhou X, et al. Transforming growth factor-β in stem cells and tissue homeostasis. *Bone Res.* 2018;6:2.

26. Wang M-K, Sun H-Q, Xiang Y-C, Jiang F, Su Y-P, Zou Z-M. Different roles of TGF-β in the multi-lineage differentiation of stem cells. *World J Stem Cells.* 2012;4:28–34.

27. Lin S-K. *The Fourth Phase of Water: Beyond Solid, Liquid, and Vapor.* By Gerald H. Pollack, Ebner & Sons Publishers, 2013; Water (Basel). 2013;5:638–9.

28. Elton DC, Spencer PD, Riches JD, Williams ED. Exclusion zone phenomena in water—A critical review of experimental findings and theories. *Int J Mol Sci.* 2020;21:5041.

29. Sommer AP, Haddad MK, Fecht H-J. Light effect on water viscosity: Implication for ATP biosynthesis. *Sci Rep.* 2015;5:12029.

30. Sommer AP, Schemmer P, Pavláth AE, Försterling H-D, Mester ÁR, Trelles MA. Quantum

biology in low level light therapy: Death of a dogma. *Ann Transl Med.* 2020;8:440.

31. Sommer AP. Mitochondrial cytochrome c oxidase is not the primary acceptor for near-infrared light—it is mitochondrial bound water: the principles of low-level light therapy. *Ann Transl Med.* 2019;7:S13.

32. Hamblin MR. Mechanisms and applications of the anti-inflammatory effects of photobiomodulation. *AIMS Biophys.* 2017;4:337–61.

33. Salman S, Guermonprez C, Peno-Mazzarino L, Lati E, Rousseaud A, Declercq L, et al. Photobiomodulation controls keratinocytes inflammatory response through Nrf2 and reduces Langerhans cells activation. *Antioxidants* (Basel). 2023;12:766.

34. Evangelista AN, Dos Santos FF, de Oliveira Martins LP, Gaiad TP, Machado ASD, Rocha-Vieira E, et al. Photobiomodulation therapy on expression of HSP70 protein and tissue repair in experimental acute Achilles tendinitis. *Lasers Med Sci.* 2021;36:1201–8.

35. Leyane TS, Jere SW, Houreld NN. Cellular signalling and photobiomodulation in chronic wound repair. *Int J Mol Sci.* 2021;22:11223.

36. Pilar EFS, Brochado FT, Schmidt TR, Leite AC, Deluca AA, Mármora BC, et al. Modulation of gene expression in skin wound healing by photobiomodulation therapy: A systematic review in vivo studies. *Photodermatol Photoimmunol Photomed.* 2024;40:e12990.

37. Peplow PV, Chung T-Y, Ryan B, Baxter GD. Laser photobiomodulation of gene expression and release of growth factors and cytokines from cells in culture: a review of human and animal studies. *Photomed Laser Surg.* 2011;29:285–304.

38. Barolet AC, Germain L, Barolet D. In vivo measurement of nitric oxide release from intact human skin post photobiomodulation using visible and near-infrared light: A chemiluminescence detection study. *Journal of Photochemistry and Photobiology.* 2024;24:100250.

39. Feng Y, Huang Z, Ma X, Zong X, Tesic V, Ding B, et al. Photobiomodulation inhibits ischemia-induced brain endothelial senescence via endothelial nitric oxide synthase. *Antioxidants* (Basel). 2024;13:633.

40. Kashiwagi S, Morita A, Yokomizo S,

Ogawa E, Komai E, Huang PL, et al. Photobiomodulation and nitric oxide signaling. *Nitric Oxide.* 2023;130:58–68.

41. Lohr NL, Keszler A, Pratt P, Bienengraber M, Warltier DC, Hogg N. Enhancement of nitric oxide release from nitrosyl hemoglobin and nitrosyl myoglobin by red/near infrared radiation: potential role in cardioprotection. *J Mol Cell Cardiol.* 2009;47:256–63.

42. Ball KA, Castello PR, Poyton RO. Low intensity light stimulates nitrite-dependent nitric oxide synthesis but not oxygen consumption by cytochrome c oxidase: Implications for phototherapy. *J Photochem Photobiol B.* 2011;102:182–91.

43. Lee HI, Lee S-W, Kim SY, Kim NG, Park K-J, Choi BT, et al. Pretreatment with light-emitting diode therapy reduces ischemic brain injury in mice through endothelial nitric oxide synthase-dependent mechanisms. *Biochem Biophys Res Commun.* 2017;486:945–50.

44. Miyamoto T, Petrus MJ, Dubin AE, Patapoutian A. TRPV3 regulates nitric oxide synthase-independent nitric oxide synthesis in the skin. *Nat Commun.* 2011;2:369.

45. Reiter RJ, Rosales-Corral S, Tan DX, Jou MJ, Galano A, Xu B. Melatonin as a mitochondria-targeted antioxidant: one of evolution's best ideas. *Cell Mol Life Sci.* 2017;74:3863–81.

46. Manchester LC, Coto-Montes A, Boga JA, Andersen LPH, Zhou Z, Galano A, et al. Melatonin: an ancient molecule that makes oxygen metabolically tolerable. *J Pineal Res.* 2015;59:403–19.

47. Venegas C, García JA, Escames G, Ortiz F, López A, Doerrier C, et al. Extrapineal melatonin: analysis of its subcellular distribution and daily fluctuations. *J Pineal Res.* 2012;52:217–27.

48. Tan D-X, Manchester LC, Qin L, Reiter RJ. Melatonin: A Mitochondrial Targeting Molecule Involving Mitochondrial Protection and Dynamics. *Int J Mol Sci* [Internet]. 2016;17.

49. Tan D-X, Reiter RJ, Zimmerman S, Hardeland R. Melatonin: Both a messenger of darkness and a participant in the cellular actions of non-visible solar radiation of near infrared light. *Biology* (Basel). 2023;12:89.

50. Zimmerman S, Reiter RJ. Transient responses

of melatonin to stress. *Melatonin Res.* 2022;5:295–303.

51. Sofic E, Rimpapa Z, Kundurovic Z, Sapcanin A, Tahirovic I, Rustembegovic A, et al. Antioxidant capacity of the neurohormone melatonin. *J Neural Transm* (Vienna). 2005;112:349–58.

52. Tan D-X, Manchester LC, Terron MP, Flores LJ, Reiter RJ. One molecule, many derivatives: a never-ending interaction of melatonin with reactive oxygen and nitrogen species? *J Pineal Res.* 2007;42:28–42.

53. Srinivasan V, Spence DW, Pandi-Perumal SR, Brown GM, Cardinali DP. Melatonin in mitochondrial dysfunction and related disorders. *Int J Alzheimers Dis.* 2011;2011:326320.

54. Leon J, Acuña-Castroviejo D, Sainz RM, Mayo JC, Tan D-X, Reiter RJ. Melatonin and mitochondrial function. *Life Sci.* 2004;75:765–90.

55. Lee JG, Woo YS, Park SW, Seog D-H, Seo MK, Bahk W-M. The neuroprotective effects of melatonin: Possible role in the pathophysiology of neuropsychiatric disease. *Brain Sci.* 2019;9:285.

56. Rodríguez MI, Escames G, López LC, López A, García JA, Ortiz F, et al. Improved mitochondrial function and increased life span after chronic melatonin treatment in senescent prone mice. *Exp Gerontol.* 2008;43:749–56.

57. Reiter RJ, Tan D-X, Mayo JC, Sainz RM, Leon J, Czarnocki Z. Melatonin as an antioxidant: biochemical mechanisms and pathophysiological implications in humans. *Acta Biochim Pol.* 2003;50:1129–46.

58. Sofic E, Rimpapa Z, Kundurovic Z, Sapcanin A, Tahirovic I, Rustembegovic A, et al. Antioxidant capacity of the neurohormone melatonin. *J Neural Transm* (Vienna). 2005;112:349–58.

59. Lowes DA, Webster NR, Murphy MP, Galley HF. Antioxidants that protect mitochondria reduce interleukin-6 and oxidative stress, improve mitochondrial function, and reduce biochemical markers of organ dysfunction in a rat model of acute sepsis. *Br J Anaesth.* 2013;110:472–80.

60. Rodriguez C, Mayo JC, Sainz RM, Antolín I, Herrera F, Martín V, et al. Regulation of antioxidant enzymes: a significant role for melatonin. *J Pineal Res.* 2004;36:1–9.

61. D'Aquila P, Bellizzi D, Passarino G. Mitochondria in health, aging and diseases: The epigenetic perspective. *Biogerontology.* 2015;16:569–85.

62. Vinck EM, Cagnie BJ, Cornelissen MJ, Declercq HA, Cambier DC. Increased fibroblast proliferation induced by light emitting diode and low power laser irradiation. *Lasers Med Sci.* 2003;18:95–9.

63. Stepanov YV, Golovynska I, Golovynskyi S, Garmanchuk LV, Gorbach O, Stepanova LI, et al. Red and near infrared light-stimulated angiogenesis mediated via Ca2+ influx, VEGF production and NO synthesis in endothelial cells in macrophage or malignant environments. *J Photochem Photobiol B.* 2022;227:112388.

64. Meng C, He Z, Xing D. Low-level laser therapy rescues dendrite atrophy via upregulating BDNF expression: implications for Alzheimer's disease. *J Neurosci.* 2013;33:13505–17.

65. Chen X, Zhou Y, Huang J, An D, Li L, Dong Y, et al. The effects of blue and red light color combinations on the growth and immune performance of juvenile steelhead trout, Oncorhynchus mykiss. *Aquac Rep.* 2022;24:101156.

66. Drohomirecka A, Iwaszko A, Walski T, Pliszczak-Król A, Wąż G, Graczyk S, et al. Low-level light therapy reduces platelet destruction during extracorporeal circulation. *Sci Rep.* 2018;8:16963.

67. Ishiguro M, Ikeda K, Tomita K. Effect of near-infrared light-emitting diodes on nerve regeneration. *J Orthop Sci.* 2010;15:233–9.

68. Gerbi MEM, Marques AMC, Ramalho LMP, Ponzi EAC, Carvalho CM, Santos RDC, et al. Infrared laser light further improves bone healing when associated with bone morphogenic proteins: an in vivo study in a rodent model. *Photomed Laser Surg.* 2008;26:55–60.

69. Khan I, Arany PR. Photobiomodulation therapy promotes expansion of epithelial colony forming units. *Photomed Laser Surg.* 2016;34:550–5.

70. Da Silva D, Crous A, Abrahamse H. Photobiomodulation: An effective approach to en-

hance proliferation and differentiation of adipose-derived stem cells into osteoblasts. *Stem Cells Int.* 2021;2021:8843179.

71. Wang Y, Huang Y-Y, Wang Y, Lyu P, Hamblin MR. Red (660 nm) or near-infrared (810 nm) photobiomodulation stimulates, while blue (415 nm), green (540 nm) light inhibits proliferation in human adipose-derived stem cells. *Sci Rep.* 2017;7:7781.

72. Li X, Hou W, Wu X, Jiang W, Chen H, Xiao N, et al. 660 nm red light-enhanced bone marrow mesenchymal stem cell transplantation for hypoxic-ischemic brain damage treatment. *Neural Regen Res.* 2014;9:236–42.

73. Tuby H, Maltz L, Oron U. Induction of autologous mesenchymal stem cells in the bone marrow by low-level laser therapy has profound beneficial effects on the infarcted rat heart. *Lasers Surg Med.* 2011;43:401–9.

74. Abrahamse H. Regenerative medicine, stem cells, and low-level laser therapy: Future directives. *Photomed Laser Surg.* 2012;30:681–2.

75. Ganeshan V, Skladnev NV, Kim JY, Mitrofanis J, Stone J, Johnstone DM. Preconditioning with remote photobiomodulation modulates the brain transcriptome and protects against MPTP insult in mice. *Neuroscience.* 2019;400:85–97.

76. Gordon LC, Martin KL, Torres N, Benabid A-L, Mitrofanis J, Stone J, et al. Remote photobiomodulation targeted at the abdomen or legs provides effective neuroprotection against parkinsonian MPTP insult. *Eur J Neurosci.* 2023;57:1611–24.

77. Dos Santos Malavazzi TC, Fernandes KPS, Lopez TCC, Rodrigues MFSD, Horliana ACRT, Bussadori SK, et al. Effects of the invasive and non-invasive systemic photobiomodulation using low-level laser in experimental models: A systematic review. *Lasers Med Sci.* 2023;38:137.

78. Lopez TCC, Malavazzi TCDS, Rodrigues MFSD, Bach EE, Silva DT, Hi EMB, et al. Histological and biochemical effects of preventive and therapeutic vascular photobiomodulation on rat muscle injury. *J Biophotonics.* 2022;15:e202100271.

79. Tobelem D da C, Andreo L, Silva T, Mala-vazzi TCS, Martinelli A, Horliana ACRT, et al. Systemic vascular photobiomodulation accelerates the recovery of motor activity in rats following spinal cord injury. *Lasers Surg Med.* 2023;55:577–89.

80. Araujo T, Andreo L, Tobelem D da C, Silva T, Malavazzi TCDS, Martinelli A, et al. Effects of systemic vascular photobiomodulation using LED or laser on sensory-motor recovery following a peripheral nerve injury in Wistar rats. *Photochem Photobiol Sci.* 2023;22:567–77.

81. Bicknell B, Liebert A, Johnstone D, Kiat H. Photobiomodulation of the microbiome: implications for metabolic and inflammatory diseases. *Lasers Med Sci.* 2019;34:317–27.

82. Chen Q, Wu J, Dong X, Yin H, Shi X, Su S, et al. Gut flora-targeted photobiomodulation therapy improves senile dementia in an Aß-induced Alzheimer's disease animal model. *J Photochem Photobiol B.* 2021;216:112152.

83. Hopkins JT, McLoda TA, Seegmiller JG, David Baxter G. Low-level laser therapy facilitates superficial wound healing in humans: A triple-blind, sham-controlled study. *J Athl Train.* 2004;39:223–9.

84. Gabel CP, Petrie SR, Mischoulon D, Hamblin MR, Yeung A, Sangermano L, et al. A case control series for the effect of photobiomodulation in patients with low back pain and concurrent depression. *Laser Ther.* 2018;27:167–73.

85. Liebert A, Bicknell B, Laakso E-L, Jalilitabaei P, Tilley S, Kiat H, et al. Remote photobiomodulation treatment for the clinical signs of Parkinson's disease: A case series conducted during COVID-19. *Photobiomodul Photomed Laser Surg.* 2022;40:112–22.

86. Elbaz-Greener G, Sud M, Tzuman O, Leitman M, Vered Z, Ben-Dov N, et al. Adjunctive laser-stimulated stem-cells therapy to primary reperfusion in acute myocardial infarction in humans: Safety and feasibility study. *J Interv Cardiol.* 2018;31:711–6.

87. Tuby H, Maltz L, Oron U. Induction of autologous mesenchymal stem cells in the bone marrow by low-level laser therapy has profound beneficial effects on the infarcted rat heart. *Lasers Surg Med.* 2011;43:401–9.

88. Blatt A, Elbaz-Greener GA, Tuby H, Maltz L, Siman-Tov Y, Ben-Aharon G, et al. Low-level laser therapy to the bone marrow reduces scarring and improves heart function post-acute myocardial infarction in the pig. *Photomed Laser Surg.* 2016;34:516–24.

89. Oron A, Oron U. Low-level laser therapy to the bone marrow ameliorates neurodegenerative disease progression in a mouse model of Alzheimer's disease: A minireview. *Photomed Laser Surg.* 2016;34:627–30.

90. Oron U, Tuby H, Maltz L, Sagi-Assif O, Abu-Hamed R, Yaakobi T, et al. Autologous bone-marrow stem cells stimulation reverses post-ischemic-reperfusion kidney injury in rats. *Am J Nephrol.* 2014;40:425–33.

91. Momenzadeh S, Abbasi M, Ebadifar A, Aryani M, Bayrami J, Nematollahi F. The intravenous laser blood irradiation in chronic pain and fibromyalgia. *J Lasers Med Sci.* 2015;6:6–9.

92. Salehpour F, Gholipour-Khalili S, Farajdokht F, Kamari F, Walski T, Hamblin MR, et al. Therapeutic potential of intranasal photobiomodulation therapy for neurological and neuropsychiatric disorders: A narrative review. *Rev Neurosci.* 2020;31:269–86.

93. Melchinger H, Jain K, Tyagi T, Hwa J. Role of platelet mitochondria: Life in a nucleus-free zone. *Front Cardiovasc Med.* 2019;6:153.

94. Al Amir Dache Z, Otandault A, Tanos R, Pastor B, Meddeb R, Sanchez C, et al. Blood contains circulating cell-free respiratory competent mitochondria. *FASEB J.* 2020;34:3616–30.

95. Mi X-Q, Chen J-Y, Liang Z-J, Zhou L-W. In vitro effects of helium-neon laser irradiation on human blood: blood viscosity and deformability of erythrocytes. *Photomed Laser Surg.* 2004;22:477–82.

96. Arany PR, Cho A, Hunt TD, Sidhu G, Shin K, Hahm E, et al. Photoactivation of endogenous latent transforming growth factor-β1 directs dental stem cell differentiation for regeneration. *Sci Transl Med.* 2014;6:238ra69.

97. Larson C, Oronsky B, Carter CA, Oronsky A, Knox SJ, Sher D, et al. TGF-beta: a master immune regulator. *Expert Opin Ther Targets.* 2020;24:427–38.

98. Lodyga M, Hinz B. TGF-β1—A truly transforming growth factor in fibrosis and immunity. *Semin Cell Dev Biol.* 2020;101:123–39.

99. Shan Y-C, Fang W, Wu J-H. A system based on photoplethysmography and photobiomodulation for autonomic nervous system measurement and adjustment. *Life* (Basel) [Internet]. 2023;13. Available from: http://dx.doi.org/10.3390/life13020564

100. Forsey JD, Merrigan JJ, Stone JD, Stephenson MD, Ramadan J, Galster SM, et al. Whole-body photobiomodulation improves post-exercise recovery but does not affect performance or physiological response during maximal anaerobic cycling. *Lasers Med Sci.* 2023;38:111.

101. Pinto HD, Vanin AA, Miranda EF, Tomazoni SS, Johnson DS, Albuquerque-Pontes GM, et al. Photobiomodulation Therapy Improves Performance and Accelerates Recovery of High-Level Rugby Players in Field Test: A Randomized, Crossover, Double-Blind, Placebo-Controlled Clinical Study. *J Strength Cond Res.* 2016;30:3329–38.

102. Hussien H, Hanafy H, Abo Elainin M, Osman D. Effect of low level laser therapy versus pulsed electromagnetic field on cortisol level in primary dysmenorrhea: A randomized controlled trial. *Egyptian Journal of Physical Therapy.* 2022;9:15–20.

103. Lin M-L, Wu J-H, Lin C-W, Su C-T, Wu H-C, Shih Y-S, et al. Clinical effects of laser acupuncture plus Chinese cupping on the pain and plasma cortisol levels in patients with chronic nonspecific lower back pain: A randomized controlled trial. *Evid Based Complement Alternat Med.* 2017;2017:3140403.

104. Slominski AT, Slominski RM, Raman C, Chen JY, Athar M, Elmets C. Neuroendocrine signaling in the skin with a special focus on the epidermal neuropeptides. *Am J Physiol Cell Physiol.* 2022;323:C1757–76.

Chapter Three: The Benefits of Red and Near-Infrared Light Therapy

1. Pugliese LS, Medrado AP, Reis SR de A, Andrade Z de A. The influence of low-level laser therapy on biomodulation of collagen and

elastic fibers. *Pesqui Odontol Bras.* 2003;17:307–13.

2. Mamalis A, Siegel D, Jagdeo J. Visible red light emitting diode photobiomodulation for skin fibrosis: Key molecular pathways. *Curr Dermatol Rep.* 2016;5:121–8.

3. Calderhead RG, Tanaka Y. Photobiological basics and clinical indications of phototherapy for skin rejuvenation. *Photomedicine— Advances in Clinical Practice.* InTech; 2017.

4. Avci P, Gupta A, Sadasivam M, Vecchio D, Pam Z, Pam N, et al. Low-level laser (light) therapy (LLLT) in skin: Stimulating, healing, restoring. *Semin Cutan Med Surg.* 2013;32:41–52.

5. Jiang M, Yan F, Avram M, Lu Z. A prospective study of the safety and efficacy of a combined bipolar radiofrequency, intense pulsed light, and infrared diode laser treatment for global facial photoaging. *Lasers Med Sci.* 2017;32:1051–61.

6. Kim H-K, Choi J-H. Effects of radiofrequency, electroacupuncture, and low-level laser therapy on the wrinkles and moisture content of the forehead, eyes, and cheek. *J Phys Therapy Sci.* 2017;29:290–4.

7. Barolet D, Roberge CJ, Auger FA, Boucher A, Germain L. Regulation of skin collagen metabolism in vitro using a pulsed 660 nm LED light source: clinical correlation with a single-blinded study. *J Invest Dermatol.* 2009;129:2751–9.

8. Wunsch A, Matuschka K. A controlled trial to determine the efficacy of red and near-infrared light treatment in patient satisfaction, reduction of fine lines, wrinkles, skin roughness, and intradermal collagen density increase. *Photomed Laser Surg.* 2014;32:93–100.

9. Andrade F do S da SD, Clark RM de O, Ferreira ML. Effects of low-level laser therapy on wound healing. *Rev Col Bras Cir.* 2014;41:129–33.

10. Barolet D. Accelerating ablative fractional resurfacing wound healing recovery by photobiomodulation. *Curr Dermatol Rep.* 2016;5:232–8.

11. Zhang P, Wu MX. A clinical review of phototherapy for psoriasis. *Lasers Med Sci.* 2018;33:173–80.

12. Ablon G. Combination 830-nm and 633-nm light-emitting diode phototherapy shows promise in the treatment of recalcitrant psoriasis: Preliminary findings. *Photomed Laser Surg.* 2010;28:141–6.

13. Nestor MS, Swenson N, Macri A, Manway M, Paparone P. Efficacy and tolerability of a combined 445 nm and 630 nm over-the-counter light therapy mask with and without topical salicylic acid versus topical benzoyl peroxide for the treatment of mild-to-moderate acne vulgaris. *J Clin Aesthet Dermatol.* 2016;9:25–35.

14. Ng JNC, Wanitphakdeedecha R, Yan C. Efficacy of home-use light-emitting diode device at 637 and 854-nm for facial rejuvenation: A split-face pilot study. *J Cosmet Dermatol.* 2020;19:2288–94.

15. Lee YI, Lee E, Nam K-H, Shin DY, Kim J, Suk J, et al. The use of a light-emitting diode device for neck rejuvenation and its safety on thyroid glands. *J Clin Med.* 2021;10:1774.

16. Wang JY, Kabakova M, Patel P, Bitterman D, Zafar K, Philip R, et al. Outstanding user reported satisfaction for light emitting diodes under-eye rejuvenation. *Arch Derm Res.* 2024;316:511.

17. Barolet D. Dual effect of photobiomodulation on Melasma: Downregulation of hyperpigmentation and enhanced solar resistance—A pilot study. *J Clin Aesthet Dermatol.* 2018;11:28–34.

18. Mineroff J, Austin E, Feit E, Ho A, Lowe B, Marson J, et al. Male facial rejuvenation using a combination 633, 830, and 1072 nm LED face mask. *Arch Derm Res.* 2023;315:2605–11.

19. Zhang Y, Su J, Ma K, Fu X, Zhang C. Photobiomodulation therapy with different wavebands for hair loss: A systematic review and meta-analysis. *Dermatol Surg.* 2022;48:737–40.

20. Gupta AK, Carviel JL. Meta-analysis of photobiomodulation for the treatment of androgenetic alopecia. *J Dermatolog Treat.* 2021;32:643–7.

21. Gupta AK, Bamimore MA. Factors influencing the effect of photobiomodulation in the treatment of androgenetic alopecia: A systematic review and analyses of summary-level data. *Dermatol Ther.* 2020;33:e14191.

22. Suchonwanit P, Chalermroj N, Khunkhet S. Low-level laser therapy for the treatment of androgenetic alopecia in Thai men and women: a 24-week, randomized, double-blind, sham device-controlled trial. *Lasers Med Sci.* 2019;34:1107–14.

23. Lanzafame RJ, Blanche RR, Chiacchierini RP, Kazmirek ER, Sklar JA. The growth of human scalp hair in females using visible red light laser and LED sources. *Lasers Surg Med.* 2014;46:601–7.

24. Willey A, Torrontegui J, Azpiazu J, Landa N. Hair stimulation following laser and intense pulsed light photo-epilation: review of 543 cases and ways to manage it. *Lasers Surg Med.* 2007;39:297–301.

25. Jimenez JJ, Wikramanayake TC, Bergfeld W, Hordinsky M, Hickman JG, Hamblin MR, et al. Efficacy and safety of a low-level laser device in the treatment of male and female pattern hair loss: a multicenter, randomized, sham device-controlled, double-blind study. *Am J Clin Dermatol.* 2014;15:115–27.

26. Dodd EM, Winter MA, Hordinsky MK, Sadick NS, Farah RS. Photobiomodulation therapy for androgenetic alopecia: A clinician's guide to home-use devices cleared by the Federal Drug Administration. *J Cosmet Laser Ther.* 2018;20:159–67.

27. Adil A, Godwin M. The effectiveness of treatments for androgenetic alopecia: A systematic review and meta-analysis. *J Am Acad Dermatol.* 2017;77:136–41.e5.

28. Gold MH, Khatri KA, Hails K, Weiss RA, Fournier N. Reduction in thigh circumference and improvement in the appearance of cellulite with dual-wavelength, low-level laser energy and massage. *J Cosmet Laser Ther.* 2011;13:13–20.

29. Lach E. Reduction of subcutaneous fat and improvement in cellulite appearance by dual-wavelength, low-level laser energy combined with vacuum and massage. *J Cosmet Laser Ther.* 2008;10:202–9.

30. Vranova J, Remlova E, Jelinkova H, Rosina J, Dostalova T. Comparison of quality of facial scars after single low-level laser therapy and combined low-level with high-level (PDL 595 nm) laser therapy. *Dermatol Ther.* 2015;28:201–9.

31. Kim YH, Kim HK, Choi JW, Kim YC. Photobiomodulation therapy with an 830-nm light-emitting diode for the prevention of thyroidectomy scars: a randomized, double-blind, sham device-controlled clinical trial. *Lasers Med Sci.* 2022;37:3583–90.

32. Jana Neto FC, Martimbianco ALC, Mesquita-Ferrari RA, Bussadori SK, Alves GP, Almeida PVD, et al. Effects of multiwavelength photobiomodulation for the treatment of traumatic soft tissue injuries associated with bone fractures: A double-blind, randomized controlled clinical trial. *J Biophotonics.* 2023;16:e202200299.

33. Haze A, Gavish L, Elishoov O, Shorka D, Tsohar T, Gellman YN, et al. Treatment of diabetic foot ulcers in a frail population with severe co-morbidities using at-home photobiomodulation laser therapy: a double-blind, randomized, sham-controlled pilot clinical study. *Lasers Med Sci.* 2022;37:919–28.

34. Bosatra M, Jucci A, Olliaro P, Quacci D, Sacchi S. In vitro fibroblast and dermis fibroblast activation by laser irradiation at low energy. An electron microscopic study. *Dermatologica.* 1984;168:157–62.

35. Trelles MA, Allones I. Red light-emitting diode (LED) therapy accelerates wound healing post-blepharoplasty and periocular laser ablative resurfacing. *J Cosmet Laser Ther.* 2006;8:39–42.

36. de Lima FJC, Barbosa FT, de Sousa-Rodrigues CF. Use alone or in combination of red and infrared laser in skin wounds. *J Lasers Med Sci.* 2014;5:51–7.

37. Mester E, Mester AF, Mester A. The biomedical effects of laser application. *Lasers Surg Med.* 1985;5:31–9.

38. Kana JS, Hutschenreiter G, Haina D, Waidelich W. Effect of low-power density laser radiation on healing of open skin wounds in rats. *Arch Surg.* 1981;116:293–6.

39. Hamblin MR. Mechanisms and applications of the anti-inflammatory effects of photobiomodulation. *AIMS Biophys.* 2017;4:337–61.

40. Ruaro JA, Fréz AR, Ruaro MB, Nicolau RA. Low-level laser therapy to treat fibromyalgia. *Lasers Med Sci.* 2014;29:1815–9.

41. Armagan O, Tascioglu F, Ekim A, Oner C. Long-term efficacy of low level laser therapy

in women with fibromyalgia: A placebo-controlled study. *Journal of Back and Musculoskeletal Rehabilitation*. 2006;19:135–40.

42. Gür A, Karakoç M, Nas K, Cevik R, Saraç J, Demir E. Efficacy of low power laser therapy in fibromyalgia: a single-blind, placebo-controlled trial. *Lasers Med Sci*. 2002;17:57–61.

43. da Silva MM, Albertini R, de Tarso Camillo de Carvalho P, Leal-Junior ECP, Bussadori SK, Vieira SS, et al. Randomized, blinded, controlled trial on effectiveness of photobiomodulation therapy and exercise training in the fibromyalgia treatment. *Lasers Med Sci*. 2018;33:343–51.

44. Navarro-Ledesma S, Carroll J, Burton P, Ana G-M. Short-Term Effects of Whole-Body Photobiomodulation on Pain, Quality of Life and Psychological Factors in a Population Suffering from Fibromyalgia: A Triple-Blinded Randomised Clinical Trial. *Pain Ther*. 2023;12:225–39.

45. Navarro-Ledesma S, Carroll J, González-Muñoz A, Pruimboom L, Burton P. Changes in Circadian Variations in Blood Pressure, Pain Pressure Threshold and the Elasticity of Tissue after a Whole-Body Photobiomodulation Treatment in Patients with Fibromyalgia: A Tripled-Blinded Randomized Clinical Trial. *Biomedicines* [Internet]. 2022;10. Available from: http://dx.doi.org/10.3390/biomedicines10112678.

46. Komaroff AL. Inflammation correlates with symptoms in chronic fatigue syndrome. *Proc Natl Acad Sci U S A*. 2017;114:8914–6.

47. Montoya JG, Holmes TH, Anderson JN, Maecker HT, Rosenberg-Hasson Y, Valencia IJ, et al. Cytokine signature associated with disease severity in chronic fatigue syndrome patients. *Proc Natl Acad Sci U S A*. 2017;114:E7150–8.

48. Romano GF, Tomassi S, Russell A, Mondelli V, Pariante CM. Fibromyalgia and chronic fatigue: the underlying biology and related theoretical issues. *Adv Psychosom Med*. 2015;34:61–77.

49. Myhill S, Booth NE, McLaren-Howard J. Chronic fatigue syndrome and mitochondrial dysfunction. *Int J Clin Exp Med*. 2009;2:1–16.

50. Natelson BH. Brain dysfunction as one cause of CFS symptoms including difficulty with attention and concentration. *Front Physiol*. 2013;4:109.

51. Hossein-Khannazer N, Kazem Arki M, Keramatinia L, Rezaei-Tavirani M. Low-level laser therapy in the treatment of autoimmune thyroiditis. *J Lasers Med Sci*. 2022;13:e34.

52. Berisha-Muharremi V, Tahirbegolli B, Phypers R, Hanna R. Efficacy of Combined Photobiomodulation Therapy with Supplements versus Supplements alone in Restoring Thyroid Gland Homeostasis in Hashimoto Thyroiditis: A Clinical Feasibility Parallel Trial with 6-Months Follow-Up. *J Pers Med* [Internet]. 2023;13. Available from: http://dx.doi.org/10.3390/jpm13081274

53. Höfling DB, Chavantes MC, Juliano AG, Cerri GG, Knobel M, Yoshimura EM, et al. Low-level laser in the treatment of patients with hypothyroidism induced by chronic autoimmune thyroiditis: a randomized, placebo-controlled clinical trial. *Lasers Med Sci*. 2013;28:743–53.

54. Hofling D, Chavantes MC, Buchpiguel CA, Cerri GG, Carneiro PC, Marui S, et al. Long-Term Follow-up of Patients with Hypothyroidism Induced by Autoimmune Thyroiditis Submitted to Low-Level Laser Therapy. 2017 [accessed 2024 Dec 8]; available from: https://observatorio.fm.usp.br/handle/OPI/21653

55. Höfling DB, Chavantes MC, Juliano AG, Cerri GG, Romão R, Yoshimura EM, et al. Low-level laser therapy in chronic autoimmune thyroiditis: a pilot study. *Lasers Surg Med*. 2010;42:589–96.

56. Поляков АВ. Применение низкоинтенсивного лазерного излучения в комплексном лечении хронического аутоиммунного тиреоидита. 1997 [accessed 2024 Dec 8]; Available from: https://medical-diss.com/medicina/primenenie-nizkointensivnogo-lazernogo-izlucheniya-v-kompleksnom-lechenii-hronicheskogo-autoimmunnogo-tireoidita.

57. Gopkalova I, Dubovik V, Danilevsky V. Effectiveness of using laser therapy in the treatment of autoimmune thyroiditis [Internet]. [accessed 2024 Dec 8]. Available from: https://ieeexplore.ieee.org/document/1251243

58. Кривова ВА. Неинвазивная гемолазеротерапия

в системе реабилитации больных аутоиммунным тиреодитом [Internet] [кандидат медицинских наук]. [Москва]; 2010 [accessed 2024 Dec 8]. Available from: https://dissercat.com/content/neinvazivnaya -gemolazeroterapiya-v-sisteme-reabilitatsii -bolnykh-autoimmunnym-tireoditom.

59. Heiskanen V. Hypothyroidism: Could it be treated with LIGHT? [Internet]. [accessed 2024 Dec 8]. Available from: http://valtsus .blogspot.com/2015/09/hypothyroidism-could -it-be-treated-with.html

60. Myakishev-Rempel M, Stadler I, Brondon P, Axe DR, Friedman M, Nardia FB, et al. A preliminary study of the safety of red light phototherapy of tissues harboring cancer. *Photomed Laser Surg.* 2012;30:551–8.

61. Austin E, Huang A, Wang JY, Cohen M, Heilman E, Maverakis E, et al. Red light phototherapy using light-emitting diodes inhibits melanoma proliferation and alters tumor microenvironments. *Front Oncol.* 2022;12:928484.

62. Santana-Blank LA, Rodríguez-Santana E, Vargas F, Reyes H, Fernández-Andrade P, Rukos S, et al. Phase I trial of an infrared pulsed laser device in patients with advanced neoplasias. *Clin Cancer Res.* 2002;8:3082–91.

63. Santana-Blank L, Rodríguez-Santana E, Santana Rodríguez KE. Concurrence of emerging developments in photobiomodulation and cancer. *Photomed Laser Surg.* 2012;30:615–6.

64. Santana-Blank L, Rodríguez-Santana E, Reyes H, Santana-Rodríguez J, Santana-Rodríguez K. Water-light interaction: A novel pathway for multi hallmark therapy in cancer. *Int J Cancer Ther Oncol* [Internet]. 2013;2. Available from: http://dx.doi.org/10.14319 /ijcto.0201.2

65. Coussens LM, Zitvogel L, Palucka AK. Neutralizing tumor-promoting chronic inflammation: a magic bullet? *Science.* 2013;339:286–91.

66. Tanaka Y, Matsuo K, Yuzuriha S, Yan H, Nakayama J. Non-thermal cytocidal effect of infrared irradiation on cultured cancer cells using specialized device. *Cancer Sci.* 2010;101:1396–402.

67. Traitcheva N, Angelova P, Radeva M, Berg H. ELF fields and photooxidation yielding lethal effects on cancer cells. *Bioelectromagnetics.* 2003;24:148–50.

68. Radeva M, Berg H. Differences in lethality between cancer cells and human lymphocytes caused by LF-electromagnetic fields. *Bioelectromagnetics.* 2004;25:503–7.

69. Wang F, Chen T-S, Xing D, Wang J-J, Wu Y-X. Measuring dynamics of caspase-3 activity in living cells using FRET technique during apoptosis induced by high fluence low-power laser irradiation. *Lasers Surg Med.* 2005;36:2–7.

70. Robijns J, Censabella S, Claes S, Pannekoeke L, Bussé L, Colson D, et al. Prevention of acute radiodermatitis by photobiomodulation: A randomized, placebo-controlled trial in breast cancer patients (TRANSDERMIS trial). *Lasers Surg Med.* 2018;50:763–71.

71. Robijns J, Censabella S, Claes S, Pannekoeke L, Bussé L, Colson D, et al. Biophysical skin measurements to evaluate the effectiveness of photobiomodulation therapy in the prevention of acute radiation dermatitis in breast cancer patients. *Support Care Cancer.* 2019;27:1245–54.

72. Robijns J, Lodewijckx J, Claes S, Van Bever L, Pannekoeke L, Censabella S, et al. Photobiomodulation therapy for the prevention of acute radiation dermatitis in head and neck cancer patients (DERMISHEAD trial). *Radiother Oncol.* 2021;158:268–75.

73. Robijns J, Lodewijckx J, Puts S, Vanmechelen S, Van Bever L, Claes S, et al. Photobiomodulation therapy for the prevention of acute radiation dermatitis in breast cancer patients undergoing hypofractioned whole-breast irradiation (LABRA trial). *Lasers Surg Med.* 2022;54:374–83.

74. Joy L, Jolien R, Marithé C, Stijn E, Laura S, Hilde L, et al. The use of photobiomodulation therapy for the prevention of chemotherapy-induced peripheral neuropathy: a randomized, placebo-controlled pilot trial (NEUROLASER trial). *Support Care Cancer.* 2022;30:5509–17.

75. Kuhn-Dall'Magro A, Zamboni E, Fontana T, Dogenski LC, De Carli JP, Dall'Magro E, et al. Low-level laser therapy in the management of oral mucositis induced by radiotherapy: A randomized double-blind clinical trial. *J Contemp Dent Pract.* 2022;23:31–6.

76. Louzeiro GC, Teixeira D da S, Cherubini K, de Figueiredo MAZ, Salum FG. Does laser photobiomodulation prevent hyposalivation in patients undergoing head and neck radiotherapy? A systematic review and meta-analysis of controlled trials. *Crit Rev Oncol Hematol.* 2020;156:103115.

77. Ayala-Orozco C, Galvez-Aranda D, Corona A, Seminario JM, Rangel R, Myers JN, et al. Molecular jackhammers eradicate cancer cells by vibronic-driven action. *Nat Chem.* 2024;16:456–65.

78. Kazem Shakouri S, Soleimanpour J, Salekzamani Y, Oskuie MR. Effect of low-level laser therapy on the fracture healing process. *Lasers Med Sci.* 2010;25:73–7.

79. Zein R, Selting W, Benedicenti S. Effect of low-level laser therapy on bone regeneration during osseointegration and bone graft. *Photomed Laser Surg.* 2017;35:649–58.

80. Mostafavinia A, Dehdehi L, Ghoreishi SK, Hajihossainlou B, Bayat M. Effect of in vivo low-level laser therapy on bone marrow-derived mesenchymal stem cells in ovariectomy-induced osteoporosis of rats. *J Photochem Photobiol B.* 2017;175:29–36.

81. Pinheiro ALB, Gerbi MEMM. Photoengineering of bone repair processes. *Photomed Laser Surg.* 2006;24:169–78.

82. Saebø H, Naterstad IF, Bjordal JM, Stausholm MB, Joensen J. Treatment of distal radius fracture during immobilization with an orthopedic cast: A double-blinded randomized controlled trial of photobiomodulation therapy. *Photobiomodul Photomed Laser Surg.* 2021;39:280–8.

83. Sæbø H, Naterstad IF, Joensen J, Stausholm MB, Bjordal JM. Pain and disability of conservatively treated distal radius fracture: A triple-blinded randomized placebo-controlled trial of photobiomodulation therapy. *Photobiomodul Photomed Laser Surg.* 2022;40:33–41.

84. Albarracin R, Eells J, Valter K. Photobiomodulation protects the retina from light-induced photoreceptor degeneration. *Invest Ophthalmol Vis Sci.* 2011;52:3582–92.

85. Ivandic BT, Ivandic T. Low-level laser therapy improves vision in patients with age-related macular degeneration. *Photomed Laser Surg.* 2008;26:241–5.

86. Markowitz SN, Devenyi RG, Munk MR, Croissant CL, Tedford SE, Rückert R, et al. A double-masked, randomized, sham-controlled, single-center study with photobiomodulation for the treatment of dry age-related macular degeneration. *Retina.* 2020;40:1471–82.

87. Shen W, Teo KYC, Wood JPM, Vaze A, Chidlow G, Ao J, et al. Preclinical and clinical studies of photobiomodulation therapy for macular oedema. *Diabetologia.* 2020;63:1900–15.

88. Montazeri K, Farhadi M, Fekrazad R, Chaibakhsh S, Mahmoudian S. Photobiomodulation therapy in mood disorders: a systematic review. *Lasers Med Sci.* 2022;37:3343–51.

89. Cassano P, Petrie SR, Hamblin MR, Henderson TA, Iosifescu DV. Review of transcranial photobiomodulation for major depressive disorder: targeting brain metabolism, inflammation, oxidative stress, and neurogenesis. *Neurophotonics.* 2016;3:031404.

90. Cassano P, Petrie SR, Mischoulon D, Cusin C, Katnani H, Yeung A, et al. Transcranial photobiomodulation for the treatment of major depressive disorder. The ELATED-2 pilot trial. *Photomed Laser Surg.* 2018;36:634–46.

91. Cassano P, Dording C, Thomas G, Foster S, Yeung A, Uchida M, et al. Effects of transcranial photobiomodulation with near-infrared light on sexual dysfunction. *Lasers Surg Med.* 2019;51:127–35.

92. Fahim C, Stip E, Mancini-Marie A, Mensour B, Leroux J-M, Beaudoin G, et al. Abnormal prefrontal and anterior cingulate activation in major depressive disorder during episodic memory encoding of sad stimuli. *Brain Cogn.* 2004;54:161–3.

93. Schaffer M, Bonel H, Sroka R, Schaffer PM, Busch M, Reiser M, et al. Effects of 780 nm diode laser irradiation on blood microcirculation: preliminary findings on time-dependent T1-weighted contrast-enhanced magnetic resonance imaging (MRI). *J Photochem Photobiol B.* 2000;54:55–60.

94. Schiffer F, Johnston AL, Ravichandran C, Polcari A, Teicher MH, Webb RH, et al. Psychological benefits two and four weeks after a single treatment with near-infrared light to the

forehead: a pilot study of 10 patients with major depression and anxiety. *Behav Brain Funct.* 2009;5:46.

95. Kerppers FK, Dos Santos KMMG, Cordeiro MER, da Silva Pereira MC, Barbosa D, Pezzini AA, et al. Study of transcranial photobiomodulation at 945-nm wavelength: anxiety and depression. *Lasers Med Sci.* 2020;35:1945–54.

96. Maiello M, Losiewicz OM, Bui E, Spera V, Hamblin MR, Marques L, et al. Transcranial photobiomodulation with near-infrared light for generalized anxiety disorder: A pilot study. *Photobiomodul Photomed Laser Surg.* 2019;37:644–50.

97. Disner SG, Beevers CG, Gonzalez-Lima F. Transcranial laser stimulation as neuroenhancement for attention bias modification in adults with elevated depression symptoms. *Brain Stimul.* 2016;9:780–7.

98. Mohammed HS. Transcranial low-level infrared laser irradiation ameliorates depression induced by reserpine in rats. *Lasers Med Sci.* 2016;31:1651–6.

99. Xu Z, Guo X, Yang Y, Tucker D, Lu Y, Xin N, et al. Low-level laser irradiation improves depression-like behaviors in mice. *Mol Neurobiol.* 2017;54:4551–9.

100. Salehpour F, Rasta SH, Mohaddes G, Sadigh-Eteghad S, Salarirad S. Therapeutic effects of 10-HzPulsed wave lasers in rat depression model: A comparison between near-infrared and red wavelengths. *Lasers Surg Med.* 2016;48:695–705.

101. Wu X, Alberico SL, Moges H, De Taboada L, Tedford CE, Anders JJ. Pulsed light irradiation improves behavioral outcome in a rat model of chronic mild stress. *Lasers Surg Med.* 2012;44:227–32.

102. Tanaka Y, Akiyoshi J, Kawahara Y, Ishitobi Y, Hatano K, Hoaki N, et al. Infrared radiation has potential antidepressant and anxiolytic effects in animal model of depression and anxiety. *Brain Stimul.* 2011;4:71–6.

103. Henderson TA, Morries LD. Multi-Watt near-infrared phototherapy for the treatment of comorbid depression: An open-label single-arm study. *Front Psychiatry.* 2017;8:187.

104. Henderson TA, Morries LD. Near-infrared photonic energy penetration: Can infrared phototherapy effectively reach the human brain? *Neuropsychiatr Dis Treat.* 2015;11:2191–208.

105. Lee T-L, Ding Z, Chan AS. Can transcranial photobiomodulation improve cognitive function? A systematic review of human studies. *Ageing Res Rev.* 2023;83:101786.

106. Hwang J, Castelli DM, Gonzalez-Lima F. Cognitive enhancement by transcranial laser stimulation and acute aerobic exercise. *Lasers Med Sci.* 2016;31:1151–60.

107. Blanco NJ, Maddox WT, Gonzalez-Lima F. Improving executive function using transcranial infrared laser stimulation. *J Neuropsychol.* 2017;11:14–25.

108. Vargas E, Barrett DW, Saucedo CL, Huang L-D, Abraham JA, Tanaka H, et al. Beneficial neurocognitive effects of transcranial laser in older adults. *Lasers Med Sci.* 2017;32:1153–62.

109. Chan AS, Lee T-L, Hamblin MR, Cheung M-C. Photobiomodulation enhances memory processing in older adults with mild cognitive impairment: A functional near-infrared spectroscopy study. *J Alzheimers Dis.* 2021;83:1471–80.

110. Baik JS, Lee TY, Kim NG, Pak K, Ko S-H, Min JH, et al. Effects of photobiomodulation on changes in cognitive function and regional cerebral blood flow in patients with mild cognitive impairment: A pilot uncontrolled trial. *J Alzheimers Dis.* 2021;83:1513–9.

111. Salehpour F, Majdi A, Pazhuhi M, Ghasemi F, Khademi M, Pashazadeh F, et al. Transcranial photobiomodulation improves cognitive performance in young healthy adults: A systematic review and meta-analysis. *Photobiomodul Photomed Laser Surg.* 2019;37:635–43.

112. Tumilty S, Munn J, McDonough S, Hurley DA, Basford JR, Baxter GD. Low level laser treatment of tendinopathy: a systematic review with meta-analysis. *Photomed Laser Surg.* 2010;28:3–16.

113. Bjordal JM, Lopes-Martins RAB, Iversen VV. A randomised, placebo controlled trial of low level laser therapy for activated Achilles tendinitis with microdialysis measurement of peritendinous prostaglandin E2 concentrations. *Br J Sports Med.* 2006;40:76–80; discussion 76–80.

114. de Oliveira PR, Arrebola LS, Stéfani KC, Pinfildi CE. Photobiomodulation associated with conservative treatment for Achilles tendon rupture: A double-blind, superiority, randomized controlled trial. *Arch Rehabil Res Clin Transl.* 2022;4:100219.

115. Martins JPS, de Lima CJ, Fernandes AB, Alves LP, Neto OP, Villaverde AB. Analysis of pain relief and functional recovery in patients with rotator cuff tendinopathy through therapeutic ultrasound and photobiomodulation therapy: a comparative study. *Lasers Med Sci.* 2022;37:3155–67.

116. Tumilty S, Munn J, Abbott JH, McDonough S, Hurley DA, Baxter GD. Laser therapy in the treatment of achilles tendinopathy: A pilot study. *Photomed Laser Surg.* 2008;26:25–30.

117. de Jesus JF, Spadacci-Morena DD, Rabelo ND dos A, Pinfildi CE, Fukuda TY, Plapler H. Low-level laser therapy on tissue repair of partially injured achilles tendon in rats. *Photomed Laser Surg.* 2014;32:345–50.

118. Grinsted A. Laser therapy for female and male infertility [Internet]. [accessed 2024 Dec 9]. Available from: https://www.laserannals.com/2016/12/04/laser-therapy-for-female-and-male-infertility/

119. Ohshiro T. Personal Overview of the Application of LLLT in Severely Infertile Japanese Females. *Laser Ther.* 2012;21:97–103.

120. Lanzafame RJ, de la Torre S, Leibaschoff GH. The rationale for photobiomodulation therapy of vaginal tissue for treatment of genitourinary syndrome of menopause: An analysis of its mechanism of action, and current clinical outcomes. *Photobiomodul Photomed Laser Surg.* 2019;37:395–407.

121. de la Torre S, Miller LE. Multimodal vaginal toning for bladder symptoms and quality of life in stress urinary incontinence. *Int Urogynecol J.* 2017;28:1201–7.

122. Salman Yazdi R, Bakhshi S, Jannat Alipoor F, Akhoond MR, Borhani S, Farrahi F, et al. Effect of 830-nm diode laser irradiation on human sperm motility. *Lasers Med Sci.* 2014;29:97–104.

123. Iurshin VV, Sergienko NF, Illarionov VE. Etiopathogenetic basis for using magnetolaser therapy in the complex treatment of male infertility. *Urologiia.* 2003;23–5.

124. Espey BT, Kielwein K, van der Ven H, Steger K, Allam J-P, Paradowska-Dogan A, et al. Effects of pulsed-wave photobiomodulation therapy on human spermatozoa. *Lasers Surg Med.* 2022;54:540–53.

125. Gabel CP, Carroll J, Harrison K. Sperm motility is enhanced by Low Level Laser and Light Emitting Diode photobiomodulation with a dose-dependent response and differential effects in fresh and frozen samples. *Laser Ther.* 2018;27:131–6.

126. Ahn J, Kim Y-H, Rhee C. The effects of low level laser therapy (LLLT) on the testis in elevating serum testosterone level in rats. 2013 [accessed 2024 Dec 9]; Available from: https://www.semanticscholar.org/paper/The-effects-of-low-level-laser-therapy-(LLLT)-on-th-Ahn-Kim/e437801422be789aa616b40368d17c03e47a831f.

127. Alves MBR, de Arruda RP, Batissaco L, Florez-Rodriguez SA, de Oliveira BMM, Torres MA, et al. Low-level laser therapy to recovery testicular degeneration in rams: effects on seminal characteristics, scrotal temperature, plasma testosterone concentration, and testes histopathology. *Lasers Med Sci.* 2016;31:695–704.

128. Zagatto AM, Dutra YM, Lira FS, Antunes BM, Faustini JB, Malta E de S, et al. Full body photobiomodulation therapy to induce faster muscle recovery in water polo athletes: Preliminary results. *Photobiomodul Photomed Laser Surg.* 2020;38:766–72.

129. Wehr E, Pilz S, Boehm BO, März W, Obermayer-Pietsch B. Association of vitamin D status with serum androgen levels in men. *Clin Endocrinol.* 2010;73:243–8.

130. Nimptsch K, Platz EA, Willett WC, Giovannucci E. Association between plasma 25-OH vitamin D and testosterone levels in men. *Clin Endocrinol (Oxf).* 2012;77:106–12.

131. Hegedus B, Viharos L, Gervain M, Gálfi M. The effect of low-level laser in knee osteoarthritis: A double-blind, randomized, placebo-controlled trial. *Photomed Laser Surg.* 2009;27:577–84.

132. Soleimanpour H, Gahramani K, Taheri R, Golzari SEJ, Safari S, Esfanjani RM, et al. The effect of low-level laser therapy on knee osteoarthritis: prospective, descriptive study. *Lasers Med Sci.* 2014;29:1695–700.

133. Elnaggar RK, Mahmoud WS, Abdelbasset WK, Alqahtani BA, Alrawaili SM, Elfakharany MS. Low-energy laser therapy application on knee joints as an auxiliary treatment in patients with polyarticular juvenile idiopathic arthritis: a dual-arm randomized clinical trial. *Lasers Med Sci.* 2022;37:1737–46.

134. Hamblin MR. Can osteoarthritis be treated with light? *Arthritis Res Ther.* 2013;15:120.

135. Alves AC, Vieira R, Leal-Junior E, dos Santos S, Ligeiro AP, Albertini R, et al. Effect of low-level laser therapy on the expression of inflammatory mediators and on neutrophils and macrophages in acute joint inflammation. *Arthritis Res Ther.* 2013;15:R116.

136. Khumaidi MA, Paturusi I, Nusdwinuringtyas N, Islam AA, Gunawan WB, Nurkolis F, et al. Is low-level laser therapy effective for patients with knee joint osteoarthritis? Implications and strategies to promote laser therapy usage. *Front Bioeng Biotechnol.* 2022;10:1089035.

137. Houreld NN. Shedding light on a new treatment for diabetic wound healing: A review on phototherapy. *ScientificWorldJournal.* 2014;2014:398412.

138. Feitosa MCP, Carvalho AFM de, Feitosa VC, Coelho IM, Oliveira RA de, Arisawa EÂL. Effects of the Low-Level Laser Therapy (LLLT) in the process of healing diabetic foot ulcers. *Acta Cir Bras.* 2015;30:852–7.

139. Houreld NN. Healing of diabetic ulcers using photobiomodulation. *Photomed Laser Surg.* 2015;33:237–9.

140. Maltese G, Karalliedde J, Rapley H, Amor T, Lakhani A, Gnudi L. A pilot study to evaluate the efficacy of class IV lasers on nonhealing neuroischemic diabetic foot ulcers in patients with type 2 diabetes. *Diabetes Care.* 2015;38:e152–3.

141. Cg SK, Maiya AG, Hande HM, Vidyasagar S, Rao K, Rajagopal KV. Efficacy of low level laser therapy on painful diabetic peripheral neuropathy. *Laser Ther.* 2015;24:195–200.

142. Bashiri H. Evaluation of low level laser therapy in reducing diabetic polyneuropathy related pain and sensorimotor disorders. *Acta Med Iran.* 2013;51:543–7.

143. Yamany AA, Sayed HM. Effect of low level laser therapy on neurovascular function of diabetic peripheral neuropathy. *J Adv Res.* 2012;3:21–8.

144. Powner MB, Jeffery G. Light stimulation of mitochondria reduces blood glucose levels. *J Biophotonics.* 2024;17:e202300521.

145. Linares SN, Beltrame T, Galdino GAM, Frade MCM, Milan-Mattos JC, Gois MO, et al. Dose response effect of photobiomodulation on hemodynamic responses and glucose levels in men with type 2 diabetes: A randomized, crossover, double-blind, sham-controlled trial. *Photonics.* 2022;9:481.

146. Silva G, Silva SS da, Guimarães DSPSF, Cruz MV da, Silveira LR, Rocha-Vieira E, et al. The dose-effect response of combined red and infrared photobiomodulation on insulin resistance in skeletal muscle cells. *Biochem Biophys Rep.* 2024;40:101831.

147. Silva G, Ferraresi C, de Almeida RT, Motta ML, Paixão T, Ottone VO, et al. Infrared photobiomodulation (PBM) therapy improves glucose metabolism and intracellular insulin pathway in adipose tissue of high-fat fed mice. *Lasers Med Sci.* 2018;33:559–71.

148. Zohreh V, Mokmeli S. Application of low level laser therapy (LLLT) in treatment of chronic tonsillitis: (case series). 12th International European Medical Laser Association congress (EMLA) [Internet]. Unknown; 2007. Available from: https://www.researchgate.net/publication/266675684_APPLICATION_OF_LOW_LEVEL_LASER_THERAPY_LLLT_IN_TREATMENT_OF_CHRONIC_TONSILLITIS_CASE_SERIES

149. Aggarwal H, Singh MP, Nahar P, Mathur H, Gv S. Efficacy of low-level laser therapy in treatment of recurrent aphthous ulcers—a sham controlled, split mouth follow up study. *J Clin Diagn Res.* 2014;8:218–21.

150. Ferreira DC, Reis HLB, Cavalcante FS, Santos KRND, Passos MRL. Recurrent herpes simplex infections: Laser therapy as a potential tool for long-term successful treatment. *Rev Soc Bras Med Trop.* 2011;44:397–9.

151. Genc G, Kocadereli I, Tasar F, Kilinc K, El S, Sarkarati B. Effect of low-level laser therapy (LLLT) on orthodontic tooth movement. *Lasers Med Sci.* 2013;28:41–7.

152. Seifi M, Atri F, Yazdani MM. Effects of low-level laser therapy on orthodontic tooth

movement and root resorption after artificial socket preservation. *Dent Res J* (Isfahan). 2014;11:61–6.

153. Yassaei S, Fekrazad R, Shahraki N. Effect of low level laser therapy on orthodontic tooth movement: a review article. *J Dent* (Tehran). 2013;10:264–72.

154. Maver-Biscanin M, Mravak-Stipetic M, Jerolimov V. Effect of low-level laser therapy on Candida albicans growth in patients with denture stomatitis. *Photomed Laser Surg.* 2005;23:328–32.

155. Teichert MC, Jones JW, Usacheva MN, Biel MA. Treatment of oral candidiasis with methylene blue-mediated photodynamic therapy in an immunodeficient murine model. *Oral Surg Oral Med Oral Pathol Oral Radiol Endod.* 2002;93:155–60.

156. Gerschman JA, Ruben J, Gebart-Eaglemont J. Low level laser therapy for dentinal tooth hypersensitivity. *Aust Dent* J. 1994;39:353–7.

157. Orhan K, Aksoy U, Can-Karabulut DC, Kalender A. Low-level laser therapy of dentin hypersensitivity: A short-term clinical trial. *Lasers Med Sci.* 2011;26:591–8.

158. Basso FG, Oliveira CF, Fontana A, Kurachi C, Bagnato VS, Spolidório DMP, et al. In Vitro effect of low-level laser therapy on typical oral microbial biofilms. *Braz Dent J.* 2011;22:502–10.

159. Asnaashari M, Mojahedi SM, Asadi Z, Azari-Marhabi S, Maleki A. A comparison of the antibacterial activity of the two methods of photodynamic therapy (using diode laser 810 nm and LED lamp 630 nm) against Enterococcus faecalis in extracted human anterior teeth. *Photodiagnosis Photodyn Ther.* 2016;13:233–7.

160. Rios A, He J, Glickman GN, Spears R, Schneiderman ED, Honeyman AL. Evaluation of photodynamic therapy using a light-emitting diode lamp against Enterococcus faecalis in extracted human teeth. *J Endod.* 2011;37:856–9.

161. Vieru D, Cortez M, Clayman L, Dumitriu AS. Low level laser therapy in the treatment of periodontal disease. *Laser Ther.* 2007;16:199–206.

162. Obradović R, Kesić L, Mihailović D, Jovanović G, Antić S, Brkić Z. Low-level la-

sers as an adjunct in periodontal therapy in patients with diabetes mellitus. *Diabetes Technol Ther.* 2012;14:799–803.

163. Hamblin MR, Carroll JD, de Freitas LF, Huang Y-Y, Ferraresi C. Low-level light therapy: Photobiomodulation. *SPIE*; 2018.

164. Abellán R, Gómez C, Palma JC. Effects of photobiomodulation on the upper first molar intrusion movement using mini-screws anchorage: A randomized controlled trial. *Photobiomodul Photomed Laser Surg.* 2021;39:518–27.

165. Rosero KAV, Sampaio RMF, Deboni MCZ, Corrêa L, Marques MM, Ferraz EP, et al. Photobiomodulation as an adjunctive therapy for alveolar socket preservation: a preliminary study in humans. *Lasers Med Sci.* 2020;35:1711–20.

166. Singh V, Garg A, Bhagol A, Savarna S, Agarwal SK. Photobiomodulation alleviates postoperative discomfort after mandibular third molar surgery. *J Oral Maxillofac Surg.* 2019;77:2412–21.

167. Sharifi R, Fekrazad R, Taheri MM, Kasaeian A, Babaei A. Effect of photobiomodulation on recovery from neurosensory disturbances after sagittal split ramus osteotomy: A triple-blind randomised controlled trial. *Br J Oral Maxillofac Surg.* 2020;58:535–41.

168. Hanna R, Dalvi S, Bensadoun RJ, Raber-Durlacher JE, Benedicenti S. Role of photobiomodulation therapy in neurological primary burning mouth syndrome. A systematic review and meta-analysis of human randomised controlled clinical trials. *Pharmaceutics.* 2021;13:1838.

169. Cronshaw M, Parker S, Anagnostaki E, Mylona V, Lynch E, Grootveld M. Photobiomodulation dose parameters in dentistry: A systematic review and meta-analysis. *Dent J.* 2020;8:114.

170. Mohamed AR, Shaban MM. Role of laser acupuncture in chronic respiratory diseases. *Egypt J Chest Dis Tuberc.* 2014;63:1065–70.

171. Landyshev IS, Avdeeva NV, Goborov ND, Krasavina NP, Tikhonova GA, Tkacheva SI. Efficacy of low intensity laser irradiation and sodium nedocromil in the complex treatment of patients with bronchial asthma. *Ter Arkh.* 2002;74:25–8.

172. Faradzheva NA. Efficiency of a combination of haloaerosols and helium-neon laser in the multimodality treatment of patients with bronchial asthma. *Probl Tuberk Bolezn Legk*. 2007;50–3.

173. de Lima FM, Moreira LM, Villaverde AB, Albertini R, Castro-Faria-Neto HC, Aimbire F. Low-level laser therapy (LLLT) acts as cAMP-elevating agent in acute respiratory distress syndrome. *Lasers Med Sci*. 2011;26:389–400.

174. Kashanskaia EP, Fedorov AA. Low-intensity laser radiation in the combined treatment of patients with chronic obstructive bronchitis. *Vopr Kurortol Fizioter Lech Fiz Kult*. 2009;19–22.

175. Miranda da Silva C, Peres Leal M, Brochetti RA, Braga T, Vitoretti LB, Saraiva Câmara NO, et al. Low Level Laser Therapy reduces the development of lung inflammation induced by formaldehyde exposure. *PLoS One*. 2015;10:e0142816.

176. Naghdi S, Ansari NN, Varedi M, Fathali M, Zarrin M, Kashi-Alashti M, et al. Use of low-level laser therapy for patients with chronic rhinosinusitis: A single-blind, sham-controlled clinical trial. *Lasers Med Sci*. 2022;38:5.

177. Williams RK, Raimondo J, Cahn D, Williams A, Schell D. Whole-organ transdermal photobiomodulation (PBM) of COVID-19: A 50-patient case study. *J Biophotonics*. 2022;15:e202100194.

178. Raji H, Arjmand B, Rahim F. The probable protective effect of photobiomodulation on the inflammation of the airway and lung in COVID-19 treatment: A preclinical and clinical meta-analysis. *Adv Exp Med Biol*. 2022;1376:29–44.

179. Pereira PC, de Lima CJ, Fernandes AB, Zângaro RA, Villaverde AB. Cardiopulmonary and hematological effects of infrared LED photobiomodulation in the treatment of SARS-COV2. *J Photochem Photobiol B*. 2023;238:112619.

180. Marashian SM, Hashemian M, Pourabdollah M, Nasseri M, Mahmoudian S, Reinhart F, et al. Photobiomodulation improves serum cytokine response in mild to moderate COVID-19: The first randomized, double-blind, Placebo controlled, pilot study. *Front Immunol*. 2022;13:929837.

181. Lim L, Hosseinkhah N, Van Buskirk M, Berk A, Loheswaran G, Abbaspour Z, et al. Photobiomodulation treatment with a home-use device for COVID-19: A randomized controlled trial for efficacy and safety. *Photobiomodul Photomed Laser Surg*. 2024;42:393–403.

182. Pacheco JA, Molena KF, Martins CROG, Corona SAM, Borsatto MC. Photobiomodulation (PBMT) and antimicrobial photodynamic therapy (aPDT) in oral manifestations of patients infected with Sars-CoV-2: systematic review and meta-analysis. *Bull Natl Res Cent*. 2022;46:140.

183. de Souza VB, Ferreira LT, Sene-Fiorese M, Garcia V, Rodrigues TZ, de Aquino Junior AE, et al. Photobiomodulation therapy for treatment olfactory and taste dysfunction COVID-19-related: A case report. *J Biophotonics*. 2022;15:e202200058.

184. Campos L, Soares LES, Berlingieri G, Ramires MCCH, Guirado MMG, Lyra LA de OP, et al. A Brazilian multicenter pilot case series on the efficacy of photobiomodulation therapy for COVID-19-related taste dysfunction. *Photodiagnosis Photodyn Ther*. 2022;37:102643.

185. Liebert A, Krause A, Goonetilleke N, Bicknell B, Kiat H. A role for photobiomodulation in the prevention of myocardial ischemic reperfusion injury: A systematic review and potential molecular mechanisms. *Sci Rep*. 2017;7:42386.

186. Gao X, Zhang W, Yang F, Ma W, Cai B. Photobiomodulation regulation as one promising therapeutic approach for myocardial infarction. *Oxid Med Cell Longev*. 2021;2021:9962922.

187. Hentschke VS, Jaenisch RB, Schmeing LA, Cavinato PR, Xavier LL, Dal Lago P. Low-level laser therapy improves the inflammatory profile of rats with heart failure. *Lasers Med Sci*. 2013;28:1007–16.

188. Tuby H, Maltz L, Oron U. Induction of autologous mesenchymal stem cells in the bone marrow by low-level laser therapy has profound beneficial effects on the infarcted rat heart. *Lasers Surg Med*. 2011;43:401–9.

189. Khanna A, Shankar LR, Keelan MH, Kornowski R, Leon M, Moses J, et al. Augmentation of the expression of proangiogenic genes

in cardiomyocytes with low dose laser irradiation in vitro. *Cardiovasc Radiat Med.* 1999;1:265–9.

190. Blatt A, Elbaz-Greener GA, Tuby H, Maltz L, Siman-Tov Y, Ben-Aharon G, et al. Low-level laser therapy to the bone marrow reduces scarring and improves heart function post-acute myocardial infarction in the pig. *Photomed Laser Surg.* 2016;34:516–24.

191. Carlos FP, Gradinetti V, Manchini M, de Tarso Camillo de Carvalho P, Silva JA Jr, Girardi ACC, et al. Role of low-level laser therapy on the cardiac remodeling after myocardial infarction: A systematic review of experimental studies. *Life Sci.* 2016;151:109–14.

192. Manchini MT, Serra AJ, Feliciano R dos S, Santana ET, Antônio EL, de Tarso Camillo de Carvalho P, et al. Amelioration of cardiac function and activation of anti-inflammatory vasoactive peptides expression in the rat myocardium by low level laser therapy. *PLoS One.* 2014;9:e101270.

193. Kazemi Khoo N, Babazadeh K, Lajevardi M, Dabaghian FH, Mostafavi E. Application of low-Level Laser Therapy following coronary artery bypass grafting (CABG) surgery. *J Lasers Med Sci.* 2014;5:86–91.

194. De Scheerder IK, Wang K, Zhou XR, Szilard M, Verbeken E, Ping QB, et al. Intravascular low-power red laser light as an adjunct to coronary stent implantation: initial clinical experience. *Catheter Cardiovasc Interv.* 2000;49:468–71.

195. De Scheerder I, Wang K, Nikolaychik V, Kaul U, Singh B, Sahota H, et al. Long-term follow-up after coronary stenting and intravascular red laser therapy. *Am J Cardiol.* 2000;86:927–30.

196. Derkacz A, Protasiewicz M, Poreba R, Szuba A, Andrzejak R. Usefulness of intravascular low-power laser illumination in preventing restenosis after percutaneous coronary intervention. *Am J Cardiol.* 2010;106:1113–7.

197. Oliveira-Junior MC, Monteiro AS, Leal-Junior ECP, Munin E, Osório RAL, Ribeiro W, et al. Low-level laser therapy ameliorates CCl4-induced liver cirrhosis in rats. *Photochem Photobiol.* 2013;89:173–8.

198. Araújo TG, de Oliveira AG, Tobar N, Saad MJA, Moreira LR, Reis ER, et al. Liver regeneration following partial hepatectomy is improved by enhancing the HGF/Met axis and Akt and Erk pathways after low-power laser irradiation in rats. *Lasers Med Sci.* 2013;28:1511–7.

199. Irani S, Mohseni Salehi Monfared SS, Akbari-Kamrani M, Ostad SN, Abdollahi M, Larijani B. Effect of low-level laser irradiation on in vitro function of pancreatic islets. *Transplant Proc.* 2009;41:4313–5.

200. Tatmatsu-Rocha JC, de Castro CA, Sene-Fiorese M, Parizotto NA. Light-emitting diode modulates carbohydrate metabolism by pancreatic duct regeneration. *Lasers Med Sci.* 2017;32:1747–55.

201. Cotler HB, Chow RT, Hamblin MR, Carroll J. The Use of Low Level Laser Therapy (LLLT) For Musculoskeletal Pain. *MOJ Orthop Rheumatol* [Internet]. 2015;2. Available from: http://dx.doi.org/10.15406/mojor.2015.02.00068.

202. Kingsley JD, Demchak T, Mathis R. Low-level laser therapy as a treatment for chronic pain. *Front Physiol.* 2014;5:306.

203. Chow RT, Heller GZ, Barnsley L. The effect of 300 mW, 830 nm laser on chronic neck pain: a double-blind, randomized, placebo-controlled study. *Pain.* 2006;124:201–10.

204. Huang Z, Ma J, Chen J, Shen B, Pei F, Kraus VB. The effectiveness of low-level laser therapy for nonspecific chronic low back pain: a systematic review and meta-analysis. *Arthritis Res Ther.* 2015;17:360.

205. Okuni I, Ushigome N, Harada T, Ohshiro T, Musya Y, Sekiguchi M. Low level laser therapy (LLLT) for chronic joint pain of the elbow, wrist and fingers. *Laser Ther.* 2012;21:33–7.

206. Bjordal JM, Couppé C, Chow RT, Tunér J, Ljunggren EA. A systematic review of low level laser therapy with location-specific doses for pain from chronic joint disorders. *Aust J Physiother.* 2003;49:107–16.

207. Ohkuin I, Ushigome N, Harada T, Ohshiro T, Mizutani K, Musya Y, et al. Low level laser therapy (LLLT) for patients with sacroiliac joint pain. *Laser Ther.* 2011;20:117–21.

208. Arslan H, Doğanay E, Karataş E, Ünlü MA, Ahmed HMA. Effect of low-level laser therapy on postoperative pain after root canal re-

treatment: A preliminary placebo-controlled, triple-blind, randomized clinical trial. *J Endod*. 2017;43:1765–9.

209. Alayat MS, Elsoudany AM, Ali ME. Efficacy of multiwave locked system laser on pain and function in patients with chronic neck pain: A randomized placebo-controlled trial. *Photomed Laser Surg*. 2017;35:450–5.

210. Dima R, Tieppo Francio V, Towery C, Davani S. Review of literature on low-level laser therapy benefits for nonpharmacological pain control in chronic pain and osteoarthritis. *Altern Ther Health Med*. 2018;24:8–10.

211. Lögdberg-Andersson M, Mützell S, Hazel Å. Low level laser therapy (LLLT) of tendinitis and myofascial pains a randomized, double-blind, controlled study. *Laser Ther*. 2004;14:0_79–0_84.

212. de Rezende MU, Varone BB, Martuscelli DF, Ocampos GP, Freire GMG, Pinto NC, et al. Pilot study of the effect of therapeutic photobiomodulation on postoperative pain in knee arthroplasty. *Braz J Anesthesiol*. 2022;72:159–61.

213. Bahrami H, Moharrami A, Mirghaderi P, Mortazavi SMJ. Low-level laser and light therapy after total knee arthroplasty improves postoperative pain and functional outcomes: A three-arm randomized clinical trial. *Arthroplast Today*. 2023;19:101066.

214. Santiago R, Gomes S, Ozsarfati J, Zitney M. Photobiomodulation for modulation of neuropathic pain and improvement of scar tissue. *Scars Burn Heal*. 2022;8:20595131221134052.

215. Fulop AM, Dhimmer S, Deluca JR, Johanson DD, Lenz RV, Patel KB, et al. A meta-analysis of the efficacy of laser phototherapy on pain relief. *Clin J Pain*. 2010;26:729–36.

216. DE Oliveira MF, Johnson DS, Demchak T, Tomazoni SS, Leal-Junior EC. Low-intensity LASER and LED (photobiomodulation therapy) for pain control of the most common musculoskeletal conditions. *Eur J Phys Rehabil Med*. 2022;58:282–9.

217. Ross G. Photobiomodulation therapy: A possible answer to the opioid crisis. *Photobiomodul Photomed Laser Surg*. 2019;37:667–8.

218. Schiffer F, Reichmann W, Flynn E, Hamblin MR, McCormack H. A novel treatment of opioid cravings with an effect size of .73 for unilateral transcranial photobiomodulation over sham. *Front Psychiatry*. 2020;11:827.

219. Schiffer F, Khan A, Bolger E, Flynn E, Seltzer WP, Teicher MH. An effective and safe novel treatment of opioid use disorder: Unilateral transcranial photobiomodulation. *Front Psychiatry*. 2021;12:713686.

220. Schiffer F. Unilateral transcranial photobiomodulation for opioid addiction in a clinical practice: A clinical overview and case series. *J Psychiatr Res*. 2021;133:134–41.

221. Mikhaylov VA. The use of the infrared laser therapy of 890-910 NM for the treatment of breast cancer (experimental and clinical study). *Clin Oncol* (Las Vegas) [Internet]. 2022;06. Available from: http://dx.doi.org/10.47829/coo.2022.6103.

222. Skobelkin OK, Michailov VA, Zakharov SD. Preoperative activation of the immune system by low reactive level laser therapy (LLLT) in oncologic patients: A preliminary report. *Laser Ther*. 1991;3:169–75.

223. Pereira PR, de Paula JB, Cielinski J, Pilonetto M, Von Bahten LC. Effects of low intensity laser in in vitro bacterial culture and in vivo infected wounds. *Rev Col Bras Cir*. 2014;41:49–55.

224. Chung H, Dai T, Sharma SK, Huang Y-Y, Carroll JD, Hamblin MR. The nuts and bolts of low-level laser (light) therapy. *Ann Biomed Eng*. 2012;40:516–33.

225. Yang J, Zhang Q, Li P, Dong T, Wu MX. Low-level light treatment ameliorates immune thrombocytopenia. *Sci Rep*. 2016;6:38238.

226. Zhang Q, Dong T, Li P, Wu MX. Noninvasive low-level laser therapy for thrombocytopenia. *Sci Transl Med*. 2016;8:349ra101.

227. Lugongolo MY, Manoto SL, Ombinda-Lemboumba S, Maaza M, Mthunzi-Kufa P. The effects of low level laser therapy on both HIV-1 infected and uninfected TZM-bl cells. *J Biophotonics*. 2017;10:1335–44.

228. Novoselova EG, Glushkova OV, Cherenkov DA, Chudnovsky VM, Fesenko EE. Effects of low-power laser radiation on mice immunity. *Photodermatol Photoimmunol Photomed*. 2006;22:33–8.

229. Odinokov D, Hamblin MR. Aging of lymphoid organs: Can photobiomodulation re-

verse age-associated thymic involution via stimulation of extrapineal melatonin synthesis and bone marrow stem cells? *J Biophotonics.* 2018;11:e201700282.

230. Kut'ko II, Frolov VM, Pustovoĭ IG, Pavlenko VV, Rachkauskas GS. The effect of endovascular laser therapy and antioxidants on the immune status and energy metabolism of patients with treatment-resistant forms of schizophrenia. *Zh Nevrol Psikhiatr Im S S Korsakova.* 1996;96:34–8.

231. Lyons J-A. Light therapy to treat autoimmune disease [Internet]. spie.org. 2015 [accessed 2024 Dec 9]. Available from: https://spie.org /news/5900-light-therapy-to-treat-auto immune-disease

232. Gonçalves ED, Souza PS, Lieberknecht V, Fidelis GSP, Barbosa RI, Silveira PCL, et al. Low-level laser therapy ameliorates disease progression in a mouse model of multiple sclerosis. *Autoimmunity.* 2016;49:132–42.

233. Naeser MA, Saltmarche A, Krengel MH, Hamblin MR, Knight JA. Improved cognitive function after transcranial, light-emitting diode treatments in chronic, traumatic brain injury: two case reports. *Photomed Laser Surg.* 2011;29:351–8.

234. Hipskind SG, Grover FL Jr, Fort TR, Helffenstein D, Burke TJ, Quint SA, et al. Pulsed transcranial red/near-infrared light therapy using light-emitting diodes improves cerebral blood flow and cognitive function in Veterans with chronic traumatic brain injury: A case series. *Photobiomodul Photomed Laser Surg.* 2019;37:77–84.

235. Stevens AR, Hadis M, Milward M, Ahmed Z, Belli A, Palin W, et al. Photobiomodulation in acute traumatic brain injury: A systematic review and meta-analysis. *J Neurotrauma.* 2023;40:210–27.

236. Detaboada L, Ilic S, Leichliter-Martha S, Oron U, Oron A, Streeter J. Transcranial application of low-energy laser irradiation improves neurological deficits in rats following acute stroke. *Lasers Surg Med.* 2006;38:70–3.

237. Lapchak PA. Transcranial near-infrared laser therapy applied to promote clinical recovery in acute and chronic neurodegenerative diseases. *Expert Rev Med Devices.* 2012;9:71–83.

238. Lapchak PA, Wei J, Zivin JA. Transcranial infrared laser therapy improves clinical rating scores after embolic strokes in rabbits. *Stroke.* 2004;35:1985–8.

239. Hashmi JT, Huang Y-Y, Osmani BZ, Sharma SK, Naeser MA, Hamblin MR. Role of low-level laser therapy in neurorehabilitation. *PM R.* 2010;2:S292–305.

240. Rochkind S, Barr-Nea L, Bartal A, Nissan M, Lubart R, Razon N. New methods of treatment of severely injured sciatic nerve and spinal cord. An experimental study. *Acta Neurochir Suppl* (Wien). 1988;43:91–3.

241. Byrnes KR, Waynant RW, Ilev IK, Wu X, Barna L, Smith K, et al. Light promotes regeneration and functional recovery and alters the immune response after spinal cord injury. *Lasers Surg Med.* 2005;36:171–85.

242. Wu X, Dmitriev AE, Cardoso MJ, Viers-Costello AG, Borke RC, Streeter J, et al. 810 nm Wavelength light: an effective therapy for transected or contused rat spinal cord. *Lasers Surg Med.* 2009;41:36–41.

243. da Silva FC, Gomes AO, da Costa Palácio PR, Politti F, de Fátima Teixeira da Silva D, Mesquita-Ferrari RA, et al. Photobiomodulation improves motor response in patients with spinal cord injury submitted to electromyographic evaluation: randomized clinical trial. *Lasers Med Sci.* 2018;33:883–90.

244. Salehpour F, Gholipour-Khalili S, Farajdokht F, Kamari F, Walski T, Hamblin MR, et al. Therapeutic potential of intranasal photobiomodulation therapy for neurological and neuropsychiatric disorders: A narrative review. *Rev Neurosci.* 2020;31:269–86.

245. Meng C, He Z, Xing D. Low-level laser therapy rescues dendrite atrophy via upregulating BDNF expression: Implications for Alzheimer's disease. *J Neurosci.* 2013;33:13505–17.

246. Johnstone DM, Moro C, Stone J, Benabid A-L, Mitrofanis J. Turning on lights to stop neurodegeneration: The potential of near-infrared light therapy in Alzheimer's and Parkinson's disease. *Front Neurosci.* 2015;9:500.

247. de la Torre JC. Treating cognitive impairment with transcranial low level laser therapy. *J Photochem Photobiol B.* 2017;168:149–55.

248. Hamblin MR. Shining light on the head: Photobiomodulation for brain disorders. *BBA Clin.* 2016;6:113–24.

249. Darlot F, Moro C, El Massri N, Chabrol C, Johnstone DM, Reinhart F, et al. Near-infrared light is neuroprotective in a monkey model of Parkinson disease. *Ann Neurol.* 2016;79:59–75.

250. Chao LL. Effects of Home Photobiomodulation Treatments on Cognitive and Behavioral Function, Cerebral Perfusion, and Resting-State Functional Connectivity in Patients with Dementia: A Pilot Trial. *Photobiomodul Photomed Laser Surg.* 2019;37:133–41.

251. Saltmarche AE, Naeser MA, Ho KF, Hamblin MR, Lim L. Significant Improvement in Cognition in Mild to Moderately Severe Dementia Cases Treated with Transcranial Plus Intranasal Photobiomodulation: Case Series Report. *Photomed Laser Surg.* 2017;35:432–41.

252. Swerdlow RH, Khan SM. A "mitochondrial cascade hypothesis" for sporadic Alzheimer's disease. *Med Hypotheses.* 2004;63:8–20.

253. Chaturvedi RK, Beal MF. Mitochondrial approaches for neuroprotection. *Ann N Y Acad Sci.* 2008;1147:395–412.

254. Gonzalez-Lima F, Barksdale BR, Rojas JC. Mitochondrial respiration as a target for neuroprotection and cognitive enhancement. *Biochem Pharmacol.* 2014;88:584–93.

255. Monteiro F, Carvalho Ó, Sousa N, Silva FS, Sotiropoulos I. Photobiomodulation and visual stimulation against cognitive decline and Alzheimer's disease pathology: A systematic review. *Alzheimers Dement* (NY). 2022;8:e12249.

256. Hamblin MR. Photobiomodulation for Alzheimer's Disease: Has the Light Dawned? *Photonics* [Internet]. 2019;6. Available from: http://dx.doi.org/10.3390/photonics6030077.

257. Hamilton CL, El Khoury H, Hamilton D, Nicklason F, Mitrofanis J. "buckets": Early observations on the use of red and infrared light helmets in Parkinson's disease patients. *Photobiomodul Photomed Laser Surg.* 2019;37:615–22.

258. Hong C-T, Hu C-J, Lin H-Y, Wu D. Effects of concomitant use of hydrogen water and photobiomodulation on Parkinson's disease: A pilot study. *Medicine* (Baltimore). 2021;100:e24191.

259. Liebert A, Bicknell B, Laakso E-L, Heller G, Jalilitabaei P, Tilley S, et al. Improvements in clinical signs of Parkinson's disease using photobiomodulation: A prospective proof-of-concept study. *BMC Neurol.* 2021;21:256.

260. Liebert A, Bicknell B, Laakso E-L, Jalilitabaei P, Tilley S, Kiat H, et al. Remote photobiomodulation treatment for the clinical signs of Parkinson's disease: A case series conducted during COVID-19. *Photobiomodul Photomed Laser Surg.* 2022;40:112–22.

261. Baroni BM, Rodrigues R, Freire BB, Franke R de A, Geremia JM, Vaz MA. Effect of low-level laser therapy on muscle adaptation to knee extensor eccentric training. *Eur J Appl Physiol.* 2015;115:639–47.

262. Baroni BM, Leal Junior ECP, De Marchi T, Lopes AL, Salvador M, Vaz MA. Low level laser therapy before eccentric exercise reduces muscle damage markers in humans. *Eur J Appl Physiol.* 2010;110:789–96.

263. Baroni BM, Leal Junior ECP, Geremia JM, Diefenthaeler F, Vaz MA. Effect of light-emitting diodes therapy (LEDT) on knee extensor muscle fatigue. *Photomed Laser Surg.* 2010;28:653–8.

264. Li F-H, Liu Y-Y, Qin F, Luo Q, Yang H-P, Zhang Q-G, et al. Photobiomodulation on Bax and Bcl-2 proteins and SIRT1/PGC-1αaxis mRNA expression levels of aging rat skeletal muscle. *Int J Photoenergy.* 2014;2014:1–8.

265. Corazza AV, Paolillo FR, Groppo FC, Bagnato VS, Caria PHF. Phototherapy and resistance training prevent sarcopenia in ovariectomized rats. *Lasers Med Sci.* 2013;28:1467–74.

266. Moussa A. LED Therapy: 30-percent Increase in Max. # of Reps in New Study, Increased Stamina and More Recent LLLT / LEDT Data [Internet]. Blogger; 2016 [cited 2024 Dec 10]. Available from: https://suppversity.blogspot.com/2016/07/led-therapy-30-increase-in-max-of-reps.html

267. Leal-Junior ECP, Lopes-Martins RÁB, Bjordal JM. Clinical and scientific recommendations for the use of photobiomodulation therapy in exercise performance enhancement and post-exercise recovery: Current evidence and future directions. *Braz J Phys Ther.* 2019;23:71–5.

268. de Almeida P, Lopes-Martins RAB, De Marchi T, Tomazoni SS, Albertini R, Corrêa JCF,

et al. Red (660 nm) and infrared (830 nm) low-level laser therapy in skeletal muscle fatigue in humans: what is better? *Lasers Med Sci.* 2012;27:453–8.

269. Avni D, Levkovitz S, Maltz L, Oron U. Protection of skeletal muscles from ischemic injury: low-level laser therapy increases antioxidant activity. *Photomed Laser Surg.* 2005;23:273–7.

270. Rizzi CF, Mauriz JL, Freitas Corrêa DS, Moreira AJ, Zettler CG, Filippin LI, et al. Effects of low-level laser therapy (LLLT) on the nuclear factor (NF)-kappaB signaling pathway in traumatized muscle. *Lasers Surg Med.* 2006;38:704–13.

271. Sene-Fiorese M, Duarte FO, de Aquino Junior AE, Campos RM da S, Masquio DCL, Tock L, et al. The potential of phototherapy to reduce body fat, insulin resistance and "metabolic inflexibility" related to obesity in women undergoing weight loss treatment. *Lasers Surg Med.* 2015;47:634–42.

272. Hemmings TJ, Kendall KL, Dobson JL. Identifying dosage effect of light-emitting diode therapy on muscular fatigue in quadriceps. *J Strength Cond Res.* 2017;31:395–402.

273. Vieira WH de B, Ferraresi C, Perez SE de A, Baldissera V, Parizotto NA. Effects of low-level laser therapy (808 nm) on isokinetic muscle performance of young women submitted to endurance training: a randomized controlled clinical trial. *Lasers Med Sci.* 2012;27:497–504.

274. Nampo FK, Cavalheri V, Dos Santos Soares F, de Paula Ramos S, Camargo EA. Low-level phototherapy to improve exercise capacity and muscle performance: a systematic review and meta-analysis. *Lasers Med Sci.* 2016;31:1957–70.

275. Leal-Junior ECP, Vanin AA, Miranda EF, de Carvalho P de TC, Dal Corso S, Bjordal JM. Effect of phototherapy (low-level laser therapy and light-emitting diode therapy) on exercise performance and markers of exercise recovery: A systematic review with meta-analysis. *Lasers Med Sci.* 2015;30:925–39.

276. Vanin AA, Verhagen E, Barboza SD, Costa LOP, Leal-Junior ECP. Photobiomodulation therapy for the improvement of muscular performance and reduction of muscular fatigue associated with exercise in healthy people: A systematic review and meta-analysis. *Lasers Med Sci.* 2018;33:181–214.

277. Aimbire F, Albertini R, Pacheco MTT, Castro-Faria-Neto HC, Leonardo PSLM, Iversen VV, et al. Low-level laser therapy induces dose-dependent reduction of TNFalpha levels in acute inflammation. *Photomed Laser Surg.* 2006;24:33–7.

278. Leal Junior ECP, Lopes-Martins RAB, Baroni BM, De Marchi T, Rossi RP, Grosselli D, et al. Comparison between single-diode low-level laser therapy (LLLT) and LED multi-diode (cluster) therapy (LEDT) applications before high-intensity exercise. *Photomed Laser Surg.* 2009;27:617–23.

279. Borsa PA, Larkin KA, True JM. Does phototherapy enhance skeletal muscle contractile function and postexercise recovery? A systematic review. *J Athl Train.* 2013;48:57–67.

280. De Marchi T, Leal Junior ECP, Bortoli C, Tomazoni SS, Lopes-Martins RAB, Salvador M. Low-level laser therapy (LLLT) in human progressive-intensity running: effects on exercise performance, skeletal muscle status, and oxidative stress. *Lasers Med Sci.* 2012;27:231–6.

281. Leal Junior EC, de Godoi V, Mancalossi JL, Rossi RP, De Marchi T, Parente M, et al. Comparison between cold water immersion therapy (CWIT) and light emitting diode therapy (LEDT) in short-term skeletal muscle recovery after high-intensity exercise in athletes—preliminary results. *Lasers Med Sci.* 2011;26:493–501.

282. Jackson RF, Dedo DD, Roche GC, Turok DI, Maloney RJ. Low-level laser therapy as a non-invasive approach for body contouring: a randomized, controlled study. *Lasers Surg Med.* 2009;41:799–809.

283. Jackson RF, Stern FA, Neira R, Ortiz-Neira CL, Maloney J. Application of low-level laser therapy for noninvasive body contouring. *Lasers Surg Med.* 2012;44:211–7.

284. McRae E, Boris J. Independent evaluation of low-level laser therapy at 635 nm for non-invasive body contouring of the waist, hips, and thighs. *Lasers Surg Med.* 2013;45:1–7.

285. Caruso-Davis MK, Guillot TS, Podichetty VK, Mashtalir N, Dhurandhar NV, Dubuis-

son O, et al. Efficacy of low-level laser therapy for body contouring and spot fat reduction. *Obes Surg.* 2011;21:722–9.

286. Nestor MS, Zarraga MB, Park H. Effect of 635 nm low-level laser therapy on upper arm circumference reduction: A double-blind, randomized, sham-controlled trial. *J Clin Aesthet Dermatol.* 2012;5:42–8.

287. Thornfeldt CR, Thaxton PM, Hornfeldt CS. A six-week low-level laser therapy protocol is effective for reducing waist, hip, thigh, and upper abdomen circumference. *J Clin Aesthet Dermatol.* 2016;9:31–5.

288. Möckel F, Hoffmann G, Obermüller R, Drobnik W, Schmitz G. Influence of water-filtered infrared-A (wIRA) on reduction of local fat and body weight by physical exercise. *Ger Med Sci.* 2006;4:Doc05.

289. Avci P, Nyame TT, Gupta GK, Sadasivam M, Hamblin MR. Low-level laser therapy for fat layer reduction: a comprehensive review. *Lasers Surg Med.* 2013;45:349–57.

290. Neira R, Arroyave J, Ramirez H, Ortiz CL, Solarte E, Sequeda F, et al. Fat liquefaction: effect of low-level laser energy on adipose tissue. *Plast Reconstr Surg.* 2002;110:912–22; discussion 923–5.

291. da Silveira Campos RM, Dâmaso AR, Masquio DCL, Duarte FO, Sene-Fiorese M, Aquino AE Jr, et al. The effects of exercise training associated with low-level laser therapy on biomarkers of adipose tissue transdifferentiation in obese women. *Lasers Med Sci.* 2018;33:1245–54.

292. Duarte FO, Sene-Fiorese M, de Aquino Junior AE, da Silveira Campos RM, Masquio DCL, Tock L, et al. Can low-level laser therapy (LLLT) associated with an aerobic plus resistance training change the cardiometabolic risk in obese women? A placebo-controlled clinical trial. *J Photochem Photobiol B.* 2015;153:103–10.

293. da Silveira Campos RM, Dâmaso AR, Masquio DCL, Aquino AE Jr, Sene-Fiorese M, Duarte FO, et al. Low-level laser therapy (LLLT) associated with aerobic plus resistance training to improve inflammatory biomarkers in obese adults. *Lasers Med Sci.* 2015;30:1553–63.

294. Gwinup G, Chelvam R, Steinberg T. Thickness of subcutaneous fat and activity of underlying muscles. *Ann Intern Med.* 1971;74:408–11.

295. Kostek MA, Pescatello LS, Seip RL, Angelopoulos TJ, Clarkson PM, Gordon PM, et al. Subcutaneous fat alterations resulting from an upper-body resistance training program. *Med Sci Sports Exerc.* 2007;39:1177–85.

296. Ramírez-Campillo R, Andrade DC, Campos-Jara C, Henríquez-Olguín C, Alvarez-Lepín C, Izquierdo M. Regional fat changes induced by localized muscle endurance resistance training. *J Strength Cond Res.* 2013;27:2219–24.

297. Frayn KN. Macronutrient metabolism of adipose tissue at rest and during exercise: A methodological viewpoint. *Proc Nutr Soc.* 1999;58:877–86.

298. Pfeifer GP. Mechanisms of UV-induced mutations and skin cancer. *Genome Instab Dis.* 2020;1:99–113.

299. Gandini S, Sera F, Cattaruzza MS, Pasquini P, Picconi O, Boyle P, et al. Meta-analysis of risk factors for cutaneous melanoma: II. Sun exposure. *Eur J Cancer.* 2005;41:45–60.

300. Elwood JM, Jopson J. Melanoma and sun exposure: An overview of published studies. *Int J Cancer.* 1997;73:198–203.

301. Nelemans PJ, Rampen FH, Ruiter DJ, Verbeek AL. An addition to the controversy on sunlight exposure and melanoma risk: A meta-analytical approach. *J Clin Epidemiol.* 1995;48:1331–42.

302. Barolet D, Christiaens F, Hamblin MR. Infrared and skin: Friend or foe. *J Photochem Photobiol B.* 2016;155:78–85.

303. Barolet D, Boucher A. LED photoprevention: reduced MED response following multiple LED exposures. *Lasers Surg Med.* 2008;40:106–12.

304. Menezes S, Coulomb B, Lebreton C, Dubertret L. Non-coherent near-infrared radiation protects normal human dermal fibroblasts from solar ultraviolet toxicity. *J Invest Dermatol.* 1998;111:629–33.

305. Belém MO, de Andrade GMM, Carlos TM, Guazelli CFS, Fattori V, Toginho Filho DO, et al. Light-emitting diodes at 940 nm attenuate colitis-induced inflammatory process in mice. *J Photochem Photobiol B.* 2016;162:367–73.

306. Bicknell B, Liebert A, Johnstone D, Kiat H. Photobiomodulation of the microbiome: implications for metabolic and inflammatory diseases. *Lasers Med Sci.* 2019;34:317–27.

307. Liebert A, Bicknell B, Johnstone DM, Gordon LC, Kiat H, Hamblin MR. "Photobiomics": Can light, including photobiomodulation, alter the microbiome? *Photobiomodul Photomed Laser Surg.* 2019;37:681–93.

308. Bicknell B, Laakso E-L, Liebert A, Kiat H. Modifying the microbiome as a potential mechanism of photobiomodulation: A case report. *Photobiomodul Photomed Laser Surg.* 2022;40:88–97.

309. Bicknell B, Liebert A, McLachlan CS, Kiat H. Microbiome changes in humans with Parkinson's disease after photobiomodulation therapy: A retrospective study. *J Pers Med.* 2022;12:49.

310. Amaroli A, Ravera S, Zekiy A, Benedicenti S, Pasquale C. A narrative review on oral and periodontal bacteria microbiota photobiomodulation, through visible and near-infrared light: From the origins to modern therapies. *Int J Mol Sci.* 2022;23:1372.

311. Zanotta N, Ottaviani G, Campisciano G, Poropat A, Bovenzi M, Rupel K, et al. Photobiomodulation modulates inflammation and oral microbiome: A pilot study. *Biomarkers.* 2020;25:677–84.

312. Ishiguro M, Ikeda K, Tomita K. Effect of near-infrared light-emitting diodes on nerve regeneration. *J Orthop Sci.* 2010;15:233–9.

313. Muraleedharan A, Ummer S V, Maiya AG, Hande M. Low level laser therapy for the patients with painful diabetic peripheral neuropathy—A systematic review. *Diabetes Metab Syndr.* 2019;13:2667–70.

314. Korada HY, Arora E, Maiya GA, Rao S, Hande M, Shetty S, et al. Effectiveness of photobiomodulation therapy on neuropathic pain, nerve conduction and plantar pressure distribution in Diabetic Peripheral Neuropathy—A systematic review. *Curr Diabetes Rev.* 2023;19:e290422204244.

315. Argenta PA, Ballman KV, Geller MA, Carson LF, Ghebre R, Mullany SA, et al. The effect of photobiomodulation on chemotherapy-induced peripheral neuropathy: A randomized, sham-controlled clinical trial. *Gynecol Oncol.* 2017;144:159–66.

316. Zinchenko E, Navolokin N, Shirokov A, Khlebtsov B, Dubrovsky A, Saranceva E, et al. Pilot study of transcranial photobiomodulation of lymphatic clearance of beta-amyloid from the mouse brain: Breakthrough strategies for non-pharmacologic therapy of Alzheimer's disease. *Biomed Opt Express.* 2019;10:4003–17.

317. Semyachkina-Glushkovskaya O, Abdurashitov A, Dubrovsky A, Klimova M, Agranovich I, Terskov A, et al. Photobiomodulation of lymphatic drainage and clearance: Perspective strategy for augmentation of meningeal lymphatic functions. *Biomed Opt Express.* 2020;11:725–34.

318. Salehpour F, Khademi M, Bragin DE, DiDuro JO. Photobiomodulation therapy and the glymphatic system: Promising applications for augmenting the brain lymphatic drainage system. *Int J Mol Sci.* 2022;23:2975.

319. Millis DL, Bergh A. A systematic literature review of complementary and alternative veterinary medicine: Laser therapy. *Animals* (Basel) [Internet]. 2023;13. Available from: http://dx.doi.org/10.3390/ani13040667.

320. Alves JC, Santos A, Jorge P, Carreira LM. A randomized double-blinded controlled trial on the effects of photobiomodulation therapy in dogs with osteoarthritis. *Am J Vet Res* [Internet]. 2022;83. Available from: http://dx.doi.org/10.2460/ajvr.22.03.0036

321. Ginimuge PR, Jyothi SD. Methylene blue: revisited. *J Anaesthesiol Clin Pharmacol.* 2010;26:517–20.

322. Schirmer RH, Adler H, Pickhardt M, Mandelkow E. "Lest we forget you—methylene blue . . ." *Neurobiol Aging.* 2011;32:2325.e7–16.

323. Tucker D, Lu Y, Zhang Q. From Mitochondrial Function to Neuroprotection—an Emerging Role for Methylene Blue. *Mol Neurobiol.* 2018;55:5137–53.

324. Stack C, Jainuddin S, Elipenahli C, Gerges M, Starkova N, Starkov AA, et al. Methylene blue upregulates Nrf2/ARE genes and prevents tau-related neurotoxicity. *Hum Mol Genet.* 2014;23:3716–32.

325. Yang L, Youngblood H, Wu C, Zhang Q. Mi-

tochondria as a target for neuroprotection: Role of methylene blue and photobiomodulation. *Transl Neurodegener.* 2020;9:19.

326. Gonzalez-Lima F, Auchter A. Protection against neurodegeneration with low-dose methylene blue and near-infrared light. *Front Cell Neurosci.* 2015;9:179.

327. Meynaghizadeh-Zargar R, Sadigh-Eteghad S, Mohaddes G, Salehpour F, Rasta SH. Effects of transcranial photobiomodulation and methylene blue on biochemical and behavioral profiles in mice stress model. *Lasers Med Sci.* 2020;35:573–84.

328. Dabholkar N, Gorantla S, Dubey SK, Alexander A, Taliyan R, Singhvi G. Repurposing methylene blue in the management of COVID-19: Mechanistic aspects and clinical investigations. *Biomed Pharmacother.* 2021;142:112023.

329. Hanna R, Dalvi S, Sălăgean T, Bordea IR, Benedicenti S. Phototherapy as a rational antioxidant treatment modality in COVID-19 management; New concept and strategic approach: Critical review. *Antioxidants* (Basel). 2020;9:875.

330. Hepburn J, Williams-Lockhart S, Bensadoun RJ, Hanna R. A novel approach of combining methylene blue photodynamic inactivation, photobiomodulation and oral ingested methylene blue in COVID-19 management: A pilot clinical study with 12-month follow-up. *Antioxidants* (Basel). 2022;11:2211.

331. Franceschi C, Campisi J. Chronic inflammation (inflammaging) and its potential contribution to age-associated diseases. *J Gerontol A Biol Sci Med Sci.* 2014;69 Suppl 1:S4–9.

332. Tian T, Wang Z, Chen L, Xu W, Wu B. Photobiomodulation activates undifferentiated macrophages and promotes M1/M2 macrophage polarization via PI3K/AKT/mTOR signaling pathway. *Lasers Med Sci.* 2023;38:86.

333. Woo K, Park SY, Padalhin A, Ryu HS, Abueva CD. Photobiomodulation enhances M2 macrophage polarization properties of tonsil-derived mesenchymal stem cells. *J Photochem Photobiol B.* 2023;246:112770.

334. Souza NHC, Mesquita-Ferrari RA, Rodrigues MFSD, da Silva DFT, Ribeiro BG, Alves AN, et al. Photobiomodulation and different mac-rophages phenotypes during muscle tissue repair. *J Cell Mol Med.* 2018;22:4922–34.

335. Brosseau L, Robinson V, Wells G, Debie R, Gam A, Harman K, et al. Low level laser therapy (Classes I, II and III) for treating rheumatoid arthritis. *Cochrane Database Syst Rev.* 2005;2010:CD002049.

336. Oron, U., Maltz, L., Tuby, H., Sorin, V., & Czerniak, A. Photobiomodulation therapy to autologous bone marrow in humans significantly increases the concentration of circulating stem cells and macrophages: A pilot study. *Photobiomodulation, Photomedicine, and Laser Surgery.* 2022; 40(2), 234-244.

337. Xu C, Wu Z, Wang L, Shang X, Li Q. 2002. The effect of endonasal low energy He-Ne laser treatment on insomnia on on sleep EEG. *Prac J Med Pharm.* 19(6): 407-408 (in Chinese).

338. Xu C, Wu Z, Wang L, Shang X, Li Q. 2002. The effect of endonasal low energy He-Ne laser treatment of insomnia on sleep EEG. *Prac J Med Pharm.* 19(6): 407-408 (in Chinese).

339. Wang F. 2006. Therapeutic effect observation and nurse of intranasal low intensity laser therapy on insomnia. *Journal of Community Medicine.* 4(3): 58 (in Chinese).

Chapter Four: The Biphasic Dose Response

1. Huang Y-Y, Chen AC-H, Carroll JD, Hamblin MR. Biphasic dose response in low level light therapy. *Dose Response.* 2009;7:358–83.

2. Hamblin MR, Ferraresi C, Huang Y-Y, Freitas de Freitas L, Carroll JD. *Low-Level Light Therapy.* Bellingham, WA: SPIE Press; 2018.

3. Barolet D, Christiaens F, Hamblin MR. Infrared and skin: Friend or foe. *J Photochem Photobiol B.* 2016;155:78–85.

4. Huang Y-Y, Sharma SK, Carroll J, Hamblin MR. Biphasic dose response in low level light therapy—an update. *Dose Response.* 2011;9:602–18.

5. Syu G-D, Chen H-I, Jen CJ. Severe exercise and exercise training exert opposite effects on human neutrophil apoptosis via altering the redox status. *PLoS One.* 2011;6:e24385.

6. Jere SW, Houreld NN. Photobiomodulation (PBM): A therapeutic technique targeting fibroblast cell regeneration and survival in diabetic wounds. *Front Photon* [Internet]. 2024;5. Available from: http://dx.doi.org/10.3389/fphot.2024.1423280

7. Ahrabi B, Rezaei Tavirani M, Khoramgah MS, Noroozian M, Darabi S, Khoshsirat S, et al. The effect of photobiomodulation therapy on the differentiation, proliferation, and migration of the mesenchymal stem cell: A review. *J Lasers Med Sci.* 2019;10:S96–103.

8. Rahbar Layegh E, Fadaei Fathabadi F, Lotfinia M, Zare F, Mohammadi Tofigh A, Abrishami S, et al. Photobiomodulation therapy improves the growth factor and cytokine secretory profile in human type 2 diabetic fibroblasts. *J Photochem Photobiol B.* 2020;210:111962.

9. PodBean Development. Illuminating the Nuances of Red Light Therapy w/ Researcher Dr. Praveen Arany [Internet]. 2023 [accessed 2025 Jan 15]. Available from: https://theredlightreport.podbean.com/e/the-radiance-revolution-unveiling-the-pioneering-work-of-dr-arany-and-the-secrets-of-red-light-therapy/.

10. Mohamad SA, Milward MR, Hadis MA, Kuehne SA, Cooper PR. Photobiomodulation of mineralisation in mesenchymal stem cells. *Photochem Photobiol Sci.* 2021;20:699–714.

11. Woodruff LD, Bounkeo JM, Brannon WM, Dawes KS, Barham CD, Waddell DL, et al. The efficacy of laser therapy in wound repair: A meta-analysis of the literature. *Photomed Laser Surg.* 2004;22:241–7.

12. Demidova-Rice TN, Salomatina EV, Yaroslavsky AN, Herman IM, Hamblin MR. Low-level light stimulates excisional wound healing in mice. *Lasers Surg Med.* 2007;39:706–15.

13. Lopes-Martins RAB, Marcos RL, Leonardo PS, Prianti AC Jr, Muscará MN, Aimbire F, et al. Effect of low-level laser (Ga-Al-As 655 nm) on skeletal muscle fatigue induced by electrical stimulation in rats. *J Appl Physiol.* 2006;101:283–8.

14. Santos LA, Marcos RL, Tomazoni SS, Vanin AA, Antonialli FC, Grandinetti V dos S, et al. Effects of pre-irradiation of low-level laser therapy with different doses and wavelengths in skeletal muscle performance, fatigue, and skeletal muscle damage induced by tetanic contractions in rats. *Lasers Med Sci.* 2014;29:1617–26.

15. Xuan W, Huang L, Hamblin MR. Repeated transcranial low-level laser therapy for traumatic brain injury in mice: Biphasic dose response and long-term treatment outcome. *J Biophotonics.* 2016;9:1263–72.

16. Oron U, Yaakobi T, Oron A, Hayam G, Gepstein L, Rubin O, et al. Attenuation of infarct size in rats and dogs after myocardial infarction by low-energy laser irradiation. *Lasers Surg Med.* 2001;28:204–11.

17. Ailioaie LM, Litscher G. Photobiomodulation and sports: Results of a narrative review. *Life* (Basel). 2021;11:1339.

18. Zhang R, Qu J. The mechanisms and efficacy of photobiomodulation therapy for arthritis: A comprehensive review. *Int J Mol Sci* [Internet]. 2023;24. Available from: http://dx.doi.org/10.3390/ijms241814293

19. Ji Q, Yan S, Ding J, Zeng X, Liu Z, Zhou T, et al. Photobiomodulation improves depression symptoms: A systematic review and meta-analysis of randomized controlled trials. *Front Psychiatry.* 2023;14:1267415.

20. Liebert A, Krause A, Goonetilleke N, Bicknell B, Kiat H. A role for photobiomodulation in the prevention of myocardial ischemic reperfusion injury: A systematic review and potential molecular mechanisms. *Sci Rep.* 2017;7:42386.

21. Tsatsakis AM, Vassilopoulou L, Kovatsi L, Tsitsimpikou C, Karamanou M, Leon G, Liesivuori J, Hayes AW, Spandidos DA. The dose response principle from philosophy to modern toxicology: The impact of ancient philosophy and medicine in modern toxicology science. *Toxicology Reports.* 2018 Jan 1;5:1107-13.

22. Cronshaw M, Parker S, Arany P. Feeling the heat: Evolutionary and microbial basis for the analgesic mechanisms of photobiomodulation therapy. *Photobiomodulation, Photomedicine, and Laser Surgery.* 2019 Sep 1;37(9):517-26.

23. Cronshaw M, Mylona V. Photobiomodulation Therapy Within Clinical Dentistry: Theoretical and Applied Concepts. In *Lasers in*

Dentistry—Current Concepts, 2024 Jan 9 (pp. 173-236). Cham: Springer International Publishing.

Chapter Five: PBM Dosing and Key Factors That Influence PBM Treatment Efficacy

1. Zein R, Selting W, Hamblin MR. Review of light parameters and photobiomodulation efficacy: Dive into complexity. *J Biomed Opt.* 2018;23:1–17.
2. Hadis MA, Zainal SA, Holder MJ, Carroll JD, Cooper PR, Milward MR, et al. The dark art of light measurement: Accurate radiometry for low-level light therapy. *Lasers Med Sci.* 2016;31:789–809.
3. Parker S, Cronshaw M, Grootveld M. Photobiomodulation delivery parameters in dentistry: An evidence-based approach. *Photobiomodul Photomed Laser Surg.* 2022;40:42–50.
4. Tanaka Y, editor. Photomedicine—Advances in clinical practice. *InTech*; 2017.
5. Barolet D, Roberge CJ, Auger FA, Boucher A, Germain L. Regulation of skin collagen metabolism in vitro using a pulsed 660 nm LED light source: Clinical correlation with a single-blinded study. *J Invest Dermatol.* 2009;129:2751–9.
6. Lee SY, Park K-H, Choi J-W, Kwon J-K, Lee DR, Shin MS, et al. A prospective, randomized, placebo-controlled, double-blinded, and split-face clinical study on LED phototherapy for skin rejuvenation: Clinical, profilometric, histologic, ultrastructural, and biochemical evaluations and comparison of three different treatment settings. *J Photochem Photobiol B.* 2007;88:51–67.
7. Silveira PCL, Ferreira KB, da Rocha FR, Pieri BLS, Pedroso GS, De Souza CT, et al. Effect of low-power laser (LPL) and light-emitting diode (LED) on inflammatory response in burn wound healing. *Inflammation.* 2016;39:1395–404.
8. Baroni BM, Rodrigues R, Freire BB, Franke R de A, Geremia JM, Vaz MA. Effect of low-level laser therapy on muscle adaptation to knee extensor eccentric training. *Eur J Appl Physiol.* 2015;115:639–47.
9. Baroni BM, Leal Junior ECP, De Marchi T, Lopes AL, Salvador M, Vaz MA. Low-level laser therapy before eccentric exercise reduces muscle damage markers in humans. *Eur J Appl Physiol.* 2010;110:789–96.
10. Baroni BM, Leal Junior ECP, Geremia JM, Diefenthaeler F, Vaz MA. Effect of light-emitting diodes therapy (LEDT) on knee extensor muscle fatigue. *Photomed Laser Surg.* 2010;28:653–8.
11. Vanin AA, Verhagen E, Barboza SD, Costa LOP, Leal-Junior ECP. Photobiomodulation therapy for the improvement of muscular performance and reduction of muscular fatigue associated with exercise in healthy people: A systematic review and meta-analysis. *Lasers Med Sci.* 2018;33:181–214.
12. Pinheiro ALB, Gerbi MEMM. Photoengineering of bone repair processes. *Photomed Laser Surg.* 2006;24:169–78.
13. Saebø H, Naterstad IF, Bjordal JM, Stausholm MB, Joensen J. Treatment of distal radius fracture during immobilization with an orthopedic cast: A double-blinded randomized controlled trial of photobiomodulation therapy. *Photobiomodul Photomed Laser Surg.* 2021;39:280–8.
14. Khumaidi MA, Paturusi I, Nusdwinuringtyas N, Islam AA, Gunawan WB, Nurkolis F, et al. Is low-level laser therapy effective for patients with knee joint osteoarthritis? Implications and strategies to promote laser therapy usage. *Front Bioeng Biotechnol.* 2022;10:1089035.
15. Chao LL. Effects of home photobiomodulation treatments on cognitive and behavioral function, cerebral perfusion, and resting-state functional connectivity in patients with dementia: A pilot trial. *Photobiomodul Photomed Laser Surg.* 2019;37:133–41.
16. Monteiro F, Carvalho Ó, Sousa N, Silva FS, Sotiropoulos I. Photobiomodulation and visual stimulation against cognitive decline and Alzheimer's disease pathology: A systematic review. *Alzheimers Dement* (NY). 2022;8:e12249.
17. Borges LS, Cerqueira MS, dos Santos Rocha JA, Conrado LAL, Machado M, Pereira R, et al. Light-emitting diode phototherapy improves muscle recovery after a damaging exercise. *Lasers Med Sci.* 2014;29:1139–44.

18. Leal Junior ECP, Lopes-Martins RAB, Dalan F, Ferrari M, Sbabo FM, Generosi RA, et al. Effect of 655-nm low-level laser therapy on exercise-induced skeletal muscle fatigue in humans. *Photomed Laser Surg.* 2008;26:419–24.

19. Stelian J, Gil I, Habot B, Rosenthal M, Abramovici I, Kutok N, et al. Improvement of pain and disability in elderly patients with degenerative osteoarthritis of the knee treated with narrow-band light therapy. *J Am Geriatr Soc.* 1992;40:23–6.

20. Ishiguro M, Ikeda K, Tomita K. Effect of near-infrared light-emitting diodes on nerve regeneration. *J Orthop Sci.* 2010;15:233–9.

21. Ash C, Dubec M, Donne K, Bashford T. Effect of wavelength and beam width on penetration in light-tissue interaction using computational methods. *Lasers Med Sci.* 2017;32:1909–18.

22. Bashkatov AN, Genina EA, Kochubey VI, Tuchin VV. Optical properties of human skin, subcutaneous and mucous tissues in the wavelength range from 400 to 2,000 nm. *J Phys D Appl Phys.* 2005;38:2543–55.

23. Hu D, van Zeyl M, Valter K, Potas JR. Sex, but not skin tone affects penetration of red-light (660 nm) through sites susceptible to sports injury in lean live and cadaveric tissues. *J Biophotonics.* 2019;12:e201900010.

24. Allen DW, Cooksey C. Reflectance Measurements of Human Skin | NIST. 2015 [accessed 2024 Dec 18]. Available from: https://www.nist.gov/programs-projects/reflectance-measurements-human-skin.

25. Koran A, Powers JM, Raptis CN, Yu R. Reflection spectrophotometry of facial skin. *J Dent Res.* 1981;60:979–82.

26. Dianna M. Red Light Therapy Penetration Depth And More . . . With Tom Kerber [Internet]. *The Energy Blueprint—Cutting-Edge Science For Overcoming Fatigue and Increasing Your Energy.* The Energy Blueprint; 2024 [cited 2024 Dec 18]. Available from: https://theenergyblueprint.com/red-light-therapy-penetration-depth-tom-kerber/.

27. Henderson TA, Morries LD. Near-infrared photonic energy penetration: Can infrared phototherapy effectively reach the human brain? *Neuropsychiatr Dis Treat.* 2015;11:2191–208.

28. Cotler HB, Chow RT, Hamblin MR, Carroll J. The use of low level laser therapy (LLLT) for musculoskeletal pain. *MOJ Orthop Rheumatol* [Internet]. 2015;2. Available from: http://dx.doi.org/10.15406/mojor.2015.02.00068.

29. Hipskind SG, Grover FL Jr, Fort TR, Helffenstein D, Burke TJ, Quint SA, et al. Pulsed transcranial red/near-infrared light therapy using light-emitting diodes improves cerebral blood flow and cognitive function in veterans with chronic traumatic brain injury: A case series. *Photobiomodul Photomed Laser Surg.* 2019;37:77–84.

30. Chan AS, Lee T-L, Hamblin MR, Cheung M-C. Photobiomodulation enhances memory processing in older adults with mild cognitive impairment: A functional near-infrared spectroscopy study. *J Alzheimers Dis.* 2021;83:1471–80.

31. Hamilton CL, El Khoury H, Hamilton D, Nicklason F, Mitrofanis J. "buckets": Early observations on the use of red and infrared light helmets in Parkinson's disease patients. *Photobiomodul Photomed Laser Surg.* 2019;37:615–22.

32. Gordon LC, Martin KL, Torres N, Benabid A-L, Mitrofanis J, Stone J, et al. Remote photobiomodulation targeted at the abdomen or legs provides effective neuroprotection against parkinsonian MPTP insult. *Eur J Neurosci.* 2023;57:1611–24.

33. Schindl A, Rosado-Schlosser B, Trautinger F. [Reciprocity regulation in photobiology. An overview]. *Hautarzt.* 2001;52:779–85.

34. Castano AP, Dai T, Yaroslavsky I, Cohen R, Apruzzese WA, Smotrich MH, et al. Low-level laser therapy for zymosan-induced arthritis in rats: Importance of illumination time. *Lasers Surg Med.* 2007;39:543–50.

35. Dos Santos Mendes-Costa L, de Lima VG, Barbosa MPR, Dos Santos LE, de Siqueira Rodrigues Fleury Rosa S, Tatmatsu-Rocha JC. Photobiomodulation: Systematic review and meta-analysis of the most used parameters in the resolution diabetic foot ulcers. *Lasers Med Sci.* 2021;36:1129–38.

36. Why Light Therapy Works [Internet]. Mercola.com. [accessed 2024 Dec 22]. Available from: https://articles.mercola.com/sites/articles/archive/2017/11/12/photobiomodulation-light-therapy.aspx.

37. Huang Y-Y, Chen AC-H, Carroll JD, Hamblin MR. Biphasic dose response in low level light therapy. *Dose Response.* 2009;7:358–83.

38. Kampa N, Jitpean S, Seesupa S, Hoisang S. Penetration depth study of 830 nm low-intensity laser therapy on living dog tissue. *Vet World.* 2020;13:1417–22.

39. Piao D, Sypniewski LA, Dugat D, Bailey C, Burba DJ, DeTaboada L. Transcutaneous transmission of photobiomodulation light to the spinal canal of dog as measured from cadaver dogs using a multi-channel intra-spinal probe. *Lasers Med Sci.* 2019;34:1645–54.

40. Hoisang S, Seesupa S, Jitpean S, Kampa N. Transcutaneous light penetration of simultaneous superpulsed and multiple wavelength photobiomodulation therapy in living dog tissue. *The Thai Journal of Veterinary Medicine.* 2022;52:23–31.

41. Joensen J, Ovsthus K, Reed RK, Hummelsund S, Iversen VV, Lopes-Martins RÁB, et al. Skin penetration time-profiles for continuous 810 nm and Superpulsed 904 nm lasers in a rat model. *Photomed Laser Surg.* 2012;30:688–94.

42. Ash C, Dubec M, Donne K, Bashford T. Effect of wavelength and beam width on penetration in light-tissue interaction using computational methods. *Lasers Med Sci.* 2017;32:1909–18.

43. Jacques SL. Optical properties of biological tissues: A review. *Phys Med Biol.* 2013;58:R37–61.

44. Haslerud S, Naterstad IF, Bjordal JM, Lopes-Martins RAB, Magnussen LH, Leonardo PS, et al. Achilles tendon penetration for continuous 810 nm and superpulsed 904 nm lasers before and after ice application: An in situ study on healthy young adults. *Photomed Laser Surg.* 2017;35:567–75.

45. Kim S, Jeong S. Effects of temperature-dependent optical properties on the fluence rate and temperature of biological tissue during low-level laser therapy. *Lasers Med Sci.* 2014;29:637–44.

46. Sommer AP, Pinheiro AL, Mester AR, Franke RP, Whelan HT. Biostimulatory windows in low-intensity laser activation: lasers, scanners, and NASA's light-emitting diode array system. *J Clin Laser Med Surg.* 2001;19:29–33.

47. Whelan HT, Smits RL Jr, Buchman EV, Whelan NT, Turner SG, Margolis DA, et al. Effect of NASA light-emitting diode irradiation on wound healing. *J Clin Laser Med Surg.* 2001;19:305–14.

48. Wong-Riley MT, Bai X, Buchmann E, Whelan HT. Light-emitting diode treatment reverses the effect of TTX on cytochrome oxidase in neurons. *Neuroreport.* 2001;12:3033–7.

49. Heiskanen V, Hamblin MR. Photobiomodulation: Lasers vs. light emitting diodes? *Photochem Photobiol Sci.* 2018;17:1003–17.

50. Jagdeo JR, Adams LE, Brody NI, Siegel DM. Transcranial red and near infrared light transmission in a cadaveric model. *PLoS ONE* 2012; 7(10): e47460.

51. Greguss P. Low-level laser therapy—reality or myth? *Opt Laser Technol.* 1984;16:81–5.

52. Laakso L, Richardson C, Cramond T. Quality of light—is laser necessary for effective photobiostimulation? *Aust J Physiother.* 1993;39:87–92.

53. Anders JJ, Lanzafame RJ, Arany PR. Low-level light/laser therapy versus photobiomodulation therapy. *Photomed Laser Surg.* 2015;33:183–4.

54. Sobral A-P-T, Sobral SS, Campos T-M, Horliana A-C-R-T, Fernandes K-P-S, Bussadori S-K, et al. Photobiomodulation and myofascial temporomandibular disorder: Systematic review and meta-analysis followed by cost-effectiveness analysis. *J Clin Exp Dent.* 2021;13:e724–32.

55. Farshidfar N, Farzinnia G, Samiraninezhad N, Assar S, Firoozi P, Rezazadeh F, et al. The effect of photobiomodulation on temporomandibular pain and functions in patients with temporomandibular disorders: an updated systematic review of the current randomized controlled trials. *J Lasers Med Sci.* 2023;14:e24.

56. Zhang Y, Ji Q. Current advances of photobiomodulation therapy in treating knee osteoarthritis. *Front Cell Dev Biol.* 2023;11:1286025.

57. Couturaud V, Le Fur M, Pelletier M, Granotier F. Reverse skin aging signs by red light photobiomodulation. *Skin Res Technol.* 2023;29:e13391.

58. Jagdeo J, Austin E, Mamalis A, Wong C, Ho D, Siegel DM. Light-emitting diodes in dermatology: A systematic review of ran-

domized controlled trials. *Lasers Surg Med.* 2018;50:613–28.

59. Ngoc LTN, Moon J-Y, Lee Y-C. Utilization of light-emitting diodes for skin therapy: Systematic review and meta-analysis. *Photodermatology, Photoimmunology & Photomedicine.* 2023;39:303–17.

60. Pruitt T, Carter C, Wang X, Wu A, Liu H. Photobiomodulation at different wavelengths boosts mitochondrial redox metabolism and hemoglobin oxygenation: Lasers vs. Light-emitting diodes in vivo. *Metabolites.* 2022;12:103.

61. Al-Quisi AF, Jamil FA, Abdulhadi BN, Muhsen SJ. The reliability of using light therapy compared with LASER in pain reduction of temporomandibular disorders: A randomized controlled trial. BMC oral health [Internet]. 2023 [accessed 2024 Dec 6];23. Available from: https://pubmed.ncbi.nlm.nih.gov /36782179/.

62. Ammar TAR. Monochromatic infrared photo energy versus low level laser therapy in patients with knee osteoarthritis. *Journal of Lasers in Medical Sciences.* 2014;5:176.

63. Alster TS, Wanitphakdeedecha R. Improvement of postfractional laser erythema with light-emitting diode photomodulation. *Dermatol Surg.* 2009;35:813–5.

64. Khoury JG, Goldman MP. Use of light-emitting diode photomodulation to reduce erythema and discomfort after intense pulsed light treatment of photodamage. *J Cosmet Dermatol.* 2008;7:30–4.

65. Koster PM. Near Infrared Light Penetration in Human Tissue: An Analysis of Tissue Structure and Heterogeneities [Internet] [Master's Thesis]. Marquette University; 2022 [accessed 2024 Dec 6]. Available from: https:// epublications.marquette.edu/cgi/viewcontent .cgi?article=1741&context=theses_open

66. Huang Y-Y, Gupta A, Vecchio D, de Arce VJB, Huang S-F, Xuan W, et al. Transcranial low-level laser (light) therapy for traumatic brain injury. *J Biophotonics.* 2012;5:827–37.

67. Agger MP, Danielsen ER, Carstensen MS, Nguyen NM, Horning M, Henney MA, et al. Safety, feasibility, and potential clinical efficacy of 40 Hz Invisible Spectral Flicker versus placebo in patients with mild-to-moderate Alzheimer's disease: A randomized, placebo-controlled, double-blinded, pilot study. *J Alzheimers Dis.* 2023;92:653–65.

68. Agger MP, Horning M, Carstensen MS, Danielsen ER, Baandrup AO, Nguyen M, et al. Study on the effect of 40 Hz non-invasive light therapy system. A protocol for a randomized, double-blinded, placebo-controlled clinical trial. *Front Aging Neurosci.* 2023;15:1250626.

69. International Agency for Research on Cancer. Non-ionizing radiation: Static and extremely low-frequency (ELF) electric and magnetic fields pt. 1. Genève, Switzerland: World Health Organization; 2002.

70. Karimi A, Ghadiri Moghaddam F, Valipour M. Insights in the biology of extremely low-frequency magnetic fields exposure on human health. *Mol Biol Rep.* 2020;47:5621–33.

71. OSHA. Extremely Low Frequency (ELF) Radiation—Health Effects [Internet]. [accessed 2024 Dec 22]. Available from: https:// www.osha.gov/elf-radiation/health-effects.

72. McNamee DA, Legros AG, Krewski DR, Wisenberg G, Prato FS, Thomas AW. A literature review: The cardiovascular effects of exposure to extremely low frequency electromagnetic fields. *Int Arch Occup Environ Health.* 2009;82:919–33.

73. Lai H. Neurological effects of static and extremely-low frequency electromagnetic fields. *Electromagn Biol Med.* 2022;41:201–21.

74. Gye MC, Park CJ. Effect of electromagnetic field exposure on the reproductive system. *Clin Exp Reprod Med.* 2012;39:1–9.

75. Mahaki H, Tanzadehpanah H, Jabarivasal N, Sardanian K, Zamani A. A review on the effects of extremely low frequency electromagnetic field (ELF-EMF) on cytokines of innate and adaptive immunity. *Electromagn Biol Med.* 2019;38:84–95.

76. Barati M, Darvishi B, Javidi MA, Mohammadian A, Shariatpanahi SP, Eisavand MR, et al. Cellular stress response to extremely low-frequency electromagnetic fields (ELF-EMF): An explanation for controversial effects of ELF-EMF on apoptosis. *Cell Prolif.* 2021;54:e13154.

77. Karbalay-Doust S, Darabyan M, Sisakht M,

Haddadi G, Sotoudeh N, Haghani M, et al. Extremely low frequency-electromagnetic fields (ELF-EMF) can decrease spermatocyte count and motility and change testicular tissue. *J Biomed Phys Eng.* 2023;13:135–46.

78. Guidelines for limiting exposure to electromagnetic fields (100 kHz to 300 GHz). *Health Phys.* 2020;118:483–524.

79. Hawkins D, Abrahamse H. Effect of multiple exposures of low-level laser therapy on the cellular responses of wounded human skin fibroblasts. *Photomed Laser Surg.* 2006;24:705–14.

80. Shinhmar H, Hogg C, Neveu M, Jeffery G. Weeklong improved colour contrasts sensitivity after single 670 nm exposures associated with enhanced mitochondrial function. *Sci Rep.* 2021;11:22872.

81. Giménez MC, Luxwolda M, Van Stipriaan EG, Bollen PP, Hoekman RL, Koopmans MA, et al. Effects of near-infrared light on well-being and health in human subjects with mild sleep-related complaints: A double-blind, randomized, placebo-controlled study. *Biology* (Basel). 2022;12:60.

82. Isobe Y, Hida H, Nishino H. Circadian rhythm of metabolic oscillation in suprachiasmatic nucleus depends on the mitochondrial oxidation state, reflected by cytochrome C oxidase and lactate dehydrogenase. *J Neurosci Res.* 2011;89:929–35.

83. Manella G, Asher G. The Circadian Nature of Mitochondrial Biology. *Front Endocrinol.* 2016;7:162.

84. Begum R, Powner MB, Hudson N, Hogg C, Jeffery G. Treatment with 670 nm light up regulates cytochrome C oxidase expression and reduces inflammation in an age-related macular degeneration model. *PLoS One.* 2013;8:e57828.

85. Figueiro MG, Sahin L, Roohan C, Kalsher M, Plitnick B, Rea MS. Effects of red light on sleep inertia. *Nat Sci Sleep.* 2019;11:45–57.

86. Zhao J, Tian Y, Nie J, Xu J, Liu D. Red light and the sleep quality and endurance performance of Chinese female basketball players. *J Athl Train.* 2012;47:673–8.

87. Petrowski K, Bührer S, Albus C, Schmalbach B. Increase in cortisol concentration due to standardized bright and blue light exposure on saliva cortisol in the morning following sleep laboratory. *Stress.* 2021;24:331–7.

88. Petrowski K, Buehrer S, Niedling M, Schmalbach B. The effects of light exposure on the cortisol stress response in human males. *Stress.* 2021;24:29–35.

89. Robertson-Dixon I, Murphy MJ, Crewther SG, Riddell N. The influence of light wavelength on human HPA axis rhythms: A systematic review. *Life* (Basel) [Internet]. 2023;13. Available from: http://dx.doi.org/10.3390/life13101968

90. Vanin AA, Miranda EF, Machado CSM, de Paiva PRV, Albuquerque-Pontes GM, Casalechi HL, et al. What is the best moment to apply phototherapy when associated to a strength training program? A randomized, double-blinded, placebo-controlled trial: Phototherapy in association to strength training. *Lasers Med Sci.* 2016;31:1555–64.

91. Leal-Junior ECP, Lopes-Martins RÁB, Bjordal JM. Clinical and scientific recommendations for the use of photobiomodulation therapy in exercise performance enhancement and post-exercise recovery: Current evidence and future directions. *Braz J Phys Ther.* 2019;23:71–5.

92. de Almeida P, Lopes-Martins RAB, De Marchi T, Tomazoni SS, Albertini R, Corrêa JCF, et al. Red (660 nm) and infrared (830 nm) low-level laser therapy in skeletal muscle fatigue in humans: What is better? *Lasers Med Sci.* 2012;27:453–8.

93. Avni D, Levkovitz S, Maltz L, Oron U. Protection of skeletal muscles from ischemic injury: low-level laser therapy increases antioxidant activity. *Photomed Laser Surg.* 2005;23:273–7.

94. Rizzi CF, Mauriz JL, Freitas Corrêa DS, Moreira AJ, Zettler CG, Filippin LI, et al. Effects of low-level laser therapy (LLLT) on the nuclear factor (NF)-kappaB signaling pathway in traumatized muscle. *Lasers Surg Med.* 2006;38:704–13.

95. Sene-Fiorese M, Duarte FO, de Aquino Junior AE, Campos RM da S, Masquio DCL, Tock L, et al. The potential of phototherapy to reduce body fat, insulin resistance and "metabolic inflexibility" related to obesity in women undergoing weight loss treatment. *Lasers Surg Med.* 2015;47:634–42.

96. Hemmings TJ, Kendall KL, Dobson JL. Identifying dosage effect of light-emitting diode therapy on muscular fatigue in quadriceps. *J Strength Cond Res.* 2017;31:395–402.

97. Vieira WH de B, Ferraresi C, Perez SE de A, Baldissera V, Parizotto NA. Effects of low-level laser therapy (808 nm) on isokinetic muscle performance of young women submitted to endurance training: a randomized controlled clinical trial. *Lasers Med Sci.* 2012;27:497–504.

98. Nampo FK, Cavalheri V, Dos Santos Soares F, de Paula Ramos S, Camargo EA. Low-level phototherapy to improve exercise capacity and muscle performance: A systematic review and meta-analysis. *Lasers Med Sci.* 2016;31:1957–70.

99. Gao Y, An R, Huang X, Liu W, Yang C, Wan Q. Effectiveness of photobiomodulation for people with age-related cognitive impairment: A systematic review and meta-analysis. *Lasers Med Sci.* 2023;38:237.

100. Lee T-L, Chan AS. Dose response of transcranial photobiomodulation on cognitive efficiency in healthy older adults: A task-related functional near-infrared spectroscopy study. *J Alzheimers Dis.* 2024;101:321–35.

101. da Silveira Campos RM, Dâmaso AR, Masquio DCL, Duarte FO, Sene-Fiorese M, Aquino AE Jr, et al. The effects of exercise training associated with low-level laser therapy on biomarkers of adipose tissue transdifferentiation in obese women. *Lasers Med Sci.* 2018;33:1245–54.

102. Duarte FO, Sene-Fiorese M, de Aquino Junior AE, da Silveira Campos RM, Masquio DCL, Tock L, et al. Can low-level laser therapy (LLLT) associated with an aerobic plus resistance training change the cardiometabolic risk in obese women? A placebo-controlled clinical trial. *J Photochem Photobiol B.* 2015;153:103–10.

103. da Silveira Campos RM, Dâmaso AR, Masquio DCL, Aquino AE Jr, Sene-Fiorese M, Duarte FO, et al. Low-level laser therapy (LLLT) associated with aerobic plus resistance training to improve inflammatory biomarkers in obese adults. *Lasers Med Sci.* 2015;30:1553–63.

104. Jeffery G, Fosbury R, Barrett E, Hogg C, Carmona MR, Powner MB. Longer wavelengths in sunlight pass through the human body and have a systemic impact which improves vision. *Sci Rep.* 2025;15:24435.

Chapter Six: Guide to Red and Near-Infrared Photobiomodulation Devices

1. Barolet D, Christiaens F, Hamblin MR. Infrared and skin: Friend or foe. *J Photochem Photobiol B.* 2016;155:78–85.

2. Alfredsson L, Armstrong BK, Butterfield DA, Chowdhury R, de Gruijl FR, Feelisch M, et al. Insufficient sun exposure has become a real public health problem. *Int J Environ Res Public Health.* 2020;17:5014.

3. Arany PR. Photoimmunotherapy: A novel field with overlapping light treatment approaches. *Photobiomodul Photomed Laser Surg* [Internet]. 2020; Available from: http://dx.doi.org/10.1089/photob.2020.4877

Index

animal studies/research (*cont'd*):
  on PBM preconditioning, 243
  on PBM's benefits for domestic animals, 107–108
  on systemic effects of PBM, 36–37, 169
anti-aging, xxv. *See also* skin aging/anti-aging
  blue light and, 186
  FDA approval for red and NIR light therapy devices for, 11
  irradiances and, 170–171
  melatonin and, 31
  stem cell production and, 113
  sunlight and, 258
antioxidant defenses, 25
  hormesis and, 118
  melatonin and, 27, 29–32
  reactive oxygen species (ROS) increases and, 19
antioxidant production, cellular stress and, 24
anti-tumor activity, 60
anti-tumor effects, 59–60
anxiety, 63–65, 72, 78
apoptosis (programmed cell death), 120
Arany, Praveen
  on biphasic dose response, 123
  on ELF electromagnetic fields (EMFs), 234
  on skin contact *vs.* non-contact, 201
  on systemic effects, 172
  on TGF-Beta 1, 21–22
  on tissue heating, 172, 273–274
Arndt, Rudolf, 117
Arndt-Schulz law, 117, 127. *See also* biphasic dose response
arthritis and arthritic joints, 36, 111, 130
  juvenile idiopathic, 70
  osteoarthritis, 70, 108, 122, 219, 220
  rheumatoid, 111
  studies on PBM's impact on, 70–71
  targeted treatment/devices for, 265
artificial light, xvii–xviii, 258
asthma, 73
Atapaseva (sunbathing), 4
Atharva Veda (Hindu text), 3
ATP. *See* adenosine triphosphate (ATP)
Aurelianus, Caelius, 4
Australian studies, 36–37
autoimmune diseases, 79–80, 81–82, 111
autoimmune hypothyroidism, 57–59
autonomic nervous system, 42–43
Ayurvedic medicine, 4

B
bacteria
  blue light and, xxiii, 149
  gut, 42, 105, 106
bacterial infections, 72
basic fibroblast growth factor (bFGF), 32, 33, 35
Battle Creek Sanitarium, Michigan, 7, 8
BDNF. *See* brain-derived neurotrophic factor (BDNF)
beam convergence, 208, 211–212
beams of light
  overlapping, 207–208
  size, 206–207
beam types, lasers *vs.* LEDs on, 217
Bernhard, Oskar, 8
Bestqool Y-200, 289
beta-endorphins, xxii
beta waves, 224
bFGF. *See* basic fibroblast growth factor (bFGF)
Biard, Robert, 216
biblical texts, healing power of sunlight in, 4
bioactive light, five types of, *xxii. See also* blue light; far-infrared (FIR) light; NIR light and NIR light therapy; red light and red-light therapy; ultraviolet (UV) light
Biolase, 243
biological clock, xxiii
biological effects, xvii, xix, xxii, xxiii, 14
  irradiance and, 162, 165–166, 194
  TRPV1 activation and, 20–21
biphasic dose response, 117–126
  differences in opinion of, 123–125
  evidence supporting, 120–126
  explained, 117
  factors contributing to, 129–131
  frequency of treatment and, 238
  in PBM, 118–120
  represented by an inverted U-shaped curve, 119
Bled, Slovenia, 7
blood glucose, 40, 71–72, 115
blood-mediated systemic effects, 40–42
blood vessels and blood flow
  brain health and, 243
  collagen and, 49
  nitric oxide (NO) and, 27, 120, 149
  optical challenges of, 215
  stubborn fat and, 99, 100–101
  targeted treatment devices for, 272
  TGF-beta 1 and, 22

duration of treatment (*cont'd*):
    examples for calculating, 196–197
    for facial skin, 262
    for superficial tissue, 260
    for system effects, 53
    tissue heating and, 182

E

Edison, Thomas, 7
efficacy of photobiomodulation (PBM)
    distance from the device and, 227–228
    dose per area/total dose and, 133, 134–145
    duration of treatment and, 191–198
    EMFs (electromagnetic fields) and, 230–236
    irradiance and. *See* irradiance(s)
    laser *vs.* LED and, 133, 215–222
    light convergence, 206–212
    method of applying a PBM device and, 198–205
    misrepresentation about irradiance of devices
      and, 187–188
    optical properties of tissues and, 133, 214
    pulsing *vs.* continuous wave and, 133, 223–227
    skin contact *vs.* non-contact, 198–204
    spot size and, 206–208
    tissue-specific properties and, 214–215
    treatment angle/device conformance to body
      surfaces, 133, 212–213
    treatment frequency, 133, 236–241
    treatment timing and, 133, 241–245
    using large LED panels, 288
    wavelengths of light and, 145–161
Einstein, Albert, 9
elastin, 15, 48, 53, 54
ELATED-2 trial, 63–64
electromagnetic fields. *See* EMFs (electromagnetic
    fields)
electromagnetic spectrum
    about, xx, *xxi,* xxii
    visible part of, xx, *xxi*
electron transport chain, 17, 18–19, 30
Elizabeth I, Queen, 5
EMFs (electromagnetic fields), 230–236
    in common household devices, 232
    dosage and, 232
    global standards on, 232–233
    harm from, 231–232
    LED panels and, 232
    quality of evidence on, 234–236
    researchers/experts on, 233–234
    studies on, 231–232

EMR-TEK Inc., 290
EMR-TEK Inc. Inferno, 289
endocrine glands, 261
endocrine system, xxiii, 45
epigenetics, 26
epithelial layer of the skin, 50
essential nutrients, xvi, xvi–xvii
exclusion zone water (EZ water), 23–24
exercise
    dosing measurement analogy using, 137
    as example of hormesis, 117
    fat loss and, 96–97, 100
    frequency of, 236–237
    melatonin and, 29
    NIR light therapy and fat loss from, 95
    PBM treatments after, 242, 266–268
    PBM treatments before, 242, 244,
      266–268
    preconditioning, 242–243
    Quad belt used during, 273
    recovery, 121, 122, 288
    red and NIR light helping with performance and
      recovery of, 87–93, 242, 266
    therapeutic window and, 131
    using PBM *during,* 244–245
exogen (hair growth cycle), 53
extracellular matrix, 22, 35, 49, 53–54, 125
extra-pineal melatonin, 27–32
extremely low frequency (ELF) electromagnetic
    fields, 230–231
eye health
    studies on PBM's benefits for, 62–63
    targeted treatment/devices for, 268–269
eyes/eye exposure
    evening PBM treatments and, 242
    laser light damaging the, 221
    lower irradiances for, 170
    photosensitivity and, 261

F

fabrics, containing FIR-emitting minerals,
    274
face masks, 285–286
    for acne, 50
    for aging skin, 51
    for direct skin contact, 228
    distance from the device and, 228
    eye health and, 269
    recommended, 262
    selecting, 261

PDGF. *See* platelet-derived growth factor (PDGF)

penetration depth

1/e method measurement approach, 154–158

biological effect and, 145–146

of blue light, 148, 149, *153*, 163

definition, 154

of green light, 148, 149, *153*, 163

influencing factors for, 161–162

irradiance and, 162–165

lasers *vs.* LEDs and, 217, 218

maximal, 164

method of applying a PBM device and, 198, *199*

of NIR light, 148, 152–153, *153*, 157, 159, 160–161, 162

overlapping beams of light and, 208

of red light, 148, 152–153, *153*, 157–160, 161, 162, 163

red light irradiance and, 180

of red *versus* NIR light, 150, 159, 160

research on red light, 158–160

studies on, 158–159, 160–161

sunlight spectrum, 159

of UV light, 148, 149, *153*, 163

wavelength of light and, 148–149, 162

periodontal disease, 72

peripheral nervous system/peripheral nerves, 44, 83, 106

peripheral neuropathy, 60, 106, 272

pets, PBM to help your, 107–108

Pharaoh Amhotep IV, 4

photobiology, xix, xxiv, 145–146

photobiomics, 105

photobiomodulation (PBM), vii. *See also* PBM devices; PBM mechanism(s); PBM treatment(s)

about, xix

ancient roots of, 3–4

benefits of, xv, xxv

birth of, 9–11

cascading effects of, 45–47, *46*

cellular stress and, 24–25

combined with methylene blue, 108–109

differences of opinions on, x

efficacy of. *See* efficacy of photobiomodulation (PBM)

final thoughts on, 293–294

hormetic response to, 25–26

improving brain health and cognitive performance, 85–87

local effects of. *See* local effects/treatments

as "non-thermal," 171–176

for pain management, 76–78

red and NIR light as primary focus of, xxiv

systemic effects of. *See* systemic (whole-body) effects/benefits

therapeutic outcomes. *See* efficacy of photobiomodulation (PBM)

photobiomodulation therapy (PBMT), 10

Photomedicine-Advances in Clinical Practice (Calderhead and Tanaka), 145–146, 165

photons

Bunsen-Roscoe law of reciprocity and, 192

overlapping beams and, 208

rate of delivery of, 194–195

TRPV1 and, 20

"photopuncture," 282

photosensitivity

biphasic dose response and, 125, 130

the eyes and, 269

fertility treatment and, 270

internal organs and, 132

targeted treatment and, 251, 261

photostimulation, 219

phototherapeutic window, 146. *See also* optical window

phototherapy

effect on exercise performance, 92

for psoriasis, 50

physical performance and recovery, xxv. *See also* exercise

pineal melatonin, 27, 28, 83, 111

Pittman, Gary, 216

plaque psoriasis, 50

platelet-derived growth factor (PDGF), 32

PlatinumLED Biomax 900, 289

poisons, biphasic dose response and, 117

Pollack, Gerald, 23

population inversion and stimulated emission, 9

portable devices, 282–283

post-exercise window, for PBM treatment, 242

power density, 133. *See also* irradiance(s)

preconditioning therapy, PBM as a, 242–243

prednisone, 105

pre-exercise PBM, 266–268

pregnancy rates, PB increasing, 67–68

professional devices, 247

protein synthesis, 15, 118

psoriasis, 50

pulse structure, 135

tendinopathy, 66, 67
testicles, applying light to the, 69
Texas Instruments, 216
TGF-beta 1, 15, 18, 21, 22–23, 32
TGF-β, 42
Thailand, research in, 199–200
therapeutic window, the, xxiii, 119, 131–132, 146, 195, 274
theta waves, 224
Thor Photomedicine, 124, 188, 211, 264
thrush, 72
thymic involution, 80–81
thyroid peroxidase autoantibodies (TPO), 58
tibia bone, 38–39, 252, 256
The Times of London, 8
timing of PBM treatments, 241–245
tissue. *See* human tissue
tissue heating
  cellular damage and excessive, 172, 174
  excessive, 123–124, 129, 171–179
  factors affecting, 182
  heat lamps and, 273–274
  heat-management strategies and, 183–184
  high irradiance PBM devices and, 172–173
  internal mechanism alerting one excessive, 177, 178
  internal mechanism alerting one of excessive, 181
  irradiance and excessive, 171–180
  "non-thermal" PBM and, 171–172, 173–174
  practical guide to avoid overheating, 181–184
  temperature thresholds, 179–181
T-Nation (website), 98
TNF-α, 110
tonsillitis, 72
tooth/teeth, 72–73
torches/torch-style devices, 153, 204, 228, 266, 269, 282–283, 292
total body surface, 143
total joules measurement, 129, 135, 137, 139, 140–145, 280
toxicity zone, 118
traditional Chinese medicine, 4, 43
transcranial PBM applications, 42, 65–66, 87, 122, 264, 287
TRANSDERMIS trial, 60
transforming growth factor beta-1 (TGF-beta 1). *See* TGF-beta 1
Transient Receptor Potential Vanilloid 1 (TRPV1), 17–18, 20–21, 178

transvaginal PBM, 270
traumatic brain injury, 82–83
  biphasic dose response and, 121
  PBM combined with methylene blue and, 109
  targeted treatment/devices for, 264
treatment. *See* PBM treatment(s)
triglycerides, 98
TRPVI. *See* Transient Receptor Potential Vanilloid 1 (TRPV1)
tuberculosis, 7, 8
Tufts New England Medical Center, 9
tumor cells, red light lasers used to kill, 9–10
type 2 diabetes, 71, 112
tyrosine, 100

U
Ukraine study, 59
ulcerative colitis, 105
ulcers, 242
  diabetic, 54, 71, 264, 280
  mouth, 72
  oral, 242, 243
  therapeutic use of sunlight for leg, 5
ultraviolet (UV) light, xvii, 145, 258
  biological effects, xxii
  electromagnetic fields (EMFs) and, 231
  Finsen Lamp and, 7
  optical window and, 147
  penetration depth, 148, 149, *153, 162, 163*
  vitamin D and, xvi, 36
ultraviolet (UV) radiation, xxii
  protection against, 103–104
  repairing damage caused by, 49
  skin cancer and, 103
under-eye wrinkles, 51
UNINOVE, Brazil, 37
University College London, 159
University of Buffalo, 159
University of Connecticut, 97
University of Greifswald, 117

V
Valeda Light Delivery System, 269
varicose veins, 48
vascular endothelial growth fact (VEGF), 15, 25, 32, 33, 35
vascular health/conditions, 27, 260. *See also* blood vessels and blood flow
VEGF. *See* vascular endothelial growth fact (VEGF)
ventilation, skin, 172, 182, 183, 203

ABOUT THE AUTHOR

Ari Whitten, M.S., is the founder of the Energy Blueprint. He has been studying health science for over twenty years and is a nutrition and life-style expert with a bachelor of science in kinesiology from San Diego State University. He has completed extensive graduate training in clinical psychology and holds a master of science in human nutrition and functional medicine. He also hosts the popular *Energy Blueprint* podcast.

2 04